Recent Advances in the Neurological and Neurodevelopmental Impact of HIV

International Review of Child Neurology Series

Recent Advances in the Neurological and Neurodevelopmental Impact of HIV

Edited by

Amina Abubakar

Institute for Human Development, Aga Khan University, Nairobi, Kenya

Kirsten A Donald

Division of Developmental Paediatrics, Department of Paediatrics and Child Health, Red Cross War Memorial Children's Hospital, Neuroscience Institute, University of Cape Town, Cape Town, South Africa

Jo M Wilmshurst

Department of Paediatric Neurology, Red Cross War Memorial Children's Hospital, Neuroscience Institute, University of Cape Town, Cape Town, South Africa

Charles R Newton

Department of Psychiatry, University of Oxford, Oxford, UK

2023

Mac Keith Press

Chief Executive: Ann-Marie Halligan
Senior Publishing Manager: Sally Wilkinson
Senior Publishing Manager: Andy Booth

First published in this edition in 2023 by Mac Keith Press
2nd Floor, Rankin Building, 139–143 Bermondsey Street, London, SE1 3UW

British Library Cataloguing-in-Publication data
A catalogue record for this book is available from the British Library

Cover designer: Marten Sealby

ISBN: 978-1-911612-20-9

Typeset by Riverside Publishing Solutions Ltd
Printed by Jellyfish Solutions Ltd

INTERNATIONAL REVIEW OF CHILD NEUROLOGY SERIES

Contents

Author Appointments

Amina Abubakar Professor and Director, Institute for Human Development, Aga Khan University, Nairobi, Kenya.

Subira Anzaya MSc Clinical Neurology Graduate, UCL, London, UK; Radiology Resident, Department of Radiology, Aga Khan University, Nairobi, Kenya.

Ebrahim Banderker Consultant Paediatric Radiologist, Red Cross War Memorial Children's Hospital, University of Cape Town, Cape Town, South Africa.

Judith K Bass Professor, Department of Mental Health, Johns Hopkins Bloomberg School of Public Health, Baltimore, MD, USA.

Michael J Boivin University Distinguished Professor for the Departments of Psychiatry and Neurology & Ophthalmology, Research Director for Psychiatry, College of Osteopathic Medicine, Michigan State University, East Lansing, MI, USA; Adjunct Professor of Psychiatry, School of Medicine, University of Michigan, Ann Arbor, MI, USA.

Karen Cohen Associate Professor, Division of Clinical Pharmacology, Department of Medicine, University of Cape Town, Cape Town, South Africa.

Alan Davidson Head of Paediatric Haematology and Oncology, Red Cross War Memorial Children's Hospital, Cape Town, South Africa.

Eric Decloedt Head of Division and Clinical Pharmacologist, Division of Clinical Pharmacology, Department of Medicine, Faculty of Medicine and Health Sciences, Stellenbosch University, Cape Town, South Africa.

Kirsten A Donald Professor, Division of Developmental Paediatrics, Department of Paediatrics and Child Health, Red Cross War Memorial Children's Hospital and Neuroscience Institute, University of Cape Town, Cape Town, South Africa.

Brian Eley Professor, Department of Paediatrics and Child Health, University of Cape Town, Cape Town, South Africa.

Rajeshree Govender Consultant Paediatric Neurologist, Inkosi Albert Luthuli Central Hospital, Nelson R. Mandela School of Medicine, University of Kwa-Zulu Natal, Durban, South Africa.

Charles K Hammond Consultant Paediatric Neurologist, Komfo Anokye Teaching Hospital, Kumasi, Ghana; Senior Lecturer, School of Medicine and Dentistry, Kwame Nkrumah University of Science and Technology, Kumasi, Ghana.

Jacqueline Hoare Mental Health Researcher, Consulting Liason, Division of Psychiatry, University of Cape Town, Cape Town, South Africa.

Felix Hosea Pharmacist, Ministry of Health, Nairobi, Kenya.

Tracy Kilborn — Head of Paediatric Radiology, Red Cross War Memorial Children's Hospital, Cape Town, South Africa; Associate Professor, University of Cape Town, Cape Town, South Africa.

Nelleke G Langerak — Associate Professor, Division of Neurosurgery, University of Cape Town, Cape Town, South Africa.

Adam Mabrouk — Project Coordinator, Aga Khan University, Nairobi, Kenya.

Theresa N Mann — Research Fellow, Division of Orthopaedic Surgery, Department of Surgical Sciences, Faculty of Medicine and Health Sciences, Stellenbosch University, Tygerberg, Cape Town, South Africa.

Alliya Mohamed — Consultant Paediatrician, Aga Khan University Hospital, Nairobi, Kenya.

Louisa R Mudawarima — Lecturer, Child and Adolescent Health Unit, Department of Primary Health Care, University of Zimbabwe Faculty of Medicine and Health Sciences, Harare, Zimbabwe.

Patrick N Mwangala — Research Specialist, Institute for Human Development, Aga Khan University, Nairobi, Kenya; PhD Fellow, School of Public Health, University of the Witwatersrand, Johannesburg, South Africa.

Alvin Ndondo — Senior Specialist/Lecturer, Paediatric Neurology, Department of Paediatrics, Red Cross War Memorial Children's Hospital, University of Cape Town, Cape Town, South Africa.

Beverley G Neethling — Consultant Paediatric Haematologist, Inkosi Albert Luthuli Hospital, Durban, South Africa.

Charles R Newton — Cheryl & Reece Scott Professor of Psychiatry, Department of Psychiatry, University of Oxford, Oxford, UK.

James Nuttall — Paediatric Infectious Diseases Specialist/Senior Lecturer, Department of Paediatrics and Child Health, Red Cross War Memorial Children's Hospital, University of Cape Town, Cape Town, South Africa.

Moses K Nyongesa — Postdoctoral Research Fellow, Aga Khan University, Institute for Human Development, Nairobi, Kenya.

Babatunde O Ogunbosi — Senior Lecturer, Paediatric Infectious Disease, Department of Paediatrics, Faculty of Clinical Sciences, College of Medicine, University of Ibadan, Ibadan, Nigeria; Consultant Paediatrician, Infectious Disease Unit, Department of Paediatrics, University College Hospital, Ibadan, Nigeria.

Sevil Ozdemir — Medical Student, College of Human Medicine, Michigan State University, East Lansing, MI, USA.

Aleya Remtulla — Senior Registrar, Red Cross War Memorial Children's Hospital, Cape Town, South Africa.

Micaela Rice — Medical Student, College of Human Medicine, Michigan State University, East Lansing, MI, USA.

Pauline Samia — Associate Professor, Chair, Department of Paediatrics and Child Health, Aga Khan University, Nairobi, Kenya.

Derrick Ssewanyana

Postdoctoral Research Fellow, Temerty Faculty of Medicine, Department of Physiology, University of Toronto, Toronto, Canada.

Stanley W Wanjala

Tutorial Fellow, Department of Social Sciences, Pwani University, Kilifi, Kenya; Doctoral Student, Department of Public Health and Primary Care, Ghent University, Ghent, Belgium.

Catherine J Wedderburn

Chief Research Officer, Department of Paediatrics and Child Health and Neuroscience Institute, University of Cape Town, Cape Town, South Africa; Clinical Research Fellow, Department of Clinical Research, London School of Hygiene & Tropical Medicine, London, UK.

Nicky Wieselthaler

Department of Paediatric Radiology, University of Cape Town, Cape Town, South Africa; Institute of Child Health, Red Cross War Memorial Children's Hospital, Cape Town, South Africa.

Jo M Wilmshurst

Head of Paediatric Neurology, Red Cross War Memorial Children's Hospital, Neuroscience Institute, University of Cape Town, Cape Town, South Africa.

Shunmay Yeung

Professor and Head of Department of Clinical Research, London School of Hygiene & Tropical Medicine, London, UK.

Preface

Human immunodeficiency virus (HIV) infection still remains a significant global health issue in both adults and children, despite the reduction in transmission through the expanded and effective prenatal prevention of mother-to-child transmission (PMTCT) programme. Sub-Saharan Africa, one of the areas of the world challenged by the greatest resource limitations, carries the highest burden of HIV and tuberculosis infection. More than 38 million people are estimated to be living with HIV globally, and an excess of two-thirds lives in this region. Brain health and growth in the early years of life, which set the stage for human development, may be disrupted directly by infections such as HIV or indirectly by associated psychosocial, environmental, or other contextual factors. Children who have not met developmental expectations in their preschool years are at much higher risk of academic and socio-emotional problems in school and later in life, influencing their adult responsibilities in economic, interpersonal, social, and civic spheres. It is therefore critical and of high public health importance to address the impact of this highly neurotropic virus on neurological, neurosurgical, developmental, and psychiatric health.

Recent Advances in the Neurological and Neurodevelopmental Impact of HIV aims to outline a number of the important clinical neurological issues facing children and young adults with HIV infection. We explore the emerging understanding of the developmental impact of HIV exposure without infection on this growing group of children. Authors have drawn from experience embedded in real-world practice settings as well as scientific excellence in order to understand the presentation, complications, and practical management of these conditions.

The book begins with an overview of the current epidemiological context of the HIV epidemic and discusses the pathophysiology that underlies the neurological complications of the virus. The subsequent sections focus on the range of clinical presentations of neuro-HIV and primary complications of the virus, including the neurological manifestations of immune reconstitution and HIV encephalopathy. The following chapters address complications of HIV such as opportunistic central nervous system (CNS) infections, vascular events, seizures, and CNS tumours. Children born to mothers who are HIV infected but who remain uninfected themselves are increasingly recognised as a vulnerable group and an exploration of the current and emerging evidence in this area is provided. Practical descriptions and examples of the neuroimaging features of these different conditions are addressed. A focus on the developmental, neurocognitive, and behavioural outcomes across the lifespan is followed by a chapter focusing on current understanding of antiretroviral strategies, particularly in the context of neuro-HIV. Taken together, the insight and expertise presented in this book aims to provide a clear, problem-based approach to the impact of HIV on the nervous system, with the aim of supporting practising adult and child neurologists, physicians, paediatricians, and trainees in their identification and management of people with these conditions.

We would like to thank the authors from across the world, for generously giving their time and expertise in researching and writing their contributions, often taking time from pressurised clinical and other commitments. We would also like to thank the Mac Keith Press team, particularly Sally Wilkinson and Lucy White, who have tirelessly maintained the momentum throughout this process.

Amina Abubakar, Kirsten A Donald, Jo M Wilmshurst, and Charles R Newton

Foreword

Whenever I am asked to contribute to a new medical textbook, I always ask myself: "Why would I do that?" Nobody reads textbooks anymore. With the vast amount of information available online, what use is another textbook? And yet, when I was asked to contribute the foreword to this current volume, I thought, "Finally, a textbook I am actually excited to read!" The present volume, *Recent Advances in the Neurological and Neurodevelopmental Impact of HIV*, edited by Amina Abubakar, Kirsten A Donald, Jo M Wilmshurst, and Charles R Newton, represents quite an achievement. The editors include many of the foremost experts on neurological complications of HIV in children, and in this book the authors provide information that is literally available nowhere else. For those of us who are neurologists or child neurologists who treat children with HIV in Africa, the insights provided by these experts are truly a breakthrough. The book begins with a review of the epidemiology and pathophysiology of HIV, and moves through key complications, with chapters comprehensively reviewing HIV encephalopathy, opportunistic infections, cerebrovascular disease, central nervous system tumors, and more.

HIV remains one of the most significant public health issues in the world. HIV has resulted in the deaths of more than 35 million people, with the majority of those residing in sub-Saharan Africa, and the World Health Organization estimates that there are nearly 2 million children living with HIV worldwide. The transformation of HIV from a nearly universally fatal illness to a chronic potentially manageable condition has been one of the great scientific and public health achievements of the last century. However, as more children with HIV survive into adulthood, chronic neurological issues have become more prominent. Issues such as cognitive impairment, increased risk of cerebrovascular disease, and peripheral neuropathies have in many locales eclipsed opportunistic infections as the most common complications seen. However, in many African countries, opportunistic infections remain a major cause of morbidity and mortality.

The editors are to be congratulated on bringing together an impressive group of experts for the current book, which is both comprehensive and also very readable. This book belongs on the shelf of anyone who cares for children with HIV.

David Bearden MD MSCE
Associate Professor of Neurology and Pediatrics,
University of Rochester School of Medicine, Rochester, NY, USA
Visiting Lecturer, University of Zambia, Lusaka, Zambia

CHAPTER 1

Epidemiology of HIV

Charles R Newton

INTRODUCTION

Human immunodeficiency virus type 1 (HIV-1) is the cause of acquired immune deficiency syndrome (AIDS) and it continues to be a major global public health problem, particularly in sub-Saharan Africa (SSA).

PREVALENCE AND INCIDENCE

Since the start of the epidemic in the 1980s, more than 76 million people have become infected with HIV-1, of whom 35 million have died. The World Health Organization (WHO 2020a) estimated in 2020 that 38 million people (95% confidence intervals: 31.6–44.5 million) were living with HIV-1, with 1.5 (1.0–2.0) million new infections and 0.7 (0.5–1.0) million people dying from AIDS-related illnesses in that year. The new infections and deaths have decreased by 39% and 51% respectively since 2000, mainly due to the implementation of antiretroviral therapy (ART; WHO 2020b). It is estimated that 68% of infections occur in SSA, with a 35% reduction in new infections and 46% reduction in deaths since 2010.

The WHO (2020b) has estimated that in 2019 there were 1.8 (1.3–2.2) million children (<15 years) living with HIV-1, with 150 000 (94 000–240 000) new infections and 95 000 (61 000–150 000) deaths, of whom 74% live in SSA. Most children acquire HIV from maternal transmission, either during pregnancy or birth, or through breast milk. There has been a 56% decline in new HIV infections in this region. Most of this reduction in childhood infections has come from preventing maternal transmission of HIV, with 85% of HIV-positive pregnant females having access to ART in 2019 (WHO 2020b).

GLOBAL BURDEN OF HIV

The global burden of disease is now expressed in disability adjusted life years (DALYs), which is the sum of the years lost of life (YLL) due to premature mortality and years living with disability (YLD) i.e. DALYS = YLL + YLD. The YLD is based upon the formula: YLD = Incidence × Disability Weight × Time spent living with the disability. More recently the prevalence has been used instead of incidence, since there are many more data recording prevalence. The disability weight (DW) reflects the severity of the condition, on a scale from 0 (perfect health) to 1 (equivalent to death). The most recent estimates of

DW for HIV infections were based upon surveys conducted in six countries. The DW for symptomatic, pre-AIDS patients is 0.274 (95% uncertainty intervals: 0.184–0.377). The DW for HIV/AIDS patients receiving antiretroviral treatment is 0.078 (0.052–0.111). Lastly, the DW for AIDS patients who are not receiving ART is 0.582 (0.406–0.743) (Salomon et al. 2015).

The global burden of HIV causing other diseases, for example, neurological complications, has changed considerably in terms of the DALYs and deaths, with HIV infections peaking between the years 2000 and 2005. The global burden as measured by DALYs is decreasing in younger children and has stabilised in 10 to 14-year-olds.

THE INVOLVEMENT OF THE NERVOUS SYSTEM

The HIV virus has a propensity for the nervous system, particularly the central nervous system (CNS), but estimation of the burden on the CNS is difficult to estimate, since it depends on the route and timing of the infection, the health care system, and the availability of ART, particularly highly active antiretroviral therapy (HAART). Furthermore, HIV affects the nervous system of children in a variety of ways, causing encephalopathy, opportunistic infections, behavioural and psychiatric disorders, cerebrovascular disease, epilepsy, CNS tumours, myelopathy, peripheral neuropathy, myopathies, and immune reconstitution syndrome. There are no studies that have systematically documented these complications over childhood. Most studies are hospital based cross-sectional data, from which it is difficult to derive accurate epidemiological data. The one exception is a population-based study of 1 645 515 neonates born in Florida, USA between 1998 and 2007, of whom 4698 (0.29%) were born to HIV/AIDS-positive primigravida women (Salihu et al. 2012). Intracranial haemorrhages (0.17%) and seizures (6.15%) were significantly more common in the neonates born to HIV-infected mothers, than to non-infected mothers.

Before the introduction of ART, it was estimated that up to 90% of children infected with HIV had CNS involvement (Belman et al. 1988; Epstein, Sharer, and Goudsmit 1988), usually manifesting as HIV encephalopathy. This is characterised by a progressive encephalopathy, with developmental delay, loss of skills and cognitive decline, microcephaly, and cortico-spinal dysfunction. Neuroimaging showed cerebral atrophy and basal ganglia calcifications in about one-third of children with CNS involvement. Since the advent of ART, the proportion of children with HIV encephalopathy has declined to about 13% to 23% (Lobato, Caldwell, and Oxtoby 1995; Tardieu et al. 2000), although there are few population-based studies on which to estimate this proportion.

There were few data from Africa during the 1990s, since most children were dying within the first 2 years of life (Newell, Brahmbhatt, and Ghys 2004) from opportunistic infections. The few data available were summarised in a systematic review which found that 15% to 56% of children had neurological signs in SSA, depending upon the age of assessment and the site (Abubakar et al. 2008). The median mental development index was 0.37 and 0.67 in African countries compared to 0.51 and 0.82 in North America at 6 months and 18 months respectively. The median psychomotor developmental index was similar between the studies in SSA and North America: 0.61 and 0.97 at 6 months respectively, compared to 0.64 and 0.76 at 18 months respectively (Abubakar et al. 2008). It was not possible to derive a proportion of children with development impairment from these studies. A more recent review (Donald et al. 2014) summarising mainly hospital-based data found that 12% to 23% developed encephalopathy, usually within the first year of life (Van Rie, Mupuala, and Dow 2008; Hoare et al. 2012; Ruel et al. 2012). In 18% of patients, encephalopathy was the first sign of an AIDS-defining illness and 35% to 50% of children with AIDS (Centers for Disease Control and Prevention category C) will develop encephalopathy (Kovacs 2009). Opportunistic infections occurred in about 8% to 34% of the HIV-infected children who were followed up (Tardieu and Boutet 2002; Donald et al. 2014) and behavioural and psychiatric disorders occurred in about 24% to 61% of HIV-infected children (Donald et al. 2014). Between 2.5% and 11% of HIV-infected children will develop a stroke (Govender et al. 2011; Hammond et al. 2016). Seizures occur in up to 23% of children with HIV-1 in SSA (Burman et al. 2019), but it is often not clear if this is epilepsy (i.e. unprovoked seizures) or secondary to undiagnosed opportunistic infections, tumours, or silent infarcts.

Although ART has reduced the transmission of HIV to children and improved the neurological outcome, it also contributes to the burden of HIV, since many of the drugs used to treat HIV have neurological side effects (Dalwadi et al. 2018). Some of these side effects are common, for example, peripheral neuropathy occurs in more than 10% of people on nucleoside reverse transcriptase inhibitors. However, the contribution to the burden of HIV from the neurological side effects of ART has not been determined. More recently, congenital abnormalities of the CNS were described in association with ARV therapy (Alemu and Yalew 2021).

CONCLUSION

Although the HIV epidemic appears to be decreasing, significant numbers of children are infected, particularly in SSA. These children are surviving, and thus at risk of developing neurological complications; however, there are few on which to base accurate estimates of the burden of neurological complications on HIV-infected children. Long-term follow up of well-documented cohorts is required to determine the burden in terms of the prevalence, incidence, and mortality associated with these complications. In addition, the effects of ARV needs to be monitored closely.

REFERENCES

Abubakar A, Van Baar A, Van de Vijver FJ, Holding P, Newton CR (2008) Paediatric HIV and neurodevelopment in sub-Saharan Africa: A systematic review. *Tropical Medicine & International Health*, 13(7): 880–887. Available from: doi: 10.1111/j.1365-3156.2008.02079.x.

Alemu FM, Yalew AW (2021) Does antiretroviral therapy cause congenital malformations? A systematic review and meta-analysis. *Epidemiol Health*, 43: e2021008. doi: 10.4178/epih.e2021008. Epub 2021 Feb 3. PMID: 33541012; PMCID: PMC8060528.

Belman AL, Diamond G, Dickson D et al. (1988) Pediatric acquired immunodeficiency syndrome: Neurologic syndromes. *American Journal of Diseases of Children*, 142(1): 29–35. doi: 10.1001/archpedi.1988.02150010039017.

Burman RJ, Wilmshurst JM, Gebauer S, Weise L, Walker KG, Donald KA (2019) Seizures in children with HIV infection in South Africa: A retrospective case control study. *Seizure*, 65: 159–165. doi: 10.1016/j.seizure.2019.01.023.

Dalwadi DA, Ozuna L, Harvey BH, Viljoen M, Schetz JA (2018) Adverse neuropsychiatric events and recreational use of efavirenz and other HIV-1 antiretroviral drugs. *Pharmacological Reviews*, 70(3): 684–711. doi: 10.1124/pr.117.013706.

Donald KA, Hoare J, Eley B, Wilmshurst JM (2014) Neurologic complications of pediatric human immunodeficiency virus: Implications for clinical practice and management challenges in the African setting. *Seminars in Pediatric Neurology*, 21(1): 3–11. doi: 10.1016/j.spen.2014.01.004.

Epstein LG, Sharer LR, Goudsmit J (1988) Neurological and neuropathological features of human immunodeficiency virus infection in children. *Annals of Neurology: Official Journal of the American Neurological Association and the Child Neurology Society*, 23(S1): S19–S23. doi: 10.1002/ana.410230709.

Govender R, Eley B, Walker K, Petersen R, Wilmshurst JM (2011) Neurologic and neurobehavioral sequelae in children with human immunodeficiency virus (HIV-1) infection. *Journal of Child Neurology*, 26(11): 1355–1364. doi: 10.1177/0883073811405203.

Hammond CK, Eley B, Wieselthaler N, Ndondo A, Wilmshurst JM (2016) Cerebrovascular disease in children with HIV infection. *Developmental Medicine & Child Neurology*, 58(5): 452–460. doi: 10.1111/dmcn.13080.

Hoare J, Fouche JP, Spottiswoode B et al. (2012) A diffusion tensor imaging and neurocognitive study of HIV-positive children who are HAART-naïve 'slow progressors'. *Journal of Neurovirology*, 18(3): 205–212. doi: 10.1007/s13365-012-0099-9.

Kovacs A (2009) Early immune activation predicts central nervous system disease in HIV-infected infants: Implications for early treatment. *Clinical Infectious Diseases*, 48(3): 347–349. doi: 10.1086/595886.

Lobato MN, Caldwell MB, Ng P, Oxtoby MJ, Pediatric Spectrum of Disease Clinical Consortium (1995) Encephalopathy in children with perinatally acquired human immunodeficiency virus infection. *The Journal of Pediatrics*, 126(5): 710–715. doi: 10.1016/S0022-3476(95)70397-7.

Newell ML, Brahmbhatt H, Ghys PD (2004) Child mortality and HIV infection in Africa: A review. *Aids*, 18: S27–S34. doi: 10.1097/01.aids.0000125981.71657.0d.

Ruel TD, Boivin MJ, Boal HE et al. (2012) Neurocognitive and motor deficits in HIV-infected Ugandan children with high CD4 cell counts. *Clinical Infectious Diseases*, 54(7): 1001–1009. doi: 10.1093/cid/cir1037.

Salihu HM, August EM, Aliyu M, Stanley KM, Weldeselasse H, Mbah AK (2012) Maternal HIV/AIDS status and neurological outcomes in neonates: A population-based study. *Maternal and Child Health Journal*, 16(3): 641–648. doi: 10.1007/s10995-011-0799-4.

Salomon JA, Haagsma JA, Davis A et al. (2015) Disability weights for the Global Burden of Disease 2013 study. *The Lancet Global Health*, 3(11): e712–e723. doi: 10.1016/S2214-109X(15)00069-8.

Tardieu M, Le Chenadec J, Persoz A, Meyer L, Blanche S, Mayaux MJ (2000) HIV-1–related encephalopathy in infants compared with children and adults. *Neurology*, 54(5): 1089–1095. doi: 10.1212/WNL.54.5.1089.

Tardieu M, Boutet A (2002) HIV-1 and the central nervous system. In: Dietzschold B, Richt JA, editors, *Protective and Pathological Immune Responses in the CNS*. Berlin & Heidelberg: Springer, pp. 183–195.

Van Rie A, Mupuala A, Dow A (2008) Impact of the HIV/AIDS epidemic on the neurodevelopment of preschool-aged children in Kinshasa, Democratic Republic of the Congo. *Pediatrics*, 122(1): e123–e128. doi: 10.1542/peds.2007-2558.

WHO (2020a) HIV/AIDS, 30 November 2021 [Online]. World Health Organization. [Viewed 12 February 2022]. Available at: https://www.who.int/news-room/fact-sheets/detail/hiv-aids.

WHO (2020b) HIV/AIDS: Key facts [Online]. World Health Organization. [Viewed 15 July 2020]. Available at: https://www.who.int/news-room/fact-sheets/detail/hiv-aids.

Pathogenesis of HIV Involvement in the Central Nervous System

Charles R Newton

INTRODUCTION

Human immunodeficiency virus type 1 (HIV-1) appears to invade the central nervous system (CNS) of children more easily than adults. Children often develop CNS manifestations before significant immunosuppression, even if they are infected after birth. The manifestations of direct invasion include neurodevelopmental impairment, behavioural difficulties, and cerebrovascular accidents: all of which are associated with a worse prognosis. Antiretroviral therapy (ART) has ameliorated the CNS effects, but there still remains significant morbidity associated with HIV infection of the CNS. In addition, the CNS of HIV-infected children is susceptible to opportunistic infections, tumours, and cerebrovascular disease – the pathogenesis of these complications will not be discussed in this chapter.

HUMAN IMMUNODEFICIENCY VIRUSES

HIV-1 is the most common and pathogenetic virus of humans. It is differentiated from HIV-2 by phylogenetic markers. HIV-1 is divided into a major group (M group), which is the most common, and other groups (N, O, P etc). The M group is further subdivided into subgroups (known as clades): A, B, C, D, F, G, H, J, and K based upon genotype. The distribution of the clades varies across the world, with the C clade most common in Africa and Asia, whilst the B clade is more common in Europe and North America. There are differences in transmission, viral replication, and progression of HIV disease between the clades. In particular, there is evidence that the B clade is more neurotoxic than the C clade in adults, although in some studies no difference was found (Ortega et al. 2013). However, even within a clade, neurotoxicity will vary. Hence, there are differences in the neurotoxicity of C clade variants between India and South Africa, probably related to the g120 protein (Rao et al. 2013). Most of these data come from adults, few from the paediatric populations. In one study of Ugandan children, clade A was associated with greater neurocognitive impairment. Boivin et al., observed greater neurocognitive impairment in ART-naïve subtype A Ugandan children compared to subtype D, with the degree of impairment associated with viral load (Boivin et al. 2010). However, if initiated on ART early in development, the preschool neurodevelopmental differences (Ruiseñor-Escudero et al. 2018) and school-age neurocognitive differences (Bangirana et al. 2017) were no longer significant. These were all clinically well-managed children, with good ART adherence. However, there were still long-term neurocognitive disabilities not resolved by ART and in need of behavioural intervention (Boivin et al. 2016). In contrast to adults where clade D was associated with a more rapid development of dementia, in ART-naïve immune-suppressed Ugandan adults, clade D was associated with more severe HIV-associated neurocognitive disorders HAND (Sacktor et al. 2009). However, these findings were not replicated in more moderate (clinically managed on ART) disease (Sacktor et al. 2014). One explanation was that affective ART management of adults with HIV diminished the neurocognitive disparities between greater clade A affinity to be trafficked into the CNS via macrophages, versus greater clade D affinity to lymphocyte system with greater immunocompromise from higher peripheral viral load and more poorly managed disease (Sacktor et al. 2019). Clade C (southern Africa) neurocognitive impairment seemed less virulent than clades A and D (Anderson et al. 2020).

ROUTES OF INFECTION

Most children are infected with HIV by mother-to-child transmission (MTCT). This can occur during pregnancy, at birth, or postnatally during breastfeeding. Before the introduction of ART, transmission occurred in up to 40% of infants (Lumaca et al. 2018). The risk factors for MTCT are vaginal delivery, preterm delivery, prolonged rupture of membranes, and chorioamnionitis. Maternal risk factors include malnutrition, the level of HIV-1 RNA at delivery, low maternal CD4+ cell count, and use of tobacco and illicit drugs, especially cocaine and heroin. Viral factors include clades, viral homogeneity, and rapid replication kinetics (Lumaca et al. 2018). The introduction of ART significantly reduced the transmission to 1% to 2% in resource-rich countries, although it is less effective in resource-poor environments. Children have also acquired HIV infection from contaminated blood products (either factor VIII for haemophilia, or blood transfusion which was not an uncommon route of transmission during the 1990s in Africa when blood was not screened), sexual intercourse (usually in the form of abuse) and, rarely, intravenous injections and percutaneous transmission from infected guardians. The route of infection influences the outcome, since it determines the age of exposure (the state of the child's immune system and brain development), the dose of the virus, and the presence of other susceptibility and protective factors.

INVASION OF HIV

HIV mainly infects cells expressing the CD4+ molecule, such as T lymphocytes, monocytes, and macrophages. The virus binds to the host CD4+ cells via a glycoprotein (gp160) on the virus surface. The binding of gp120 (one of the components of gp160) to the CD receptor induces a conformational change, exposing co-receptors (CCR5 and CXCR4) on the host cell wall, which allows the gp41 (another component of gp160) to insert into the host cell membrane, thus allowing viral particles to enter the cell. Viral particles release viral RNA strands and enzymes (protease, reverse transcriptase, and integrase). The viral RNA is transcribed by reverse transcriptase into pro-viral dsDNA, which is inserted into T-cell DNA by the integrase. Thus, during the transcription of the host cell DNA, the viral DNA is transcribed as well. Thereafter viral particles are produced, leading to virions, which bud from the host cell, maturing into infectious virions. This leads to the death of the CD4+ cells, which impairs cellular immunity.

The virus is spread throughout the body primarily by monocytes, particularly CD14[+] and CD16[+] T cells, and enters into the CNS (Williams et al. 2014). The HIV-1 invasion of the CNS occurs early after infection (within days) most probably via the choroid plexus and meninges, with the integrity of the blood–brain barrier compromised by inflammatory mediators such as cytokines. There is some evidence to suggest the virus may enter via other routes such as myelinated nerves and it is possible that cell-free HIV enters the brain directly. Although HIV enters the CNS most often during the early stages of the infection, further infections can occur during periods of high viral load.

Once within the immune-privileged CNS, the virus will infect other perivascular macrophages, microglia, and astrocytes. The virus particles are found more often in perivascular macrophages than in microglia, particularly those in the choroid plexus and meninges. This may be particularly important in children as lymphocytic meningitis is more often documented in children than in adults (Bell et al. 1997). The virus replicates in the macrophages and microglia, and both of these cell types are likely to be the source of the inflammatory mediators that are thought to cause neuronal damage in HIV infections. Replication of the virus in these cells is dependent on virus and host factors, with the degree of replication associated with cognitive decline in adults, although there are a few data from children. Astrocytes do not have CD4 receptors, yet up to 20% of astrocytes may contain HIV nucleic material. The mechanism by which astrocytes become infected is unclear – they may phagocytose debris from CD4+ cells. Although HIV-1 does not appear to replicate in astrocytes, these cells may be important reservoirs of HIV-1. The infection of these cells results in meningeal inflammation, microglial nodules, white matter lesions, multinucleated giant cells, myelin loss, HIV encephalitis, reactive astrogliosis, and regional atrophy, particularly in those not exposed to ART.

There is controversy as to whether HIV infects neurons that do not express CD4 receptors. There is experimental evidence that shows viral nucleic material in neurons; however, there is little evidence from human brain tissue in adults. Viral nucleic material has been found in the neuronal progenitor cells of children dying with HIV, and these cell types may act as reservoirs for HIV.

The genome of HIV integrates into the host cell genome (via reverse transcription) in some cells, after which HIV replication and destruction of the host cell may cease. This quiescent phase may last months or years before re-activation produces disease. The replication of HIV within the CNS occurs independently of that in the blood and other organs: thus, there is a partition of genetically distinct HIV clades within the CNS compared to that found in the blood. In a study of ART-naïve Malawian children, more than half had compartmentalisation of HIV-1 subtype C between the blood and cerebrospinal fluid as detected by single genome sequencing of Env (Sturdevant et al. 2012). The CNS is thought to act as a reservoir for HIV, since the infected cells have a longer half-life than those in the blood, there is a relative lack of immune surveillance, and some ART are not able to cross the blood–brain barrier. This has implications about for the effectiveness of ART.

The evaluation of clades A versus D in East Africa is important because it affords a direct comparison between the CCR5 (clade A) greater macrophage affinity for trafficking within CNS, versus CXCR4 (greater peripheral lymphocyte affinity). Such differences diminish post-ART in CNS development.

NEURONAL DAMAGE

HIV can cause neuronal damage by a multitude of mechanisms, with the products released by the virus or the cytokines and chemokines produced by the macrophages and microglia likely to be the most important. Gp120 is a potent neurotoxin, but the mechanisms of toxicity are unclear. Gp120 attaches to the CCR5 and CXCR4 receptors in CD4 negative neurons and astrocytes inducing apoptosis, possibly by the activation of p38/mitogen-activated protein kinase and c-Jun terminal kinase. The interaction of gp120 with CXCR4 receptors may also be protective, as it promotes neuronal migration and differentiation. The transactivator of transcription (*Tat*) protein in HIV-1 may also be directly neurotoxic. *Tat* protein reacts with proteins within the extracellular matrix involved in the adhesion of the neurons. In addition, it promotes apoptosis possibly via N-methyl-D-aspartate (NMDA). Both gp120 and *tat* proteins may induce the release of cytokines and glutamate, which induces apoptosis as well. In addition, *tat* protein induces nitric oxide, reactive oxygen species, and mitochondrial membrane depolarisation. Viral protein R appears to have a more direct effect by causing cell cycle arrest at the G2 stage and interactions with several candidate cellular proteins (Tungaturthi et al. 2003).

It is likely that products of the activated macrophages and microglia play a major role in the neuronal damage caused by HIV-1. HIV-1 infection in the brain causes an inflammatory response characterised by multinucleated giant cells, microglial nodules, perivascular cuffing by inflammatory cells, and gliosis. The infected and non-infected macrophages and microglia are activated, producing cytokines and chemokines. The pro-inflammatory cytokines, in particular tumour necrosis factor, interleukin (IL)-1$_\beta$ and IL-6 and the chemokines (CCL2, CXCL10, and CXCL12) produced by these cells, are thought to be the main mediators of neuronal damage (Nickoloff-Bybel et al. 2020).

More recent neuroinflammatory biomarkers predictive of progressive encephalopathy in children are identified. CD163 and its relationship to neurofilaments is strategic in the neurocognitive progression of even very early well-managed children on ART (Benki-Nugent et al. 2019). Also, neuroinflammatory array as it relates to neurocognitive effects in a multi-site neuropsychological study of virally suppressed African children identifies CD163 and other strategic biomarkers.

The patterns of neuronal damage are dependent on the expression of the chemokine and cytokine receptors. For example, the pyramidal neurons in the neocortex are susceptible to HIV damage since they express receptors, not only for chemokine and cytokine receptors, but also for glutamate, neurofilament, and microtubule associated protein-2. The expression of these and other receptors in the neurons and interneurons varies according to the region of the brain. Other types of neurons in the basal ganglia, and interneurons in the CA3 region of the hippocampus, are particularly prone to HIV-1 mediated damage. This may lead to dendritic simplification, aberrant sprouting, pruning, and dystrophic synaptodendritic connectivity, such as the connections between the left inferior frontal gyrus and caudate nucleus, in HIV-associated neurocognitive disorders in adults (du Plessis et al. 2017).

The pathogenesis of HIV infection on the CNS may be affected by comorbid conditions, in particular exposure to other neurotoxins such as illicit drugs and ART. Maternal drug abuse is likely to increase the transmission of the HIV to the foetus during birth and to the child during breastfeeding. This may be related to an increased viral load; but illicit drugs such as morphine, opioids, methamphetamine, and cocaine also enhance replication and spread of HIV (Wang and Ho 2011). ART has significantly reduced maternal transmission of HIV-1 and has altered the pathogenesis of HIV infection of the CNS. Despite the increasing use of ART to prevent MTCT, there is increasing evidence that such prophylactic treatment does not prevent HIV-1 entering the CNS, where it may reside for life.

CONCLUSION

HIV-1 causes neuronal injury through a variety of mechanisms, including damage induced by HIV proteins and inflammatory mediators, and is likely to be influenced by different clades, host genetics, comorbid conditions, and ART. Many of the data on the effect of HIV on the CNS have been derived from adults, and there are a few data on the pathogenesis of neuronal damage in children.

REFERENCES

Anderson SG, McCaul M, Khoo S et al. (2020) The neurologic phenotype of South African patients with HIV-associated neurocognitive impairment. *Neurol Clin Pract*, 10(1): 15–22. doi: 10.1212/CPJ.0000000000000.
Bangirana P, Ruel TD, Boivin MJ et al. (2017) Absence of neurocognitive disadvantage associated with paediatric HIV subtype A infection in children on antiretroviral therapy. *J Int AIDS Soc*, October, 20(2): e25015. doi: 10.1002/jia2.25015.

Bell, JE, Lowrie S, Koffi K et al. (1997) The neuropathology of HIV-infected African children in Abidjan, Cote d'Ivoire. *J Neuropathol Exp Neurol*, 56(6): 686–692.

Benki-Nugent SF, Martopullo I, Laboso T et al. (2019) High plasma soluble CD163 during infancy is a marker for neurocognitive outcomes in early-treated HIV-infected children. *J Acquir Immune Defic Synd*, May 1, 81(1): 102–109. doi: 10.1097/QAI.0000000000001979.

Boivin MJ, Ruel TD, Boal H et al. (2010) HIV-subtype A is associated with poorer neuropsychological performance compared to subtype D in ART-naïve Ugandan children. *AIDS*, 24(8): 1163–1170.

Boivin MJ, Ruiseñor-Escudero H, Familiar-Lopez I (2016) CNS impact of perinatal HIV infection and early treatment: The need for behavioral rehabilitative interventions along with medical treatment and care. *Curr HIV/AIDS Rep*, December, 13(6): 318–327. doi: 10.1007/s11904-016-0342-8.

du Plessis L, Paul RH, Hoare J et al. (2017) Resting-state functional magnetic resonance imaging in clade C HIV: Within-group association with neurocognitive function. *J Neurovirol*, 23(6): 875–885.

Lumaca A, Galli L, de Martino M, Chiappini E (2018) Paediatric HIV-1 infection: Updated strategies of prevention of mother-to-child transmission. *J Chemother*, 30(4): 193–202.

Nickoloff-Bybel EA, Calderon TM, Gaskill PJ, Berman JW (2020) HIV neuropathogenesis in the presence of a disrupted dopamine system. *J Neuroimmune Pharmacol*, 15(4): 729–742.

Ortega M, Heaps JM, Joska J et al. (2013) HIV clades B and C are associated with reduced brain volumetrics. *J Neurovirol*, 19(5): 479–487.

Rao VR, Neogi U, Talboom JS et al. (2013) Clade C HIV-1 isolates circulating in Southern Africa exhibit a greater frequency of dicysteine motif-containing Tat variants than those in Southeast Asia and cause increased neurovirulence. *Retrovirology*, 10: 61. doi: 10.1186/1742-4690-10-61; PMC3686704.

Ruiseñor-Escudero H, Sikorskii A, Familiar-Lopez I et al. (2018) Neurodevelopmental outcomes in preschool children living with HIV-1 subtypes A and D in Uganda. *Pediatr Infect Dis J*, December, 37(12): e298–e303. doi: 10.1097/INF.0000000000002097.

Sacktor N, Nakasujja N, Skolasky RL et al. (2009) HIV subtype D is associated with dementia, compared with subtype A, in immunosuppressed individuals at risk of cognitive impairment in Kampala, Uganda. *Clin Infect Dis*, September 1, 49(5): 780–786. doi: 10.1086/605284.

Sacktor N, Nakasujja N, Redd AD et al. (2014) HIV subtype is not associated with dementia among individuals with moderate and advanced immunosuppression in Kampala, Uganda. *Metab Brain Dis*, June, 29(2): 261–268. doi: 10.1007/s11011-014-9498-3. Epub 2014 Feb 12.

Sacktor N, Saylor D, Nakigozi G et al. (2019) Effect of HIV subtype and antiretroviral therapy on HIV-associated neurocognitive disorder stage in Rakai, Uganda. *J Acquir Immune Defic Syndr*, June 1, 81(2): 216–223. doi: 10.1097/QAI.0000000000001992.

Sturdevant CB, Dow A, Jabara CB et al. (2012) Central nervous system compartmentalization of HIV-1 subtype C variants early and late in infection in young children. *PLoS Pathog*, 8(12): e1003094.

Tungaturthi PK, Sawaya BE, Singh SP et al. (2003) Role of HIV-1 Vpr in AIDS pathogenesis: Relevance and implications of intravirion, intracellular and free Vpr. *Biomedicine & Pharmacotherapy*, 57(1): 20–24.

Wang X, Ho WZ (2011) Drugs of abuse and HIV infection/replication: Implications for mother-fetus transmission. *Life Sci*, 88(21–22): 972–979.

Williams DW, Veenstra M, Gaskill P et al. (2014) Monocytes mediate HIV neuropathogenesis: Mechanisms that contribute to HIV-associated neurocognitive disorders. *Curr HIV Res*, 12(2): 85–96.

Neurological Manifestations of HIV Infection

Charles K Hammond and Jo M Wilmshurst

INTRODUCTION

The human immunodeficiency virus type 1 (HIV-1) is highly neurotropic. It enters the central nervous system (CNS) compartment within the first few weeks of systemic infection and may cause a spectrum of neurological complications in both the CNS and peripheral nervous system (PNS), collectively referred to as neuroAIDS. The CNS may serve as a reservoir for HIV-1, as latent viral DNA may persist in the CNS, preventing the eradication of HIV. In children infected through vertical (mother-to-child) transmission who are left untreated, up to 60% will develop progressive HIV encephalopathy (HIVE), a severe manifestation of neuroAIDS (Donald et al. 2015). Most of these children acquire this condition during their first year of life (Van Rie et al. 2007). In older persons, severe neurocognitive difficulties are seen if the HIV infection is left untreated (Clifford and Ances 2013).

Since 2008, the World Health Organization (WHO) has recommended that all HIV-infected children less than 1 year of age should be treated with combination antiretroviral therapy (cART) (WHO 2008). However, in low- and middle-income countries (LMICs), particularly in sub-Saharan Africa and Southeast Asia, where most HIV-infected children reside, there is limited access to health care. This results in significant delays in initiating cART during early childhood (Davies et al. 2013), allowing neuroAIDS to manifest.

In a clinical trial in HIV-infected infants, there was evidence that early initiation of ART significantly reduced the progression of the infection to severe forms such as neuroAIDS (Violari et al. 2008). In a similar study conducted in HIV-infected adults, there were improved outcomes in asymptomatic patients who were treated early with antiretroviral drugs as compared to those who received deferred treatment (INSIGHT START Study Group 2015). These studies, among others, have informed the current standard of care for early start of cART among both children and adults with HIV infection.

In managing a child with neuroAIDS, it is important to have a broader view of not just the HIV infection and the specific neurological complication identified, but also of other possible undiagnosed neurological complications, the host's immune response to treatment, adverse effects of antiretroviral drugs (ARVs), and possible drug-to-drug interactions. In LMICs, it is also important to consider the multiple socioeconomic challenges faced by HIV-infected children, leading to anaemia, protein energy malnutrition, and micronutrient deficiencies.

This chapter gives an overview of the neurological complications of HIV-1 infection in children and adolescents, including HIVE, HIV-associated neurocognitive disorder (HAND), opportunistic neuroinfections, neuro-oncologic complications, seizures and epilepsy, cerebrovascular diseases, and peripheral nerve disease, as well as neurocognitive and neuropsychiatric complications. All these topics are elaborated upon in the subsequent chapters.

HIV ENCEPHALOPATHY

In children infected in utero or in the perinatal period, early invasion of the CNS by HIV affects the developing foetal or infant brain, exposing the child to the potential risk of developing HIVE if the infection is left untreated (Van Rie et al. 2007). The Centers for Disease Control and Prevention (CDC) criteria for the diagnosis of HIVE (CDC 1994) requires the presence of at least one of the following for 2 or more months:

- Loss of, or failure to reach, developmental milestones, or loss of intellectual ability.
- Impaired brain growth or acquired microcephaly.
- Acquired systemic motor deficit manifested by two or more of the following: paresis, pathologic reflexes, ataxia, or gait disturbance.

HIVE is the most common primary HIV-related CNS complication, with a reported prevalence in non-treated, vertically-infected children ranging from 20% to 60% (Donald et al. 2015). In the pre-ART era, the most severe form of this disorder typically occurred among young children who were infected in utero and developed rapidly progressing disease associated with profound immunosuppression (Mitchell 2006). In the era of cART, there has been a significant decrease in the incidence, prevalence, and severity of HIVE, with improved outcomes in most children who are treated early (Czornyj 2006; Moulignier 2006). Recent reports quote the prevalence of HIVE to be about 18% among HIV-infected children (Donald et al. 2014).

The most remarkable results in children who received cART treatment compared to children who did not receive treatment in the pre-ART era are:

1. A remission or noteworthy improvement of progressive and non-progressive encephalopathy.
2. Conversion of the most severe cases of progressive encephalopathy (severe developmental delay, acquired microcephaly, spastic quadriparesis, and fatal progression) into a more moderate phenotype (less developmental delay, normal head growth, spastic paraparesis, and chronic evolution of the disease).
3. Reversion of acquired microcephaly observed in the early years of the AIDS epidemic (Czornyj 2006).

The introduction of cART alone cannot explain the decline in the global incidence of HIVE. This is because in LMICs where most of the affected children reside, there is still reduced access to cART. Thus, it is suggested that other factors, including improved global health care, have contributed to the decline in HIVE in these regions (Donald et al. 2015).

HIV-ASSOCIATED NEUROCOGNITIVE DISORDER

In older persons living with HIV, significant impairment in cognition may develop. This is known as HAND. The typical manifestations include difficulties with attention, concentration, and memory, as well as slowed movements. In the pre-cART era, HIV-associated dementia (HAD) was the most common form of HAND. However, in the cART era, HAD has declined substantially, and milder forms – namely asymptomatic neurocognitive impairment and mild neurocognitive disorder – predominate. While patients with HAD had marked impairments in activities of daily living, patients with asymptomatic neurocognitive impairment and mild neurocognitive disorder have no and mild impairments respectively (Clifford and Ances 2013; Sacktor 2018), indicating that cART is beneficial in the prevention and treatment of HAND.

NEUROINFECTIONS

The incidence of CNS opportunistic infections among HIV-infected children is reported to range from 8% to 34% (Donald et al. 2014). This includes bacterial, viral, fungal, and parasitic (predominantly toxoplasmosis) infections. The neurologic outcome of infections such as measles in the HIV-infected child is also noteworthy. In South Africa, there was an outbreak of measles from 2009 to 2011, affecting up to 37 per 100 000 individuals, including both HIV-infected and uninfected children and adults (Ntshoe et al. 2013). However, there are differences between the HIV-infected and uninfected children in the presentation of some long-term neurologic outcomes.

Bacterial Meningitis

The most common bacterial pathogens causing meningitis in HIV-infected children are *Streptococcus pneumoniae* and *Haemophilus influenzae* type B, primarily affecting unvaccinated children (Madhi et al. 2001; Molyneux et al. 2003). Their presentation is like that of HIV seronegative children, but HIV-infected children are more likely to be in shock on arrival at the hospital, and they often have a focal site of infection (Molyneux et al. 2003). Management should include standard comprehensive infection workup and appropriate antibiotic treatment. Compared to HIV negative children, there is a higher rate of recurrence and an increased mortality among HIV-infected children (Molyneux et al. 2003). Immunisation and long-term antibiotic (e.g. co-trimoxazole) prophylaxis are important interventions for preventing both primary and recurrent bacterial infections in HIV-infected children (Bwakura-Dangarembizi et al. 2014; Wilmshurst, Donald, and Eley 2014). Specific immunisations useful in this cohort include pneumococcal conjugate vaccine, *Haemophilus influenzae* B vaccine, and meningococcal vaccines (Hoffmann and Cennimo 2021).

Tuberculous Meningitis

Tuberculous meningitis (TBM) is common in high tuberculosis (TB) endemic regions. Clinical presentations may include nonspecific findings, such as a low-grade fever, night sweats, failure to thrive, seizures, and encephalopathy. In HIV-infected children, TBM may present as a diagnostic and therapeutic challenge, because the typical basal meningeal enhancement and hydrocephalus seen on neuroimaging in immuno-competent individuals with TBM (see Figure 4.9d, Chapter 4) may be subtle or absent (see Figures 4.9a and 4.9b, Chapter 4) (van der Weert et al. 2006). This is because HIV-infected children lack the immunologic response required to produce these changes shown on neuroimaging. Similarly, responses from TB skin tests may not be as definitive as in immuno-competent children (Lancella et al. 2016). As such, a low threshold for diagnostic consideration is necessary when analysing this demographic.

HIV-TBM coinfection also presents unique therapeutic challenges. TB granulomas may be poorly organised due to impaired cellular recruitment and this increases the susceptibility to both active and disseminated TB disease. This may lead to the persistence of an *M. tuberculosis* infection despite optimal treatment (Diedrich, O'Hern, and Wilkinson 2016). The WHO recommends a 12-month anti-TB treatment regimen, where children with suspected or confirmed TBM are treated with a four-drug regimen comprising isoniazid, rifampicin, pyrazinamide, and ethambutol for 2 months. This is followed by a two-drug regimen comprising isoniazid and rifampicin for 10 months (WHO 2010). However, some authors recommend a shorter treatment duration of 9 months (Lancella et al. 2016). Corticosteroid treatment reduces the risk of neurodisability and death in HIV-uninfected children with TBM, and may also be used in HIV-infected children, although the benefits of this treatment in this cohort are not clearly demonstrated (van Toorn and Solomons 2014).

Significant drug–drug interactions may also complicate the management of HIV-TBM coinfection. Some antituberculous drugs induce cytochrome P450 enzymes, which tend to metabolise the ARVs leading to a significant decrease in ARV concentrations, resulting in treatment failure and the development of increased viral resistance. For example, rifampicin reduces markedly the concentration of lopinavir when coadministered, resulting in subtherapeutic lopinavir concentrations (Ren et al. 2008). There is a modest decrease in nevirapine concentrations when administered concomitantly with rifampicin-based tuberculosis treatment (Cohen et al. 2008). The effect of rifampicin-containing tuberculosis treatment on efavirenz concentrations is complex, with mid-dosing concentrations of efavirenz usually decreasing marginally when coadministered with rifampicin (Ren et al. 2009).

The timing of cART initiation in HIV-TBM coinfection is another important treatment consideration. Initiation of cART may lead to an immune reconstitution inflammatory syndrome (TBM-IRIS) with a paradoxical clinical deterioration (Kampmann et al. 2006; Schoeman and van Toorn 2014). In these children, starting cART restores immune function. In the context of an underlying opportunistic infection, this restoration in immune function may trigger an exaggerated immune response within weeks to months after cART initiation. This results in a paradoxical worsening of the patient's clinical condition. CNS IRIS may develop with or without an opportunistic infection and can range in severity. It should be suspected when new neurological signs develop shortly after initiation of cART in an HIV-infected child. Severe cases can be fatal and may require treatment with steroids (Johnson and Nath 2010; van Toorn et al. 2012).

Viral Infections

Viral infections of the CNS occur in HIV-infected children less frequently than in adults, since reactivation of prior infections is less likely in childhood. Common viruses include herpes simplex virus, varicella-zoster virus, and cytomegalovirus, causing acute, subacute, or chronic encephalitis or ventriculitis. The John Cunningham virus causes progressive multifocal leukoencephalopathy, a symmetrical white-matter disorder (see Figures 4.10a–4.10d, Chapter 4) more common in adults. In HIV-infected children, progressive multifocal leukoencephalopathy is rarely reported but may follow cART initiation due to IRIS (Nuttall et al. 2004; Wilmshurst, Eley, and Brew 2014).

CNS Complications of Measles

The CNS complications of measles include primary measles encephalitis and acute post-infectious measles encephalomyelitis, which occur within days of measles infection; measles inclusion body encephalitis (MIBE), which occurs in immunocompromised individuals within a year of measles infection or vaccination; and subacute sclerosing panencephalitis (SSPE), which may occur several years after measles infection in children, especially in the immunocompromised and those infected in the first year of life (Buchanan and Bonthius 2012).

Patients with MIBE often present with altered mental status, intractable focal seizures (epilepsia partialis continua), focal motor deficits, cortical blindness, language or articulation problems, and dysphagia.

They may also present with emotional lability, headache, vomiting, fever, hypertension, or other autonomic signs (Mustafa et al. 1993; Buchanan and Bonthius 2012). In a case series of eight patients seen in South Africa after the 2009 to 2011 measles outbreak, the affected persons were HIV-infected adolescents and adults with low CD4+ counts at the time of measles infection. Epilepsia partialis continua was a key symptom in all cases (Albertyn et al. 2011). There is no effective treatment, but intravenous and oral ribavirin have been used in some cases (Mustafa et al. 1993; Freeman et al. 2004; Buchanan and Bonthius 2012).

SSPE is due to persistent infection with defective measles virus, and it is seen in children who contract measles in infancy or early childhood (Buchanan and Bonthius 2012; Griffin 2014). HIV-infected or exposed children who contract measles may be at increased risk (Mekki et al. 2019). It manifests 6 to 15 years after the acute measles infection, but it may manifest earlier in immunocompromised children (Kija et al. 2015). Patients initially present with behavioural problems and cognitive decline, followed by motor dysfunction and myoclonic seizures. Progressive neurological deterioration leads to rigidity and later ocular manifestations, including necrotising retinitis, optic neuritis, and cortical blindness. As the disease progresses, patients lapse into a stupor, total mutism, autonomic instability, and eventual death (Buchanan and Bonthius 2012; Griffin 2014). Treatment with a combination of isoprinosine and interferon-alpha may slow disease progression (Griffin 2014). There are reports of symptomatic relief of the myoclonic jerks with antiseizure medications (ASMs) such as carbamazepine, sodium valproate and clonazepam (Yiğit and Sarikaya 2006; Ravikumar and Crawford 2013; Mekki et al. 2019). Routine measles vaccination remains the best approach for preventing both MIBE and SSPE (Buchanan and Bonthius 2012; Griffin 2014; Mekki et al. 2019).

Fungal Meningitis

Fungal meningitis may be caused by *Candida* species or *Aspergillus fumigatus*, which could be complicated by fungal abscesses (Kozlowski, Sher, and Dickson 1990). Cryptococcal meningitis and toxoplasma encephalitis may occur, but are rare in children (Simmonds and Gonzalo 1998; Wilmshurst, Eley, and Brew 2014).

NEURO-ONCOLOGY COMPLICATIONS

Primary CNS lymphoma is the most common CNS mass lesion in HIV-infected children and adults (Mikol et al. 1995; Little 2006), with an incidence rate of 0.4% to 0.56% in epidemiological studies and 7.6% in post-mortem series from the pre-cART era (Mikol et al. 1995). Tumours tend to be high-grade, multifocal B-cell tumours. Affected children present with new onset focal neurological signs, headaches, and seizures, and they may have subacute onset of changes in cognitive status or behaviour. On neuroimaging, lesions are enhanced with contrast (see Figures 4.13a and 4.13b, Chapter 4), and they are associated with mass effect and oedema. Demonstration of Epstein–Barr virus (EBV) in cerebrospinal fluid (CSF) can accurately confirm the lymphoma. The outcome of primary CNS lymphoma is usually poor (Little 2006).

SEIZURES AND EPILEPSY

The prevalence of epilepsy in HIV-infected children is quoted as between 7.6% and 14%, which is higher than in uninfected children (Govender et al. 2011; Samia et al. 2013). Seizures may result from direct viral damage done during the acute disease course, neuroinfections, or chronic encephalopathy

(Kellinghaus et al. 2008; Donald et al. 2014). Focal seizures are more common than generalised seizures in these patients (Siddiqi and Birbeck 2013).

During acute seizure presentation, a thorough assessment is necessary to identify the primary aetiology of seizure activity. Basic laboratory and radiological studies should include serum glucose, electrolytes, complete blood count, liver function tests, blood and urine cultures, and a chest X-ray. An initial cranial computed tomography (CT) scan may help rule out a mass lesion prior to a lumbar puncture. CSF examination is recommended in all immunocompromised patients, even if they are afebrile. These tests should include cell counts, basic chemistry, bacterial cultures, and viral studies (Siddiqi and Birbeck 2013).

The long-term management of epilepsy in HIV-infected children may be complicated by significant drug interactions between ASMs and ARVs. The enzyme-inducing ASMs – namely phenytoin, phenobarbital and carbamazepine – can have significant interactions with protease inhibitors (PIs) and non-nucleoside reverse transcriptase inhibitors (NNRTIs). This can potentially result in virologic failure, suboptimal seizure control, or drug toxicity (DiCenzo et al. 2004; Lim et al. 2004; Ji et al. 2008; Siddiqi and Birbeck 2013).

The selection of ASMs for the long-term management of seizures in HIV-infected children should be guided by the seizure types, comorbidities, cART regimen, and the current data on drug–drug interactions (University of Liverpool 2021). The recommendation is to avoid enzyme-inducing ASMs in people on cART regimens that include PIs or NNRTIs (Birbeck et al. 2012; Okulicz et al. 2013; Siddiqi and Birbeck 2013). If such ASMs are required for seizure control, patients may be monitored through pharmacokinetic assessments to ensure efficacy of the ARV regimen (Birbeck et al. 2012). In resource-poor settings where the newer ASMs are unavailable and pharmacokinetic testing is only accessible within research, sodium valproate/valproic acid remains a reasonable choice due to its broad spectrum of activity, relative affordability, and less significant interactions with PIs and NNRTIs (Birbeck et al. 2012). Where available, lamotrigine, levetiracetam, and lacosamide have been used in both children and adults. (Birbeck et al. 2012; Siddiqi and Birbeck 2013).

CEREBROVASCULAR DISEASE

Between 1.3% and 2.6% of HIV-infected children develop strokes (Park et al. 1990; Patsalides et al. 2002), although the prevalence of ischaemic infarcts at autopsy is higher (Park et al. 1990; Qureshi et al. 1997). Strokes may be ischaemic or haemorrhagic, the former being more common. Haemorrhagic strokes are usually intracerebral or subarachnoid bleeds (Hammond et al. 2016a).

Stroke in HIV-infected children may result directly from viral invasion of the cerebral blood vessels, known as HIV-associated cerebral vasculopathy, or indirectly from opportunistic vasculitides, primary CNS lymphomas, coagulopathy, or cardio-embolisms (Hammond et al. 2016a). HIV-associated cerebral vasculopathy predominantly affects medium-sized vessels with radiological evidence of vessel stenosis, occlusion, or aneurysmal dilatation (see Figures 4.6a–4.6f, Chapter 4) that appears without any identifiable cause other than the HIV infection (Connor 2009; Benjamin et al. 2012).

HIV directly infects the vascular wall, leading to damage to the endothelium, smooth muscle, and connective tissue, with resultant stenosis, occlusion, or dilatation of the vessels, increasing the risk of thrombosis and ischaemic strokes (Hammond et al. 2016a). This is more frequently reported in individuals with active infection (low CD4 counts or high viral loads) (Chow et al. 2014). The systemic infection may also trigger an autoimmune vasculopathy, leading to endothelial cell damage and, subsequently, stroke (Hammond et al. 2016a).

In settings with limited access to cARTs, strokes may result from opportunistic vasculitides secondary to varicella-zoster virus, cytomegalovirus, mycobacterium, candida, cryptococcal, or treponemal infections (Pinto 1996). In patients with primary CNS lymphomas, strokes are the result of either direct vascular injury caused by focal infiltration, or ischaemia following focal thrombosis (Kieburtz et al. 1993).

Stroke in HIV-infected children is reported to follow deficiencies in proteins S and/or C because of consumptive coagulopathy in response to the systemic infection. Cardio-embolism usually results from bacterial endocarditis, and, in rare cases, from opportunistic infections (marantic endocarditis) or cardiac infection with HIV itself (Hammond et al. 2016a).

Prolonged use of cART, which includes PIs in adults, is reported to result in elevated cholesterol and triglyceride levels, which increases the risk of stroke (d'Arminio et al. 2004). Cerebral vasculopathy is also reported in individuals with rapid immune restoration following the initiation of cART (Bonkowsky et al. 2002).

Cerebrovascular disease in HIV-infected children may present clinically as overt motor manifestations, transient ischaemic attacks, or subtle behavioural or cognitive changes that can often be confused with HIVE. Cases of silent progression to moyamoya syndrome, a vasculopathy in which there is progressive occlusion of the major vessels in the circle of Willis with development of collateral circulation (see Figures 4.7a–4.7e, Chapter 4) have been reported (Hammond et al. 2016b).

The basic workup of an HIV-infected child presenting with a stroke should include complete blood counts, glucose level, and electrolytes, as well as CD4 counts and HIV RNA viral load. Blood and CSF samples should be sent for infectious screenings. Basic imaging should include a brain CT scan, chest radiographs, and an echocardiograph. Where available, magnetic resonance imaging or magnetic resonance angiography should be undertaken as well as screening for opportunistic vasculitis, coagulopathy, and cardio-embolism (Benjamin et al. 2012; Hammond et al. 2016a).

Management priorities should include optimising virologic suppression, correcting anaemia, controlling seizures, and initiating aspirin prophylaxis (Hammond et al. 2016a).

PERIPHERAL NERVE DISEASE

HIV-associated distal symmetrical polyneuropathy (HIV-DSP) is the most common presentation of peripheral nerve disease in HIV. Other forms of neuropathies include acute inflammatory demyelinating polyneuropathy (Guillain-Barré syndrome), chronic inflammatory demyelinating polyneuropathy, autonomic neuropathy, mononeuropathies, and cranial neuropathies (Kaku and Simpson 2014).

HIV-DSP has been reported in both children and adults, and it is mainly caused by the direct effect of HIV infection on the PNS or by the toxic effect of ART on the PNS (such as the dideoxynucleoside analogues stavudine and didanosine, also called the d-drugs). It may be asymptomatic or present with distal, symmetric symptoms in a stocking-glove distribution. Poor nutritional state and global muscle wasting may dominate the clinical picture, masking focal wasting due to underlying peripheral neuropathy (Donald et al. 2014; Kaku and Simpson 2014). Thus, unless accompanied by pain, the clinical signs are often subtle in a chronically unwell child and can be easily missed. Acute inflammatory demyelinating polyradiculoneuropathy (AIDP) typically presents with ascending muscle weakness and loss of reflexes with sparing of sensory symptoms (Kaku and Simpson 2014).

The evaluation of peripheral nerve disease in HIV-infected children should include a clinical neurological examination and basic laboratory investigations, such as blood counts and a CSF examination, and, where available, nerve conduction studies and an electromyography (Kaku and Simpson 2014). Blood counts should aim to exclude other forms of neuropathy such as vitamin B12 deficiency. In patients with high CD4 counts presenting with AIDP or chronic inflammatory demyelinating polyneuropathy (CIDP), CSF should be interpreted with caution, as it tends to show elevated protein with mild lymphocytic pleocytosis even in steady states. CSF studies should also include polymerase chain reaction (PCR) assays for cytomegalovirus and other viruses.

Available treatment options focus on symptomatic pain management. Several agents have been used with limited success. They include topical capsaicin, recombinant human nerve growth factor, gabapentin, pregabalin, lamotrigine, amitriptyline, cannabis, prosaptide, peptide-T, and acetyl-L-carnitine (Kaku and Simpson 2014; Wilmshurst, Eley, and Brew 2014). AIDP and CIDP are typically treated with intravenous immunoglobulin or plasmapheresis. The use of corticosteroids in HIV-infected patients should be undertaken with caution because of immunosuppression (Kaku and Simpson 2014). In antiretroviral toxic neuropathy, management may require termination of the culprit ARV. With the shift away from d-drugs, there has been a decrease in the incidence of peripheral nerve disease in HIV-infected individuals (Machado-Alba 2013).

NEUROCOGNITIVE AND NEUROPSYCHIATRIC MANIFESTATIONS IN ADOLESCENTS

As more children gain access to cART, they are surviving longer and living into adolescence and adulthood. The prolonged survival comes with the specific issues of adolescence in addition to the neurocognitive and neuropsychiatric challenges from the HIV infection. Inflammatory cytokines and immune activation play important roles in the progression of neurocognitive impairment (Buch et al. 2016). The neurocognitive and psychiatric manifestations seen in HIV-infected adolescents are the results of several factors. These include the direct effect of the virus on the brain, the psychosocial stressors of the disease, and the behavioural issues related to adolescence. The spectrum of neurocognitive and behavioural manifestations ranges from mild neurocognitive impairment to severe disabilities, and includes:

1. Poor performance in general intelligence testing, in specific cognitive domains like executive function, and in academic challenges (Hoare et al. 2015, 2016).
2. Mental health problems, such as attention deficit hyperactivity disorder, depression, anxiety, and conduct disorders (Scharko 2006; Mellins and Malee 2013).
3. Behavioural issues associated with adolescence, such as risk-taking, poor cART adherence, peer relationship problems, and experimentation with drugs, alcohol, and sex (Battles and Wiener 2002; Mellins and Malee 2013).
4. Psychosocial stressors, including stigmatisation, post-traumatic stress following the loss of parents or siblings to AIDS, the fear of death from AIDS or AIDS-related conditions, and issues of disclosure (Battles and Wiener 2002).
5. Some neuropsychiatric manifestations in adolescents, such as depression, paranoia, hallucinations, and suicidal ideation may be related to the effects of ARVs such as efavirenz (Hammond, Eley, and Wilmshurst 2016).

SUMMARY

HIV-1 is highly neurotropic and may cause a spectrum of neurological complications collectively known as neuroAIDS. In children infected through vertical (mother-to-child) transmission, the neurological manifestations may display a more complex phenotype because of the effects of the virus on the immature brain. With the early initiation of cART, there has been an improvement in the overall health of children with vertically transmitted HIV infection. HIVE, which previously presented with severe neurodisability and demise, now presents with a more insidious phenotype in association with prolonged survival.

However, in many parts of sub-Saharan Africa and Southeast Asia, where prevalence of HIV in children remains high, there are multiple factors that allow neuroAIDS to persist. These include limited access to cART, and socioeconomic challenges such as being orphaned, being born into child-led households, and inadequate nutrition. Prevention of mother-to-child transmission, early initiation of cART, appropriate immunisations and prophylaxis, and improvement in general health and nutrition are important interventions in the prevention of neuroAIDS.

Clinicians should have a high index of suspicion to accurately diagnose and treat these complications, as they often present with subtle signs and elude definitive diagnosis. Appropriate surveillance and follow-up measures are necessary in HIV-infected children because some neurological manifestations may evolve silently over time.

As a result of improvement in the general health care of perinatally-infected children, many more children are surviving into adolescence and adulthood. These persons often present with cognitive and psychiatric complications that require active intervention from health-care services. Clinicians should be prepared for changes in the clinical manifestations of neuroAIDS in these adolescents.

This chapter has provided a general overview of the neurological complications in children and adolescents with HIV infection, describing many recent developments that have broadened our understanding of the impact that HIV-1 infection has on the brain during childhood and adolescence. Subsequent chapters provide more detailed descriptions of these complications.

REFERENCES

Albertyn C, van der Plas H, Hardie D et al. (2011) Silent casualties from the measles outbreak in South Africa. *South African Medical Journal = Suid-Afrikaanse Tydskrif Vir Geneeskunde*, 101(5): 313–314, 316–317. https://doi.org/10.7196/samj.4616.

Battles HB, Wiener LS (2002) From adolescence through young adulthood: Psychosocial adjustment associated with long-term survival of HIV. *The Journal of Adolescent Health: Official Publication of the Society for Adolescent Medicine*, 30(3): 161–168.

Benjamin LA, Bryer A, Emsley HCA, Khoo S, Solomon T, Connor MD (2012) HIV infection and stroke: Current perspectives and future directions. *The Lancet. Neurology*, 11(10): 878–890. https://doi.org/10.1016/S1474-4422(12)70205-3.

Birbeck GL, French JA, Perucca E et al. (2012) Antiepileptic drug selection for people with HIV/AIDS: Evidence-based guidelines from the ILAE and AAN. *Epilepsia*, 53(1): 207–314. https://doi.org/10.1111/j.1528-1167.2011.03335.x.

Bonkowsky JL, Christenson JC, Nixon GW, Pavia AT (2002) Cerebral aneurysms in a child with acquired immune deficiency syndrome during rapid immune reconstitution. *Journal of Child Neurology*, 17(6): 457–460.

Buch S, Chivero ET, Hoare J et al. (2016) Proceedings from the NIMH Symposium on 'NeuroAIDS in Africa: Neurological and Neuropsychiatric Complications of HIV'. *Journal of Neurovirology*, 22(5): 699–702. https://doi.org/10.1007/s13365-016-0467-y.

Buchanan R, Bonthius DJ (2012) Measles virus and associated central nervous system sequelae. *Seminars in Pediatric Neurology*, 19(3): 107–114. https://doi.org/10.1016/j.spen.2012.02.003.

Bwakura-Dangarembizi M, Kendall L, Bakeera-Kitaka S et al. (2014) A randomized trial of prolonged co-trimoxazole in HIV-infected children in Africa. *The New England Journal of Medicine*, 370(1): 41–53. https://doi.org/10.1056/NEJMoa1214901.

CDC (1994) Revised classification system for human immunodeficiency virus infection in children less than 13 years of age. https://www.cdc.gov/MMWR/preview/mmwrhtml/00032890.htm.

Chow FC, Bacchetti P, Kim AS, Price RW, Hsue PY (2014) Effect of CD4+ cell count and viral suppression on risk of ischemic stroke in HIV infection. *AIDS (London, England)*, 28(17): 2573–2577. https://doi.org/10.1097/QAD.0000000000000452.

Clifford DB, Ances BM (2013) HIV-associated neurocognitive disorder. *The Lancet. Infectious Diseases*, 13(11): 976–986. https://doi.org/10.1016/S1473-3099(13)70269-X.

Cohen K, van Cutsem G, Boulle A et al. (2008) Effect of rifampicin-based antitubercular therapy on nevirapine plasma concentrations in South African adults with HIV-associated tuberculosis. *The Journal of Antimicrobial Chemotherapy*, 61(2): 389–393. https://doi.org/10.1093/jac/dkm484.

Connor M (2009) Treatment of HIV-associated cerebral vasculopathy. *Journal of Neurology, Neurosurgery, and Psychiatry* 80(8): 831. https://doi.org/10.1136/jnnp.2008.169490.

Czorny LA (2006) [Encephalopathy in children infected by vertically transmitted human immunodeficiency virus] [Article in Spanish]. *Revista De Neurologia*, 42(12): 743–753.

d'Arminio A, Sabin CA, Phillips AN et al. (2004) Cardio- and cerebrovascular events in HIV-infected persons. *AIDS*, 18(13): 1811–1817.

Davies M-A, Phiri S, Wood R et al. (2013) Temporal trends in the characteristics of children at antiretroviral therapy initiation in Southern Africa: The IeDEA-SA collaboration. *PloS One*, 8(12): e81037. https://doi.org/10.1371/journal.pone.0081037.

DiCenzo R, Peterson D, Cruttenden K et al. (2004) Effects of valproic acid coadministration on plasma efavirenz and lopinavir concentrations in human immunodeficiency virus-infected adults. *Antimicrobial Agents and Chemotherapy*, 48(11): 4328–4331. https://doi.org/10.1128/AAC.48.11.4328-4331.2004.

Diedrich CR, O'Hern J, Wilkinson RJ (2016) HIV-1 and the mycobacterium tuberculosis granuloma: A systematic review and meta-analysis. *Tuberculosis (Edinburgh, Scotland)*, 98(May): 62–76. https://doi.org/10.1016/j.tube.2016.02.010.

Donald KA, Hoare J, Eley B, Wilmshurst JM (2014) Neurologic complications of pediatric human immunodeficiency virus: Implications for clinical practice and management challenges in the African setting. *Seminars in Pediatric Neurology*, 21(1): 3–11. https://doi.org/10.1016/j.spen.2014.01.004.

Donald KA, Walker KG, Kilborn T et al. (2015) HIV encephalopathy: Pediatric case series description and insights from the clinic coalface. *AIDS Research and Therapy*, 12(1) (January): 2. https://doi.org/10.1186/s12981-014-0042-7.

Freeman AF, Jacobsohn DA, Shulman ST et al. (2004) A new complication of stem cell transplantation: Measles inclusion body encephalitis. *Pediatrics*, 114(5): e657–e660. https://doi.org/10.1542/peds.2004-0949.

Govender R, Eley B, Walker K, Petersen R, Wilmshurst JM (2011) Neurologic and neurobehavioral sequelae in children with human immunodeficiency virus (HIV-1) infection. *Journal of Child Neurology*, 26(11): 1355–1364. https://doi.org/10.1177/0883073811405203.

Griffin DE (2014) Measles virus and the nervous system. *Handbook of Clinical Neurology*, 123: 577–590. https://doi.org/10.1016/B978-0-444-53488-0.00027-4.

Hammond CK, Eley B, Wilmshurst JM (2016) Neuropsychiatric complications of efavirenz in children with HIV infection. *Future Virology*, 11(6): 469–480. https://doi.org/10.2217/fvl-2016-0030.

Hammond CK, Eley B, Wieselthaler N, Ndondo A, Wilmshurst JM (2016a) Cerebrovascular disease in children with HIV-1 infection. *Developmental Medicine and Child Neurology*, 58(5)(February): 452–460. https://doi.org/10.1111/dmcn.13080.

Hammond CK, Shapson-Coe A, Govender R et al. (2016b) Moyamoya syndrome in South African children with HIV-1 infection. *Journal of Child Neurology*, 31(8)(March): 1010–1017. https://doi.org/10.1177/0883073816635747.

Hoare J, Fouche J-P, Phillips N et al. (2015) White matter micro-structural changes in ART-naïve and ART-treated children and adolescents infected with HIV in South Africa. *AIDS (London, England)*, 29(14): 1793–1801. https://doi.org/10.1097/QAD.0000000000000766.

Hoare J, Phillips N, Joska JA et al. (2016) Applying the HIV-associated neurocognitive disorder diagnostic criteria to HIV-infected youth. *Neurology*, 87(1): 86–93. https://doi.org/10.1212/WNL.0000000000002669.

Hoffmann JR, Cennimo DJ (2021) Prevention of opportunistic infections (OI) in patients with HIV infection: General guidelines for prophylaxis, exposure avoidance, initiation of prophylaxis and treatment. Edited by Mary L Windle and John Bartlett. July 2021. https://emedicine.medscape.com/article/1529727-overview#a5.

INSIGHT START Study Group, Lundgren JD, Babiker AG et al. (2015) Initiation of antiretroviral therapy in early asymptomatic HIV infection. *The New England Journal of Medicine*, 373(9): 795–807. https://doi.org/10.1056/NEJMoa1506816.

Ji P, Damle B, Xie J, Unger SE, Grasela DM, Kaul S (2008) Pharmacokinetic interaction between efavirenz and carbamazepine after multiple-dose administration in healthy subjects. *Journal of Clinical Pharmacology*, 48(8): 948–956. https://doi.org/10.1177/0091270008319792.

Johnson T, Nath A (2010) Neurological complications of immune reconstitution in HIV-infected populations. *Annals of the New York Academy of Sciences*, 1184 (January): 106–120. https://doi.org/10.1111/j.1749-6632.2009.05111.x.

Kaku M, Simpson DM (2014) HIV neuropathy. *Current Opinion in HIV and AIDS*, 9(6): 521–526. https://doi.org/10.1097/COH.0000000000000103.

Kampmann B, Tena-Coki GN, Nicol MP, Levin M, Eley B (2006) Reconstitution of antimycobacterial immune responses in HIV-infected children receiving HAART. *AIDS (London, England)*, 20(7): 1011–1018. https://doi.org/10.1097/01.aids.0000222073.45372.ce.

Kellinghaus C, Engbring C, Kovac S et al. (2008) Frequency of seizures and epilepsy in neurological HIV-infected patients. *Seizure*, 17(1): 27–33. https://doi.org/10.1016/j.seizure.2007.05.017.

Kieburtz KD, Eskin TA, Ketonen L, Tuite MJ (1993) Opportunistic cerebral vasculopathy and stroke in patients with the acquired immunodeficiency syndrome. *Archives of Neurology*, 50(4): 430–432.

Kija E, Ndondo A, Spittal G, Hardie DR, Eley B, Wilmshurst JM (2015) Subacute sclerosing panencephalitis in South African children following the measles outbreak between 2009 and 2011. *South African Medical Journal = Suid-Afrikaanse Tydskrif Vir Geneeskunde*, 105(9): 713–718.

Kozlowski PB, Sher JH, Dickson D (1990) CNS infections in paediatric HIV infection: A multicentre study. In: Kozlowski PB, Snider DA, Vietze PM, Wisniewski HM, editors, *Brain in Pediatric AIDS*. Basel: Karger, pp. 132–146.

Lancella L, Galli L, Chiappini E et al. (2016) Recommendations concerning the therapeutic approach to immunocompromised children with tuberculosis. *Clinical Therapeutics*, 38(1): 180–190. https://doi.org/10.1016/j.clinthera.2015.10.012.

Lim ML, Min SS, Eron JJ et al. (2004) Coadministration of lopinavir/ritonavir and phenytoin results in two-way drug interaction through cytochrome P-450 induction. *Journal of Acquired Immune Deficiency Syndromes (1999)*, 36(5): 1034–1040.

Little R (2006) Neoplastic disease in pediatric HIV infection. In: Zeichner SL, Read JS, editors, *Handbook of Pediatric HIV Care*. Cambridge: Cambridge University Press, pp. 637–649.

Machado-Alba JE (2013) Pharmacosurveillance regarding Colombian patients being treated with stavudine. *Revista De Salud Pública (Bogotá, Colombia)*, 15(3): 446–454.

Madhi SA, Madhi A, Petersen K, Khoosal M, Klugman KP (2001) Impact of human immunodeficiency virus type 1 infection on the epidemiology and outcome of bacterial meningitis in South African children. *International Journal of Infectious Diseases: IJID: Official Publication of the International Society for Infectious Diseases*, 5(3): 119–125.

Mekki M, Eley B, Hardie D, Wilmshurst JM (2019) Subacute sclerosing panencephalitis: Clinical phenotype, epidemiology, and preventive interventions. *Developmental Medicine and Child Neurology*, 61(10): 1139–1144. https://doi.org/10.1111/dmcn.14166.

Mellins CA, Malee KM (2013) Understanding the mental health of youth living with perinatal HIV infection: Lessons learned and current challenges. *Journal of the International AIDS Society*, 16(1): 18593.

Mikol J, Costagliola D, Polivka M, Thiebaut JB, Trotot P (1995) The epidemiology of cerebral lymphoma in AIDS. *Journal of Neuroradiology. Journal De Neuroradiologie*, 22(3): 204–206.

Mitchell CD (2006) HIV-1 encephalopathy among perinatally infected children: Neuropathogenesis and response to highly active antiretroviral therapy. *Mental Retardation and Developmental Disabilities Research Reviews*, 12(3): 216–222. https://doi.org/10.1002/mrdd.20111.

Molyneux EM, Tembo M, Kayira K et al. (2003) The effect of HIV infection on paediatric bacterial meningitis in Blantyre, Malawi. *Archives of Disease in Childhood*, 88(12): 1112–1118.

Moulignier A (2006) [HIV and the central nervous system][Article in French]. *Revue Neurologique* 162(1): 22–42.

Mustafa MM, Weitman SD, Winick NJ, Bellini WJ, Timmons CF, Siegel JD (1993) Subacute measles encephalitis in the young immunocompromised host: Report of two cases diagnosed by polymerase chain reaction and treated with ribavirin and review of the literature. *Clinical Infectious Diseases: An Official Publication of the Infectious Diseases Society of America*, 16(5): 654–660.

Ntshoe GM, McAnerney JM, Archer BN et al. (2013) Measles outbreak in South Africa: Epidemiology of laboratory-confirmed measles cases and assessment of intervention, 2009–2011. *PloS One*, 8(2): e55682. https://doi.org/10.1371/journal.pone.0055682.

Nuttall JJC, Wilmshurst JM, Ndondo AP et al. (2004) Progressive multifocal leukoencephalopathy after initiation of highly active Aatiretroviral therapy in a child with advanced human immunodeficiency virus infection: A case of immune reconstitution inflammatory syndrome. *The Pediatric Infectious Disease Journal*, 23(7): 683–685.

Okuliz JF, Grandits GA, French JA et al. (2013) The impact of enzyme-inducing antiepileptic drugs on antiretroviral drug levels: A case-control study. *Epilepsy Research*, 103(2–3): 245–253. https://doi.org/10.1016/j.eplepsyres.2012.07.009.

Park YD, Belman AL, Kim TS et al. (1990) Stroke in pediatric acquired immunodeficiency syndrome. *Annals of Neurology* 28(3): 303–311. https://doi.org/10.1002/ana.410280302.

Patsalides AD, Wood LV, Atac GK, Sandifer E, Butman JA, Patronas NJ (2002) Cerebrovascular disease in HIV-infected pediatric patients: Neuroimaging findings. *AJR. American Journal of Roentgenology*, 179(4): 999–1003. https://doi.org/10.2214/ajr.179.4.1790999.

Pinto AN (1996) AIDS and cerebrovascular disease. *Stroke; A Journal of Cerebral Circulation*, 27(3): 538–543.

Qureshi AI, Janssen RS, Karon JM et al. (1997) Human immunodeficiency virus infection and stroke in young patients. *Archives of Neurology*, 54(9): 1150–1153.

Ravikumar S, Crawford JR (2013) Role of carbamazepine in the symptomatic treatment of subacute sclerosing panencephalitis: A case report and review of the literature. *Case Reports in Neurological Medicine*, 2013(March): e327647. https://doi.org/10.1155/2013/327647.

Ren Y, Nuttall JJC, Egbers C et al. (2008) Effect of rifampicin on lopinavir pharmacokinetics in HIV-infected children with tuberculosis. *Journal of Acquired Immune Deficiency Syndromes (1999)*, 47(5): 566–569. https://doi.org/10.1097/QAI.0b013e3181642257.

Ren Y, Nuttall JJC, Eley BS et al. (2009) Effect of rifampicin on efavirenz pharmacokinetics in HIV-infected children with tuberculosis. *Journal of Acquired Immune Deficiency Syndromes (1999)*, 50(5): 439–443. https://doi.org/10.1097/QAI.0b013e31819c33a3.

Sacktor N (2018) Changing clinical phenotypes of HIV-associated neurocognitive disorders. *Journal of Neurovirology*, 24(2): 141–145. https://doi.org/10.1007/s13365-017-0556-6.

Samia P, Petersen R, Walker KG, Eley B, Wilmshurst JM (2013) Prevalence of seizures in children infected with human immunodeficiency virus. *Journal of Child Neurology*, 28(3): 297–302. https://doi.org/10.1177/0883073812446161.

Scharko AM (2006) DSM psychiatric disorders in the context of pediatric HIV/AIDS. *AIDS Care*, 18(5): 441–445. https://doi.org/10.1080/09540120500213487.

Schoeman JF, van Toorn R (2014) Tuberculosis. In: Singhi P, Griffin DE, Newton CR, editors, *Central Nervous System Infections in Childhood*. London: Mac Keith Press, pp. 202–218.

Siddiqi O, Birbeck GL (2013) Safe treatment of seizures in the setting of HIV/AIDS. *Current Treatment Options in Neurology*, 15(4): 529–543. https://doi.org/10.1007/s11940-013-0237-6.

Simmonds RJ, Gonzalo O (1998) *Pneumocystis* Carinii Pneumonia and toxoplasmosis. In: Wilfert CM, Pizzo PA, editors, *Pediatric AIDS: The Challenges of HIV Infection in Infants, Children and Adolescents*. Baltimore: Williams & Wilkins, pp. 251–265.

University of Liverpool (2021) HIV drug Interactions. 2021. https://www.hiv-druginteractions.org/prescribing_resources.

van der Weert EM, Hartgers NM, Schaaf HS et al. (2006) Comparison of diagnostic criteria of tuberculous meningitis in human immunodeficiency virus-Infected and uninfected children. *The Pediatric Infectious Disease Journal*, 25(1): 65–69.

Van Rie A, Harrington PR, Dow A, Robertson K (2007) Neurologic and neurodevelopmental manifestations of pediatric HIV/AIDS: A global perspective. *European Journal of Paediatric Neurology: EJPN: Official Journal of the European Paediatric Neurology Society*, 11(1): 1–9. https://doi.org/10.1016/j.ejpn.2006.10.006.

van Toorn R, Rabie H, Dramowski A, Schoeman JF (2012) Neurological manifestations of TB-IRIS: A report of 4 children. *European Journal of Paediatric Neurology: EJPN: Official Journal of the European Paediatric Neurology Society*, 16(6): 676–682. https://doi.org/10.1016/j.ejpn.2012.04.005.

van Toorn R, Solomons R (2014) Update on the diagnosis and management of tuberculous meningitis in children. *Seminars in Pediatric Neurology*, 21(1): 12–18. https://doi.org/10.1016/j.spen.2014.01.006.

Violari A, Cotton MF, Gibb DM et al. (2008) Early antiretroviral therapy and mortality among HIV-infected infants. *The New England Journal of Medicine*, 359(21): 2233–2244. https://doi.org/10.1056/NEJMoa0800971.

WHO (2008) 'WHO antiretroviral therapy for infants and children 2008.' Report of the WHO Technical Reference Group, Pediatric HIV/ART Care Guideline Group Meeting. http://www.who.int/hiv/pub/paediatric/WHO_Paediatric_ART_guideline_rev_mreport_2008.

WHO (2010) *Rapid Advice. Treatment of Tuberculosis in Children*. Geneva: World Health Organization.

Wilmshurst JM, Donald KA, Eley B (2014) Update on the key developments of the neurologic complications in children infected with HIV. *Current Opinion in HIV and AIDS*, 9(6): 533–538. https://doi.org/10.1097/COH.0000000000000101.

Wilmshurst JM, Eley BS, Brew BJ (2014) HIV infections. In: Singhi P, Griffin DE, Newton CR, editors, *Central Nervous System Infections in Childhood*, International Review of Child Neurology Series. London: Mac Keith Press, pp. 147–159.

Yiğit A, Sarikaya S (2006) Myoclonus relieved by carbamazepine in subacute sclerosing panencephalitis. *Epileptic Disorders*, 8(1): 77–80.

Neuroimaging in Children with HIV

Nicky Wieselthaler, Jacqueline Hoare, and Tracy Kilborn

INTRODUCTION

Neurological conditions associated with human immunodeficiency virus (HIV) infection can be divided into three main categories: HIV-associated lesions or conditions, opportunistic infections, and neoplasms. A combination of computed tomography (CT) and magnetic resonance imaging (MRI) is used to assist in the management of paediatric patients. Although there is considerable overlap in the imaging appearances of different entities, often requiring clinical and laboratory correlation, some imaging findings may be highly suggestive of a specific condition or narrow the differential diagnosis. This chapter will highlight the brain imaging findings in HIV-positive children.

CHOICE OF IMAGING MODALITY

CT is readily accessible, inexpensive, and the images are acquired rapidly, making it the ideal modality for emergent or acute presentations since in most cases no sedation is required. The concern with CT relates to radiation exposure, particularly in younger patients, who are especially vulnerable, and in those who undergo multiple examinations within a short period of time thereby being subjected to a cumulative dose. Although modern scanners have allowed us to monitor and reduce the dose, it is incumbent on all clinicians involved in the management of children to be aware of potential risk. If one uses CT, all attempts must be made to ensure that the scan is done with a dose 'as low as reasonably achievable' (the ALARA principle) and the field being scanned minimised to try and avoid the lens. Contrast-enhanced scans with iodine-based agents may provide added sensitivity and specificity in certain cases but they carry the additional risk of contrast-induced nephropathy in patients with renal dysfunction (Nickerson et al. 2012).

MRI has greatly advanced the imaging of the central nervous system (CNS). It provides excellent tissue contrast, is free of ionising radiation, and the use of different sequences is used to increase conspicuity of abnormalities. Advanced imaging techniques, including diffusion-weighted imaging (DWI), magnetic resonance spectroscopy (MRS), and diffusion tensor imaging (DTI), used together with structural imaging techniques, provide non-invasive physiological data that assist in our understanding of the pathological processes resulting from HIV infection. Even though new fast sequences have reduced scanning times, children younger than 6 years of age and older children who cannot cooperate require sedation or general anaesthesia to acquire diagnostic studies. The use of gadolinium-based contrast agents is limited in neonates, infants, and patients with renal dysfunction due to the risk of nephrogenic systemic fibrosis (Nickerson et al. 2012). Unfortunately, MRI is less readily available than CT in resource-limited settings where the prevalence of HIV is higher, and the cost is significantly more than that of a CT scan.

HIV ENCEPHALOPATHY

Neuroimaging assists in defining the spectrum of neurocognitive disorders in HIV-positive children. Conventional neuroimaging has two roles: first, the detection of cerebral atrophy and other early signs of encephalopathy; and second, to exclude or investigate secondary CNS complications of HIV that may mimic encephalopathy. Advanced techniques such as DTI and MRS aid in detecting early changes that may not be visible on conventional sequences and they may act as imaging biomarkers in the future to track disease progression.

Cerebral atrophy and ventriculomegaly are the most common reported findings in HIV-infected children and can be seen in both CT and MRI as prominence of the surface sulcal markings (grey matter volume loss) and enlargement of the ventricles (grey and white matter volume loss). Ventriculomegaly may be disproportionate to the cortical atrophy owing to the predilection of the virus for the basal ganglia (specifically caudate nuclei), periventricular white matter, and corpus callosum (Figure 4.1) (Safriel et al. 2000; Thompson et al. 2006; Ances et al. 2012). The extent of atrophy was initially thought to correlate with viral load and disease severity, but multiple studies have since challenged this. However, it may still be the case in patients who are at the more severe end of the spectrum (Donald et al. 2015). A paper from our institution documented normal neuroimaging in 29% of patients imaged with a clinical diagnosis of HIV encephalopathy (HIVE; Donald et al. 2015). It is important to realise that apparent atrophy may be multifactorial and not only due to HIV. Thus, atrophy should be seen in the context of influence from environmental and nutritional factors and may show some reversibility. We prefer the term 'shrinkage' unless the findings of atrophy can be correlated with a reduced expected head circumference and findings persist on follow-up imaging.

Basal ganglia calcification, initially regarded as a hallmark of vertical transmission, should rather be regarded as an acquired vascular injury (George et al. 2009). This calcification is usually bilateral and symmetrical and is only seen after 10 months of age (Safriel et al. 2000). The subcortical white matter

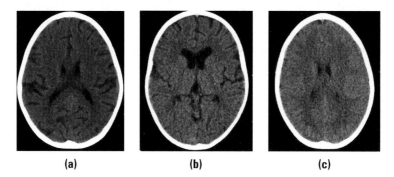

(a)   (b)   (c)

Figure 4.1 **(a)** Axial CT scan of an 8-year-old HIV-positive male demonstrating brain shrinkage with prominent surface sulcal markings. The distinction between cerebral atrophy cannot be made on the first CT scan. **(b)** Axial CT scan of a 6-year-old HIV-positive male on antiretroviral therapy demonstrating severe brain shrinkage/atrophy and ex-vacuo dilatation of the ventricles. **(c)** Axial CT scan of a normal brain at the same level as (Figure 4.1a) an 8-year-old male.

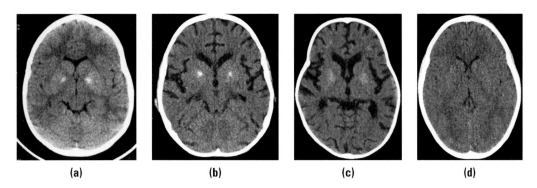

(a) (b) (c) (d)

Figure 4.2 **(a)** Axial CT scan of a 5-year-old HIV-positive female, demonstrating bilateral basal ganglia calcification with no atrophy. **(b)** Axial CT scan of a 12-year-old HIV-positive male demonstrating bilateral basal ganglia calcification and diffuse atrophy. **(c)** Axial CT scan of a 10-year-old HIV-positive male, demonstrating bilateral basal ganglia and frontal cortical calcification with severe atrophy and ex-vacuo dilatation of the ventricles. **(d)** Axial CT scan of a 9-year-old female with a normal brain and no calcification.

and cerebellum may also calcify (Kauffman et al. 1992). Although calcification is said to occur in up to 33% of HIV-infected children, in our experience it is a lot less common (Safriel et al. 2000). If calcification is seen in patients younger than 10 months of age, other causes such as congenital infection should be considered (States, Zimmerman, and Rutstein 1997). Calcification is optimally assessed using CT (Figure 4.2).

White matter signal abnormalities (WMSA) are seen in 50% of patients with HIVE (Ackermann et al. 2014). Although these areas may be recognised as hypodense areas on CT scans they are better seen on MRI as areas of high signal intensity on T2-weighted and fluid-attenuated inversion recovery (FLAIR) images and low signal intensity on T1-weighted images. These areas show no mass effect, no abnormal diffusion, and no contrast enhancement (Figure 4.3). WMSA are found in both superficial and deep white matter, and have been variably reported as predominantly located in the frontal and

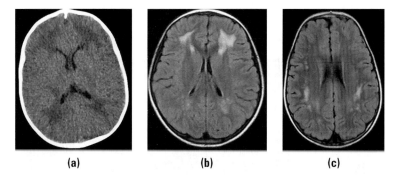

(a) (b) (c)

Figure 4.3 **(a)** Axial CT scan of a 22-month-old HIV-positive male on antiretroviral therapy who was growing well and presented with a new focal seizure, demonstrating diffuse bilateral symmetrical white matter low density consistent with HIV encephalopathy. **(b)** Axial FLAIR MRI scan of a 3-year-old HIV-positive male with HIV encephalopathy and bilateral cerebral palsy, demonstrating bilateral symmetrical predominantly frontal white matter high signal intensity consistent with HIV encephalopathy. **(c)** Axial FLAIR MRI scan of an 8-year-old HIV-positive female who presented with developmental delay, demonstrating bilateral asymmetrical patchy white matter high signal intensity lesions consistent with HIV encephalopathy.

parietal lobes of young children (Safriel et al. 2000; Ackermann et al. 2014) and more diffusely located in both juxtacortical and deep white matter in adolescents (Cohen et al. 2016). White-matter changes on MRI parallel those of neuropathological examination and represent a variable combination of myelin loss, astroglial proliferation, and infiltration by mononucleated and multinucleated macrophages (Gray et al. 2005).

White matter volumes are also reported to be lower in HIVE than in age-matched controls (States, Zimmerman, and Rutstein 1997). Using MRI to measure the volume of the corpus callosum as a surrogate marker of white matter volume is reported as a useful biomarker of HIV-related brain disease, since the authors showed correlation between degree of mental development, microcephaly, and immunity with length and segmental thickness (Andronikou et al. 2014).

Quantitative imaging techniques such as DTI can assess and quantify white matter microstructural abnormalities that are not visible using conventional MRI. DTI can examine the integrity and directionality of the white matter and provides information on the location of white matter structural changes that can be correlated with clinical variables in HIVE (Hoare et al. 2015a). Traditional scalar metrics derived from DTI include fractional anisotropy (FA), which represents axon integrity and/or packing density, mean diffusivity (MD), representing the mean water mobility within the white matter, and axial and radial diffusivity (AD and RD), which correspond to diffusion parallel and perpendicular to the direction of white matter tracts respectively (Hoare et al. 2015a, 2015b). High FA and low MD values are typically associated with a healthy microstructure, whereas low FA and high MD values represent lack of axonal integrity and are indicative of white matter damage (Hoare et al. 2015b). Myelin loss is represented by increases in RD and axonal damage is represented by increases in AD. Separate analyses of changes in these indices for clinical predictors or disease symptoms may provide insight into the underlying mechanism of white matter damage (Song et al. 2002). DTI as a measure of white matter integrity may have a role in the future, acting as an imaging biomarker to track progression of neurological disease in children living with HIV (Figure 4.4) (Hoare et al. 2014).

Proton MRS has been used to assess brain chemistry in HIVE; the commonly measured compounds N-acetyl aspartate (NAA) (a neuronal marker), creatine (CRE) (metabolite involved in energy metabolism), and choline (CHO) (a marker of cell membrane turnover, myelination, and gliosis) are expressed as ratios between areas under metabolite resonances (Prado et al. 2011). Children with HIVE have

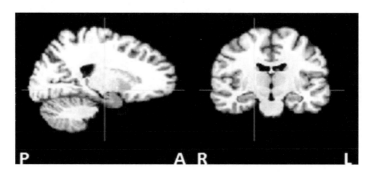

Figure 4.4 Voxelwise group analysis from a diffusion tensor imaging study reveals lower fractional anisotropy or high mean diffusivity in the right corticospinal tract in patients with HIV encephalopathy with bilateral cerebral palsy compared to patients with cerebral palsy only. Crosshairs indicate peak coordinates.

been reported to have a low NAA/CRE ratio compared to non-encephalopathic children and controls (Pavlakis et al. 1995; Lu et al. 1996). MRS may be a valuable biomarker before and after the introduction of antiretroviral therapy (ART; Prado et al. 2011).

CNS disease and mental health problems (Hoare et al. 2019) persist in young people living with HIV despite ART and viral suppression, contributing to a significant decline in functioning (Phillips et al. 2018). In both perinatally infected young people (PHIV) and adults living with HIV on ART in South Africa the prevalence of neurocognitive disorders is greater than 50% (Hoare et al. 2016; Gouse et al. 2017), with significant alterations in brain macrostructure and microstructure (Heaps et al. 2012; Hoare et al. 2018). Associations in these children of compromised neuronal integrity, cell membrane metabolism and functional connectivity with immunocompromise around birth (Mbugua et al. 2016; Toich et al. 2017; Robertson et al. 2018) point to possible long-term consequences of early damage in the CNS compartment that may impact outcomes in PHIV. In PHIV, inflammatory markers, albeit different in plasma and the cerebrospinal fluid (CSF), have been linked with white matter injury and poorer cognitive outcomes (Blokhuis et al. 2019). MRI has shown that myelinogenesis continues from childhood and that the brain's region-specific neurocircuitry remains structurally and functionally vulnerable in young people (Giedd et al. 1999; Arain et al. 2013). HIV-infected children who accessed the early antiretroviral program (CHER) at ages 5 to 9 years, had abnormalities in subcortical regions (Mbugua et al. 2016; Randall et al. 2017; Nwosu et al. 2018; Robertson et al. 2018), frontal forceps minor white matter and tracts connecting subcortical and frontal regions (Ackermann et al. 2016; Jankiewicz et al. 2017), and lower fronto-parietal functional connectivity (Toich et al. 2017). This suggests that HIV may exacerbate developmental imbalances between the limbic system and prefrontal cortex, leading to increased reward-seeking behaviours in young people living with HIV, which may further negatively impact outcomes. Work from Cape Town Adolescent Antiretroviral Cohort (CTAAC) and CHER suggests significant brain disruption in this despite intact CD4 cell counts(Hoare et al. 2018), including brain atrophy, morphometric (Sarma et al. 2014; Hoare et al. 2015a; Cohen et al. 2016) and functional changes (Heany et al. 2019; Plessis et al. 2019), altered cerebral blood flow (CBF) (Blokhuis et al. 2017) and white matter damage (Hoare, Heany et al. 2019). Studies have applied arterial spin labelling in young people living with HIV, revealing higher CBF in white matter and basal ganglia (Blokhuis et al. 2017), suggestive of increased local metabolic activity, such as glial proliferation, neuroinflammation, or compensation for injury. Of five studies examining metabolic changes in young people living with HIV using magnetic resonance spectroscopic imaging (MRSI) (Van den Hof et al. 2019), only three (Keller et al. 2004; Dalen et al. 2016; Mbugua et al. 2016) have reported regionally higher CHO and/or myoinositol indicative of glial cell proliferation, and one study has used arterial spin labelling, revealing white matter and basal ganglia CBF increases that are suggestive of blood–brain barrier compromise but unrelated to other MRI abnormalities (Blokhuis et al. 2017).

In the CTAAC cohort, high sensitivity C-reactive protein (hs-CRP), a systemic inflammatory marker, negatively correlated with general intelligence, visual spatial acuity and executive function, and whole brain MD correlated with higher hs-CRP (Hoare et al. 2020). Functional MRI studies within the CTAAC cohort showed that PHIV had decreased activation in the left superior temporal gyrus, pre- and postcentral gyri, insula, and putamen as well as bilateral hippocampus, and mid cingulum when doing a maintenance working memory task (Heany et al. 2019), and had significantly blunted proactive inhibitory behavioural responses (Plessis et al. 2019). In addition, PHIV had higher rates of depression compared to healthy controls (7% vs 2%) and displayed poorer self-concept and motivation (Hoare et al. 2019). Together, these findings from CTAAC point to an aberrant neurodevelopmental trajectory among PHIV, with cognitive and mental health challenges.

HIV-RELATED VASCULAR DISEASE

The annual risk of developing cerebrovascular disease in HIV-infected paediatric patients is reported as 1.3% (Safriel et al. 2000). Poor access to imaging in developing countries, however, means that the true incidence in areas of high prevalence of HIV is unknown. Cerebrovascular disease may be due to the primary effects of HIV. The inflammatory reaction is thought to begin in the adventitia and involve the vasa vasorum leading to ischemia of the arterial wall, or it is thought to be secondary to infectious vasculitis, thrombocytopenia, or cardiogenic emboli (Patsalides et al. 2002). Patients may present with signs and symptoms of ischaemic or haemorrhagic stroke, subarachnoid haemorrhage, or neurocognitive delay or decline because of multiple subclinical events that are due to HIVE (George et al. 2009; Hammond et al. 2016).

In the acute setting, most patients are imaged with CT. Depending on the time post infarct, a pre-contrast CT may be normal or may show areas of low density with or without high-density haemorrhage (Figure 4.5). If the infarct is subacute, cortical enhancement can be seen and should not be mistaken for an infectious process. Infarcts will proceed to form areas of encephalomalacia with volume loss in the chronic stage.

MRI is the imaging technique of choice not only in acute or subacute stroke but also in identifying cerebrovascular disease and its progression or response to treatment. A combination of multiple sequences is used to ascertain the most information relating to the cause of the stroke. Sequences worth discussing include DWI, which demonstrates restricted diffusion (representing cytotoxic oedema) in the area of infarction as early as 30 minutes after the acute event. T1-weighted images returning low signal intensity and T2/ FLAIR images returning high signal intensity may lag DWI by up to 8 hours (Safriel et al. 2000).

Time-of-flight magnetic resonance angiography (MRA) is used to visualise the circle of Willis; findings include focal stenosis, multifocal stenosis, dilatation of vessels, and aneurysms (Figure 4.6)

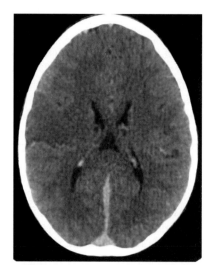

Figure 4.5 Axial CT scan with contrast of a 9-year-old HIV-positive female who had commenced antiretroviral therapy 2 weeks before and was on treatment for tuberculosis meningitis. She presented with acute left hemi-plegia. The CT scan demonstrates a wedge-shaped area of low density in the right parietal region that does not enhance post-contrast and is consistent with an infarct.

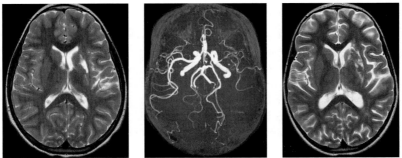

(a)   (b)   (c)

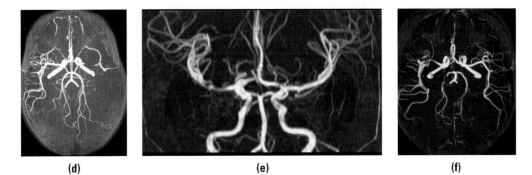

(d)   (e)   (f)

Figure 4.6   **(a)**, **(b)** Axial T2-weighted MRI scan and corresponding maximum intensity projection MRA image of an 11-year-old HIV-positive female with a chronic left basal ganglia infarct. The MRA image demonstrates attenuation and irregularity of the left M1 segment of the middle cerebral artery (MCA) with further attenuation of the M3 branches. **(c)**, **(d)** Axial T2-weighted MRI scan and corresponding maximum intensity projection MRA image of a 7-year-old HIV-positive female with a chronic left basal ganglia infarct. The MRA image demonstrates complete occlusion of the left MCA. **(e)**, **(f)** Maximum intensity projection MRA images of an 8-year-old HIV-positive male with a left hemiplegia demonstrating a right internal carotid artery–anterior cerebral artery bifurcation fusiform aneurysm as well as attenuation of the right MCA and posterior cerebral artery.

(Patsalides et al. 2002; George et al. 2009). MRA of the neck vessels is a useful adjunct to complete visualisation of the extracranial vasculature.

In the setting of stenosis or occlusion of the terminal internal carotid(s) and circle of Willis with or without collateral vessels, moyamoya syndrome should be considered since these patients are at high risk of further events (Figure 4.7) (Hammond et al. 2016). Aneurysms have been reported to be fusiform rather than saccular and multiple (Patsalides et al. 2002; George et al. 2009); however, we have found this to be a rare manifestation in our population.

Gradient echo and black blood sequences are best used to assess subarachnoid or parenchymal haemorrhage and may be from immune thrombocytopenia, haemorrhagic transformation of ischemic infarcts, or after aneurysm rupture. CT is still considered best to evaluate acute haemorrhage (Figure 4.8). T1-weighted images with contrast are used to look for vessel wall enhancement that may indicate active vasculitis.

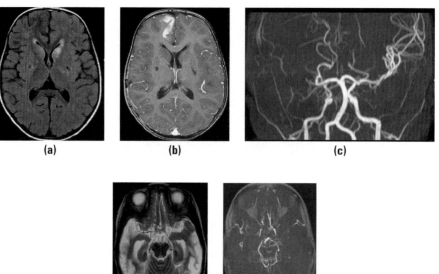

Figure 4.7 **(a)**, **(b)**, **(c)** Axial FLAIR, T1-weighted MRI scan with contrast and maximum intensity projection (MIP) MRA image of a 6-year-old HIV-positive female who presented with left hemiplegia. The images demonstrate infarcts of varying ages, including laminar necrosis in the right frontal lobe. The MIP MRA image demonstrates bilateral distal carotid artery attenuation, right worse than left, complete occlusion right middle cerebral artery (MCA) and both anterior communicating arteries with attenuated left MCA segments. Features consistent with moyamoya syndrome. **(d)**, **(e)** Axial T2-weighted MRI scan and MIP MRA image of a 3-year-old female who demonstrates features of severe moyamoya syndrome. All vessels are occluded except the attenuated posterior cerebral arteries. Note severe encephalomalacia and collateral vessel formation on T2.

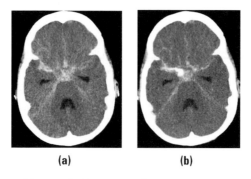

Figure 4.8 **(a)**, **(b)** Axial CT scan without and with contrast of a 9-year-old HIV-positive male who defaulted antiretroviral therapy for 1 year. He presented with seizures and decerebrate posturing. A large right internal carotid artery–anterior cerebral artery aneurysm is demonstrated on the post-contrast CT scan with extensive subarachnoid haemorrhage, hydrocephalus, and brain swelling.

INFECTIONS
Bacterial Meningitis

The imaging findings of bacterial meningitis are similar in HIV-infected and non-infected children, which is that both contrast-enhanced CT and MRI are often normal at presentation (Nickerson et al. 2012). An increased incidence of complications from meningitis is mentioned in one study (George et al. 2009) and HIV-infected children are reported to have a higher mortality rate than uninfected children (Madhi et al. 2001).

Tuberculous Meningitis

Intracranial tuberculosis (TB) is caused by haematogenous spread from elsewhere in the body such as the lungs. HIV-infected children with tuberculosis meningitis (TBM) are more likely than those who are uninfected to present with chest X-ray findings of pulmonary TB, and a chest X-ray is therefore mandatory as part of the workup of TBM (van der Weert et al. 2006). Two theories of the pathogenesis of TBM exist and impact imaging findings. First, rupture of subependymal or subpial granulomata into the CSF or, second, direct penetration of walls by haematogenous spread (van der Weert et al. 2006; Vinnard and Macgregor 2009). A cell-mediated immune response leads to the formation of the basal tuberculous exudate that causes cranial nerve palsies, obliterative vasculitis of the vessels of the circle of Willis, vertebrobasilar system, and branch vessels of the middle cerebral artery (MCA), which infarcts and obstructs CSF pathways resulting in hydrocephalus (van der Weert et al. 2006; Janse van Rensburg et al. 2008). As HIV infection primarily impairs cell-mediated immunity, the immune response to TB bacilli may be different, which results in the different radiological features (Janse van Rensburg et al. 2008).

Basal meningeal enhancement is the most characteristic and sensitive finding of paediatric TBM, reported in up to 93% of patients (Andronikou et al. 2012). The involved meninges are hyperdense relative to the CSF on pre-contrast CT and demonstrate enhancement post contrast. The contrast enhancement is seen with greater clarity on MRI due to the greater resolution and lack of artefact produced by bone (Andronikou et al. 2004). In HIV-infected children, the intense basal meningeal enhancement occurs less frequently and often the enhancement is asymmetrical and nodular (Figure 4.9) (Pienaar, Andronikou, and van Toorn 2009). Pathological correlation in adult patients has shown that the scant (thin, minimal, serous) exudates observed pathologically corresponded with minimal meningeal enhancement on imaging (Dekker et al. 2011). Parenchymal tuberculomas are found less frequently in HIV-infected children (Katrak et al. 2000; Dekker et al. 2011).

CT and MRI can show hydrocephalus in TBM by demonstrating dilated ventricles and, as pressure increases, periventricular extrusion of fluid, seen as periventricular low density on CT and as high signal on T2 and FLAIR. There is communicating hydrocephalus in 80% of paediatric TBM cases and noncommunicating hydrocephalus in the other 20% of paediatric TBM cases (Vinnard and Macgregor 2009; Andronikou et al. 2012). Communicating hydrocephalus is caused by the decreased CSF reabsorption in the presence of the inflammatory exudate, while noncommunicating hydrocephalus is caused by dense exudate interrupting CSF flow through the ventricles (Vinnard and Macgregor 2009; Andronikou et al. 2012). Obstructive hydrocephalus is a less common presentation in HIV-infected patients (Katrak et al. 2000; Marais et al. 2010). Cerebral atrophy is more common in HIV-infected children and may mask the findings of cerebral oedema associated with hydrocephalus. The decreased likelihood of developing hydrocephalus with TBM may also be a consequence of the defective host immune response (Katrak et al. 2000).

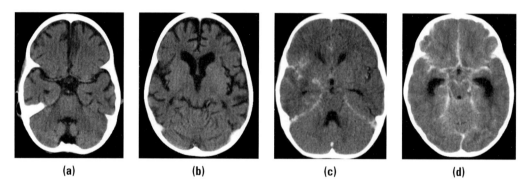

(a)   **(b)**   **(c)**   **(d)**

Figure 4.9 **(a)**, **(b)** Axial CT scan with contrast of a 5-year-old HIV-positive male with proven tuberculous meningitis. The CT scan demonstrates atrophy with ex-vacuo dilatation of the ventricles and noticeably no basal meningeal enhancement. **(c)** Axial CT scan with contrast in a 10-year-old HIV-positive female who presented with a decreased level of consciousness. The CT scan demonstrates asymmetrical right-sided Sylvian fissure and quadrigeminal plate basal meningeal enhancement with early hydrocephalus consistent with atypical tuberculosis meningitis. **(d)** Axial CT scan with contrast demonstrating the usual features of tuberculosis meningitis: bilateral symmetrical basal meningeal enhancement with hydrocephalus.

Infarction in TBM is mediated by the inflammatory exudate enveloping the vessels at the base of the brain, resulting in arteritis that in turn leads to thrombosis and occlusion causing infarcts. The vessels most commonly involved are the perforators and the lenticulostriate branches of the MCA accounting for the predominant distribution of the infarcts. Thus, the predominant areas that are infarcted in TBM are the basal ganglia (heads of caudate nuclei), anteromedial thalami, and anterior limbs of the internal capsules (Andronikou et al. 2006). HIV-infected patients have been reported as more likely to present with cortical infarcts than basal ganglia infarcts, thought to be due to less immune-mediated vasculopathy (see Figure 4.5) (Vinnard and Macgregor 2009; Garg and Sinha 2011).

CRYPTOCOCCUS NEOFORMANS MENINGITIS

Cryptococcus is an infrequent cause of meningitis in paediatric HIV. Imaging features that suggest the diagnosis are dilated perivascular spaces returning CSF signal (low signal intensity on T1-weighted MRI and high signal intensity on T2-weighted MRI) in the basal ganglia and thalami (van Toorn and Rabie 2005). These dilated spaces or pseudocysts represent mucoid material dissecting along perforating arteries and are considered characteristic of cryptococcal meningitis (CM) (Smith, Smirniotopoulos, and Rushing 2008). Other findings are granulomas that are preferentially located on the ependyma of the choroid plexus and intraparenchymal cryptococcomas (George et al. 2009). In these cases, contrast enhancement is minimal (George et al. 2009).

Toxoplasmosis

Although a leading cause of secondary protozoal infections in adults, toxoplasmosis is extremely rare in HIV-infected children. Contrast-enhanced CT shows lesion(s) with inhomogeneous or peripheral enhancement in the basal ganglia or periventricular white matter. On MRI, the lesions are of low signal intensity on T1-weighted MRI, high signal intensity on T2-weighted MRI, and enhance post contrast as with CT (Safriel et al. 2000). The differential includes tuberculoma, tuberculous abscess, bacterial abscess, and lymphoma (Safriel et al. 2000).

CEREBRAL MALARIA

Limited neuroimaging studies have been done on the effects of cerebral malaria on HIV- infected children versus those who are HIV non-infected. One study from Malawi concluded that children who were HIV positive with acute cerebral malaria demonstrated fewer white matter lesions compared to those who were HIV negative. The extent of acute ischaemic change was noted to be higher in the basal ganglia and caudate nuclei in HIV-positive children. These findings correspond to the same areas where previous studies have demonstrated microscopic ischaemic changes and a higher concentration of HIV (Potchen et al. 2016).

Progressive Multifocal Leukoencephalopathy

Progressive multifocal leukoencephalopathy (PML) is a demyelinating disease caused by the John Cunningham virus of the Papovaviridae family. Primary infection occurs in childhood and usually remains latent and, although well-reported in adults, it remains rare in children even with severe immunosuppression from HIV (Schwenk et al. 2014). In the setting of severely altered cellular immunity, the virus causes extensive myelin breakdown and white matter destruction. The involved areas are of low density on CT and of low signal intensity on T1-weighted MRI and high signal intensity on T2-weighted MRI/FLAIR (George et al. 2009; Senocak et al. 2010; Schwenk et al. 2014). The lesions most commonly involve the frontal and parieto-occipital subcortical white matter spreading to the deep white matter in a confluent pattern (George et al. 2009; Senocak et al. 2010). There is no mass effect and 84% demonstrate no contrast enhancement unless associated with immune reconstitution inflammatory syndrome (IRIS) (Figure 4.10) (Schwenk et al. 2014).

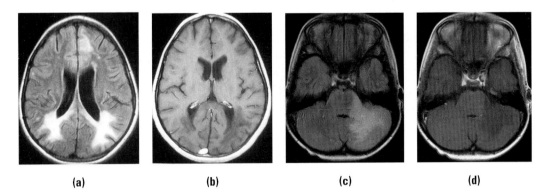

| (a) | (b) | (c) | (d) |

Figure 4.10 **(a)**, **(b)** Axial FLAIR and T1-weighted MRI scans with contrast of a 10-year-old HIV-positive male demonstrating bilateral symmetrical intense increased signal intensity in the occipital subcortical and deep white matter as well as less intense high signal in the frontal white matter. Note no contrast enhancement. Features consistent with progressive leukoencephalopathy. **(c)**, **(d)** Axial FLAIR and T1-weighted MRI scans with contrast of a 12-year-old HIV-positive female who presented with progressive leukoencephalopathy 4 weeks after commencing antiretroviral therapy. The images show high signal intensity in the left cerebellar hemisphere with minimal contrast enhancement. Marginal mass effect was noted on the brainstem. John Cunningham virus was cultured on lumbar puncture and features are consistent with progressive multifocal leukoencephalopathy-immune reconstitution inflammatory syndrome.

Immune Reconstitution Inflammatory Syndrome

In the setting of HIV, IRIS is broadly described as clinical and radiological deterioration after initiation of ART. This condition occurs within 3 months of commencing ART (range 2–31 weeks) and is a response to immune recovery. It may manifest with the unmasking of an occult subclinical infection or as an enhanced inflammatory response to a treated infection (Kilborn and Zampoli 2009). There should be evidence of immune restoration (rise in CD4+ count and fall in HIV viral load) and exclusion of alternate explanations such as drug resistance, non-compliance, or a newly acquired illness.

Mycobacterium TB is the most common pathogen associated with CNS IRIS in HIV-infected children in our institution. TBM-IRIS should be considered when new neurological signs develop after initiation of ART in patients with TBM, or in patients with pulmonary TB who may go on to manifest signs of TBM with restoration of immune function. CT and MRI show basal enhancement that may appear de novo or worsen, and previously undiagnosed tuberculomas may be unmasked (Figures 4.11 and 4.12) (Janse van Rensburg et al. 2008; Kilborn and Zampoli 2009; van Toorn et al. 2012).

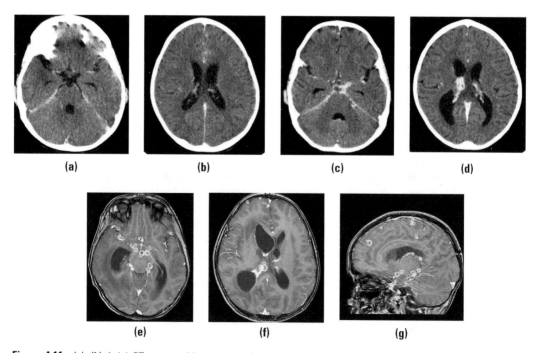

(a)   **(b)**   **(c)**   **(d)**

(e)   **(f)**   **(g)**

Figure 4.11 **(a)**, **(b)** Axial CT scans with contrast of a 6-year-old newly diagnosed HIV-positive male who was also diagnosed with TB meningitis and started on antiretroviral therapy. Interhemispheric meningeal enhancement is noted **(b)** but no tuberculomas. Note early ventricular prominence. **(c)**, **(d)** Axial CT scan with contrast in same patient as (Figure 4.11a) and (Figure 4.11b) 1 month after commencement of antiretroviral therapy. Multiple new tuberculomas are demonstrated in the suprasellar cistern and right choroid plexus with interval worsening hydrocephalus. Features are consistent with TB meningitis-immune reconstitution inflammatory syndrome. **(e)**, **(f)**, **(g)** Axial and sagittal T1-weighted MRI scans with contrast in the same patient as (Figure 4.11a–d) now 2 months after commencing antiretroviral therapy. Further deterioration with more ring-enhancing tuberculomas in the suprasellar cistern and into the quadrigeminal plate cistern as well as right choroid plexus and worsening hydrocephalus is demonstrated compared to Figure 4.11c and Figure 4.11d.

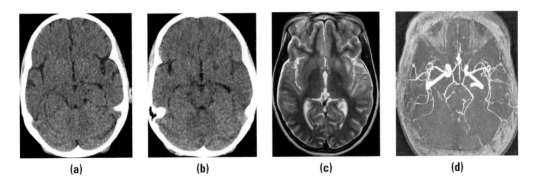

(a)   **(b)**   **(c)**   **(d)**

Figure 4.12   (a) Axial CT scan of a 9-year-old newly diagnosed HIV-positive male diagnosed with pulmonary and abdominal TB who was started on antiretroviral therapy. Patient presented with headache and fever, but the initial CT scan was normal. Chest radiograph showed interval deterioration with worsening adenopathy and TB-immune reconstitution inflammatory syndrome was diagnosed. **(b)** Axial CT scan of same patient as (Figure 4.12a), 1 month after commencement of antiretroviral therapy now shows a new left basal ganglia infarct. **(c)**, **(d)** Axial T2-weighted MRI scan and maximum intensity projection MRA image of the same patient demonstrating left basal ganglia and perisylvian infarct (pontine infarct not shown) with diffuse attenuation of posterior circulation and left A1 segment. Features consistent with HIV vasculopathy but likely secondary to TB meningitis-immune reconstitution inflammatory syndrome.

In a subset of patients with PML, inflammation and an apparent increase in John Cunningham virus-mediated tissue destruction follow suppression of HIV infection with ART. This PML-IRIS is a severe and often fatal complication. On MRI, the lesions may either show progression or be associated with new contrast enhancement – so-called 'inflammatory PML', which has been treated with steroids with limited response (see Figures 4.10c and 4.10d) (Nuttall et al. 2004; van Toorn et al. 2012; Schwenk et al. 2014).

CM-IRIS is uncommon in paediatric patients, with only a few cases in the literature (Puthanakit et al. 2006; George et al. 2009). Specific imaging findings of CM-IRIS have been reported in adults and may be of use in the diagnosis of the condition in children. Specific imaging findings of CM-IRIS typically present as intense leptomeningeal enhancement which can be accompanied by hydrocephalus, linear perivascular enhancement in the sulci, and choroid plexus enhancement (Post et al. 2013). Enhancement of distended Virchow-Robin spaces and secondary involvement of brain parenchyma with areas of high T2/FLAIR signal, restricted diffusion, and enhancement are also reported to be characteristic of CM-IRIS (Post et al. 2013). Of note, a single case series reported herpes encephalitis and Guillain-Barré syndrome as manifestations of IRIS (Puthanakit et al. 2006).

Malignancy

Primary HIV-related malignancies affecting the CNS are usually B-cell lymphomas and include primary CNS lymphoma and plasmablastic lymphoma.

PRIMARY CNS LYMPHOMA

This complication is rare with an incidence of less than 1% in HIV-infected children. Primary CNS lymphoma can involve the brain and/or leptomeninges or eyes (Abla and Weitzman 2006). Primary CNS lymphoma often has high density on pre-contrast CT because of its high nuclear/cytoplasmic ratio and hypercellularity and all lesions show contrast enhancement (Haldorsen et al. 2011). On MRI, the lesions are hypo- to isointense on T1 and iso- to hyperintense on T2 but often hypointense to grey matter (Haldorsen et al. 2011). Contrast enhancement is commonly irregular or peripheral and can be ring-like

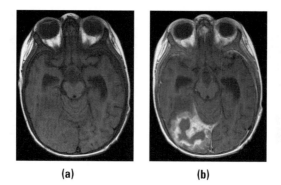

(a)   (b)

Figure 4.13 **(a)**, **(b)** Axial T1-weighted MRI scans without and with contrast in a 7-year-old HIV-positive female who presented with seizures. The MRI scan demonstrates a T1 isointense mass that irregularly ring-enhances post-contrast in the right occipital lobe. Note adjacent meningeal enhancement. Features consistent with primary CNS lymphoma.

(Figure 4.13) (Abla and Weitzman 2006; Haldorsen, Espeland, and Larsson 2011). Paediatric patients have also been reported to have leptomeningeal disease without a discrete mass (Abla and Weitzman 2006). The diagnosis may be suggested by imaging but is confirmed by biopsy as the major differential diagnoses are infectious entities such as TB, toxoplasmosis, and PML.

PLASMABLASTIC LYMPHOMA

A subtype of diffuse large B-cell lymphoma, plasmablastic lymphoma is rare and characterised by its involvement of the oral cavity in more than half the reported cases (Bibas and Castillo 2014). There is a male predominance and isolated case reports refer to extra-oral sites, including the CNS (Bibas and Castillo 2014). There is a single report from our institution documenting the MRI features: namely, T1 as isointense and T2 as hypointense masses with peripheral enhancement (du Toit and Wieselthaler 2015). We have seen a further patient who presented with large mass originating from the skull. CT showed extensive bony destruction, expansion, and infiltration with an associated enhancing soft tissue mass (Figures 4.14 and 4.15). Differential diagnosis depending on clinical context includes neuroblastoma metastases, plasmablastic Burkitt lymphoma variant, and, given the marked bone destruction, osteosarcoma.

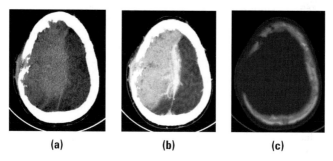

(a)   (b)   (c)

Figure 4.14 **(a)**, **(b)**, **(c)** Axial CT scans without and with contrast in a 13-year-old HIV-positive male who presented with a huge scalp mass. The CT scan demonstrates a large hyperdense extra-axial mass that enhances post-contrast with associated bone destruction and infiltration. Biopsy confirmed a plasmablastic lymphoma. Images kindly provided by Jia Fan, University of Cape Town.

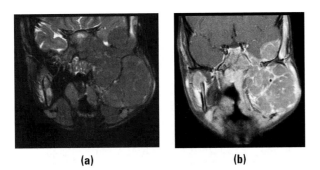

(a)   (b)

Figure 4.15   (a), (b) Coronal T2 and T1 with contrast-weighted MRI scan of the face of an 11-year-old HIV-positive female who presented with bilateral facial masses. The MRI scan demonstrates a large predominantly left-sided lobulated facial mass with intracranial extension. The mass is T2 hypointense and shows inhomogeneous, peripheral, and septated enhancement post contrast. Biopsy confirmed a plasmablastic lymphoma. Images kindly provided by Jia Fan, University of Cape Town.

CONCLUSION

This chapter provides a pictorial overview of the wide array of CNS presentations in an HIV-positive child. Patients can present with HIV-associated lesions and opportunistic infections, usually with an atypical appearance or malignancy. Imaging findings, together with clinical and laboratory investigations, can aid in the diagnosis of these often-complex presentations.

REFERENCES

Abla O, Weitzman S (2006) Primary central nervous system lymphoma in children. *Neurosurg Focus*, 21(5): E8.

Ackermann C, Andronikou S, Laughton B et al. (2014) White matter signal abnormalities in children with suspected HIV-related neurologic disease on early combination antiretroviral therapy. *The Pediatric Infectious Disease Journal*, 33(8): e207–212.

Ackermann C, Andronikou S, Saleh MG et al. (2016) Early antiretroviral therapy in HIV-infected children is associated with diffuse white matter structural abnormality and corpus callosum sparing. *American Journal of Neuroradiology*, 37(12): 2363–2369. https://doi.org/10.3174/ajnr.a4921.

Ances BM, Ortega M, Vaida F, Heaps J, Paul R (2012) Independent effects of HIV, aging, and HAART on brain volumetric measures. *Journal of Acquired Immune Deficiency Syndromes*, 59(5): 469–477.

Andronikou S, Smith B, Hatherhill M, Douis H, Wilmshurst J (2004) Definitive neuroradiological diagnostic features of tuberculous meningitis in children. *Pediatric Radiology*, 34: 876–885.

Andronikou S, Wilmshurst J, Hatherill M, Vantoorn R (2006) Distribution of brain infarction in children with tuberculous meningitis and correlation with outcome score at 6 months. *Pediatric Radiology*, 36: 1289–1294.

Andronikou S, Govender N, Ramdass A, van Toorn R (2012) MRI appearances of tuberculous meningitis in HIV-infected children: A paradoxically protective mechanism? *Imaging in Medicine*, 4(3): 359–366.

Andronikou S, Ackermann C, Laughton B et al. (2014) Correlating brain volume and callosal thickness with clinical and laboratory indicators of disease severity in children with HIV-related brain disease. *Child's Nervous System*, 30: 1549–1557.

Arain M, Haque M, Johal L et al. (2013) Maturation of the adolescent brain. *Neuropsychiatric Disease and Treatment*, 9: 449–461. https://doi.org/10.2147/ndt.s39776.

Bibas M, Castillo JJ (2014) Current knowledge on HIV-associated plasmablastic lymphoma. *Mediterranean Journal of Hematology and Infectious Diseases*, 6: e2014064.

Blokhuis C, Mutsaerts HJMM, Cohen S et al. (2017) Higher subcortical and white matter cerebral blood flow in perinatally HIV-infected children. *Medicine*, 96(7): e5891. https://doi.org/10.1097/md.0000000000005891.

Blokhuis C, Peeters CFW, Cohen S et al. (2019) Systemic and intrathecal immune activation in association with cerebral and cognitive outcomes in paediatric HIV. *Scientific Reports*, 9(1): 8004–8010. https://doi.org/10.1038/s41598-019-44198-z.

Cohen S, Caan MWA, Mutsaerts H-J et al. (2016) Cerebral injury in perinatally HIV-infected children compared to matched healthy controls. *Neurology*, 86(1): 19–27. https://doi.org/10.1212/wnl.0000000000002209.

Dalen YWV, Blokhuis C, Cohen S et al. (2016) Neurometabolite alterations associated with cognitive performance in perinatally HIV-infected children. *Medicine*, 95(12): e3093. https://doi.org/10.1097/md.0000000000003093.

Dekker G, Andronikou S, van Toorn R, Scheepers S, Brandt A, Ackermann C (2011) MRI findings in children with tuberculous meningitis: A comparison of HIV-infected and non-infected patients. *Child's Nervous System*, 27: 1943–1949.

Donald KA, Walker KG, Kilborn T et al. (2015) HIV Encephalopathy: Pediatric case series description and insights from the clinic coalface. *AIDS Research and Therapy*, 12(1): 2. doi: 10.1186/s12981-014-0042-7.

Du Toit J, Wieselthaler N (2015) Let's face it – 13 unusual causes of facial masses in children. *Insights Imaging*, 6: 519–530.

Garg RK, Sinha MK (2011) Tuberculous meningitis in patients infected with human immunodeficiency virus. *Journal of Neurology*, 258: 3–13.

George R, Andronikou S, Du Plessis J, Du Plessis AM, van Toorn R, Maydell A (2009) Central nervous system manifestations of HIV infection in children. *Pediatric Radiology*, 39: 575–585.

Giedd JN, Blumenthal J, Jeffries NO et al. (1999) Brain development during childhood and adolescence: A longitudinal MRI study. *Nature Neuroscience*, 2(10): 861–863. https://doi.org/10.1038/13158.

Gouse H, Casson-Crook M, Decloedt EH, Joska JA, Thomas KGF (2017) Adding a brief self-report cognitive tool to the IHDS improves effectiveness of identifying patients with HIV-associated dementia in South Africa. *Journal of NeuroVirology*, 23(5): 686–695. https://doi.org/10.1007/s13365-017-0551-y.

Gray L, Sterjovski J, Churchill M et al. (2005) Uncoupling coreceptor usage of human immunodeficiency virus type 1 (HIV-1) from macrophage tropism reveals biological properties of CCR5-restricted HIV-1 isolates from patients with acquired immunodeficiency syndrome. *Virology*, 337: 384–398.

Haldorsen IS, Espeland A, Larsson EM (2011) Central nervous system lymphoma: Characteristic findings on traditional and advanced imaging. *AJNR American Journal of Neuroradiology*, 32: 984–992.

Hammond CK, Shapson-Coe A, Govender R et al. (2016) Moyamoya syndrome in South African children with HIV-1 infection. *Journal of Child Neurology*, 31(8): 1010–1017.

Heany SJ, Phillips N, Brooks S et al. (2019) Neural correlates of maintenance working memory, as well as relevant structural qualities, are associated with earlier antiretroviral treatment initiation in vertically transmitted HIV. *Journal of NeuroVirology*, 6(1): 1–10. https://doi.org/10.1007/s13365-019-00792-5.

Heaps JM, Joska J, Hoare J et al. (2012) Neuroimaging markers of human immunodeficiency virus infection in South Africa. *Journal of NeuroVirology*, 18(3): 151–156. https://doi.org/10.1007/s13365-012-0090-5.

Hoare J, Ransford GL, Phillips N, Amos T, Donald K, Stein DJ (2014) Systematic review of neuroimaging studies in vertically transmitted HIV positive children and adolescents. *Metabolic Brain Disease*, 29: 221–229.

Hoare J, Fouche J-P, Phillips N et al. (2015a) Clinical associations of white matter damage in cART-treated HIV-positive children in South Africa. *Journal of NeuroVirology*, 21: 120–128.

Hoare J, Fouche J-P, Phillips N et al. (2015b) White matter micro-structural changes in ART-naive and ART-treated children and adolescents infected with HIV in South Africa. *AIDS (London, England)*, 29(14): 1793–1801. https://doi.org/10.1097/qad.0000000000000766.

Hoare J, Phillips N, Joska JA et al. (2016) Applying the HIV-associated neurocognitive disorder diagnostic criteria to HIV-infected youth. *Neurology*, 87(1): 86–93. https://doi.org/10.1212/wnl.0000000000002669.

Hoare J, Fouche J-P, Phillips N et al. (2018) Structural brain changes in perinatally HIV infected young adolescents in South Africa. *AIDS (London, England)*, 32(18): 1. https://doi.org/10.1097/qad.0000000000002024.

Hoare J, Heany SJ, Fouche J-P et al. (2019). Initiation of antiretroviral therapy after the critical neuronal developmental period of the second postnatal year affects white matter microstructure in adolescents living with HIV. *Journal of NeuroVirology*, 25(2): 254–262. https://doi.org/10.1007/s13365-018-0712-7.

Hoare J, Phillips N, Brittain K, Myer L, Zar HJ, Stein DJ (2019) Mental health and functional competence in the Cape Town Adolescent Antiretroviral Cohort. *Journal of Acquired Immune Deficiency Syndromes (1999)*, 81(4): e109–e116. https://doi.org/10.1097/qai.0000000000002068.

Hoare J, Myer L, Heany S et al. (2020) Cognition, structural brain changes and systemic inflammation in adolescents living with HIV on antiretroviral therapy. *Journal of Acquired Immune Deficiency Syndromes* 84(1): 114–121.

Jankiewicz M, Holmes MJ, Taylor PA et al. (2017) White matter abnormalities in children with HIV infection and exposure. *Frontiers in Neuroanatomy*, 11: 88. https://doi.org/10.3389/fnana.2017.00088.

Janse van Rensburg P, Andronikou S, van Toorn R, Pienaar M (2008) Magnetic resonance imaging of miliary tuberculosis of the central nervous system in children with tuberculous meningitis. *Pediatric Radiology*, 38: 1306–1313.

Katrak SM, Shembalkar PK, Bijwe SR, Bhandarkar LD (2000) The clinical, radiological and pathological profile of tuberculous meningitis in patients with and without human immunodeficiency virus infection. *Journal of the Neurological Sciences*, 181: 118–126.

Kauffman WM, Sivit CJ, Fitz CR, Rakusan TA, Herzog K, Chandra RS (1992) CT and MR evaluation of intracranial involvement in pediatric HIV infection: A clinical-imaging correlation. *AJNR American Journal of Neuroradiology*, 13: 949–957.

Keller MA, Venkatraman TN, Thomas A et al. (2004) Altered neurometabolite development in HIV-infected children: Correlation with neuropsychological tests. *Neurology*, 62(10): 1810–1817. https://doi.org/10.1212/01.wnl.0000125492.57419.25.

Kilborn T, Zampoli M (2009) Immune reconstitution inflammatory syndrome after initiating highly active antiretroviral therapy in HIV-infected children. *Pediatric Radiology*, 39: 569–574.

Lu D, Pavlakis SG, Frank Y et al. (1996) Proton MR spectroscopy of the basal ganglia in healthy children and children with AIDS. *Radiology*, 199: 423–428.

Madhi SA, Madhi A, Petersen K, Khoosal M, Klugman KP (2001) Impact of human immunodeficiency virus type 1 infection on the epidemiology and outcome of bacterial meningitis in South African children. *International Journal of Infectious Diseases: IJID: Official Publication of the International Society for Infectious Diseases*, 5: 119–125.

Marais S, Pepper DJ, Marais BJ, Török ME (2010) HIV-associated tuberculous meningitis – Diagnostic and therapeutic challenges. *Tuberculosis (Edinb)*, 90: 367–374.

Mbugua KK, Holmes MJ, Cotton MF et al. (2016) HIV-associated CD4+/CD8+ depletion in infancy is associated with neurometabolic reductions in the basal ganglia at age 5 years despite early antiretroviral therapy. *AIDS (London, England)*, 30(9): 1353–1362. https://doi.org/10.1097/qad.0000000000001082.

Nickerson JP, Richner B, Santy K et al. (2012) Neuroimaging of pediatric intracranial infection – Part 1: Techniques and bacterial infections. *J Neuroimaging*, 22: e42–51.

Nuttall JJ, Wilmshurst JM, Ndondo AP et al. (2004) Progressive multifocal leukoencephalopathy after initiation of highly active antiretroviral therapy in a child with advanced human immunodeficiency virus infection: A case of immune reconstitution inflammatory syndrome. *The Pediatric Infectious Disease Journal*, 23: 683–685.

Nwosu EC, Robertson FC, Holmes MJ et al. (2018) Altered brain morphometry in 7-year-old HIV-infected children on early ART. *Metabolic Brain Disease*, 33(2): 523–535. https://doi.org/10.1007/s11011-017-0162-6.

Patsalides AD, Wood LV, Atac GK, Sandifer E, Butman JA, Patronas NJ (2002) Cerebrovascular disease in HIV-infected pediatric patients: Neuroimaging findings. *AJR.American Journal of Roentgenology*, 179: 999–1003.

Pavlakis SG, Lu D, Frank Y et al. (1995) Magnetic resonance spectroscopy in childhood AIDS encephalopathy. *Pediatric Neurology*, 12: 277–282.

Phillips NJ, Hoare J, Stein DJ, Myer L, Zar HJ, Thomas KGF (2018) HIV-associated cognitive disorders in perinatally infected children and adolescents: A novel composite cognitive domains score. *AIDS Care*, 30(Suppl): 1–9. https://doi.org/10.1080/09540121.2018.1466982.

Pienaar M, Andronikou S, van Toorn R (2009) MRI to demonstrate diagnostic features and complications of TBM not seen with CT. *Child's Nervous System*, 25: 941–947.

Plessis SD, Perez A, Fouche J-P et al. (2019) Efavirenz is associated with altered fronto-striatal function in HIV+ adolescents. *Journal of NeuroVirology*, 41(6): 3278. https://doi.org/10.1007/s13365-019-00764-9.

Post MJ, Thurnher MM, Clifford DB et al. (2013) CNS-immune reconstitution inflammatory syndrome in the setting of HIV infection, Part 1: Overview and discussion of progressive multifocal leukoencephalopathy-immune reconstitution inflammatory syndrome and cryptococcal-immune reconstitution inflammatory syndrome. *AJNR American Journal of Neuroradiology*, 34: 1297–1307.

Potchen M, Kampondeni S, Seydel K et al. (2016) Adding malaria insult to HIV injury – A neuroimaging study. *Neurology*, April 5 (86) 16 Supplement.

Prado PT, Escorsi-Rosset S, Cervi MC, Santos AC (2011) Image evaluation of HIV encephalopathy: A multimodal approach using quantitative MR techniques. *Neuroradiology*, 53: 899–908.

Puthanakit T, Oberdorfer P, Akarathum N, Wannarit P, Sirisanthana T, Sirisanthana V (2006) Immune reconstitution syndrome after highly active antiretroviral therapy in human immunodeficiency virus-infected thai children. *The Pediatric Infectious Disease Journal*, 25: 53–58.

Randall SR, Warton CMR, Holmes MJ et al. (2017) Larger subcortical gray matter structures and smaller corpora callosa at age 5 years in HIV-infected children on early ART. *Frontiers in Neuroanatomy*, 11: 95. https://doi.org/10.3389/fnana.2017.00095.

Robertson FC, Holmes MJ, Cotton MF et al. (2018) Perinatal HIV infection or exposure is associated with low N-acetylaspartate and glutamate in basal ganglia at age 9 but not 7 years. *Frontiers in Human Neuroscience*, 12: 145. https://doi.org/10.3389/fnhum.2018.00145.

Safriel YI, Haller JO, Lefton DR, Obedian R (2000) Imaging of the brain in the HIV-positive child. *Pediatric Radiology*, 30: 725–732.

Sarma MK, Nagarajan R, Keller MA et al. (2014) Regional brain gray and white matter changes in perinatally HIV-infected adolescents. *NeuroImage. Clinical*, 4: 29–34. https://doi.org/10.1016/j.nicl.2013.10.012.

Schwenk H, Ramirez-Avila L, Sheu SH et al. (2014) Progressive multifocal leukoencephalopathy in pediatric patients: Case report and literature review. *The Pediatric Infectious Disease Journal*, 33: e99–105.

Senocak E, Oğuz KK, Ozgen B et al. (2010) Imaging features of CNS involvement in AIDS. *Diagnostic and Interventional Radiology*, 16: 193–200.

Smith AB, Smirniotopoulos JG, Rushing EJ (2008) From the archives of the AFIP: Central nervous system infections associated with human immunodeficiency virus infection: Radiologic–pathologic correlation. *Radiographics*, 28: 2033–2058.

Song SK, Sun SW, Ramsbottom MJ, Chang C, Russell J, Cross AH (2002) Dysmyelination revealed through MRI as increased radial (but unchanged axial) diffusion of water. *Neuroimage*, 17: 1429–1436.

States LJ, Zimmerman RA, Rutstein RM (1997) Imaging of pediatric central nervous system HIV infection. *Neuroimaging Clinics of North America*, 7: 321–339.

Thompson PM, Dutton RA, Hayashi KM et al. (2006) 3D mapping of ventricular and corpus callosum abnormalities in HIV/AIDS. *Neuroimage*, 31: 12–23.

Toich JTF, Taylor PA, Holmes MJ et al. (2017) Functional connectivity alterations between networks and associations with Infant immune health within networks in HIV-infected children on early treatment: A study at 7 years. *Frontiers in Human Neuroscience*, 11: 635. https://doi.org/10.3389/fnhum.2017.00635.

Van den Hof M, ter Haar AM, Caan MWA, Spijker R, van der Lee JH, Pajkrt D (2019) Brain structure of perinatally HIV-infected patients on long-term treatment: A systematic review. *Neurology. Clinical Practice*, 9(5): 433–442. https://doi.org/10.1212/cpj.0000000000000637.

van der Weert EM, Hartgers NM, Schaaf HS et al. (2006) Comparison of diagnostic criteria of tuberculous meningitis in human immunodeficiency virus-infected and uninfected children. *The Pediatric Infectious Disease Journal*, 25: 65–69.

van Toorn R, Rabie H (2005) Pseudocystic cryptococcal meningitis complicated by transient periaqueductal obstruction in a child with HIV infection. *European Journal of Paediatric Neurology*, 9: 81–84.

van Toorn R, Rabie H, Dramowski A, Schoeman JF (2012) Neurological manifestations of TB-IRIS: A report of 4 children. *European Journal of Paediatric Neurology*, 16: 676–682.

Vinnard C, Macgregor RR (2009) Tuberculous meningitis in HIV-infected individuals. *Current HIV/AIDS Reports*, 6: 139–145.

HIV Encephalopathy

Kirsten A Donald, Nelleke G Langerak, Aleya Remtulla, and Theresa N Mann

INTRODUCTION

Human immunodeficiency virus (HIV) encephalopathy (HIVE) refers to the disease, damage or malfunction of the brain caused by the invasion of the central nervous system (CNS) by HIV during early development of the foetal and infant brain (Donald et al. 2015). While the HIV virus, with its direct inflammatory and immune impact on the CNS, is the core mechanism for the clinical expression of HIVE, environmental and contextual factors also play a role. It is often difficult to tease out the extent to which different, often co-occurring factors such as nutrition, social interaction, parenting, communication, sleep, maternal health and autonomy, maternal substance abuse, and infant health, influence brain development and cognitive function in the early years. More so, in the context of real-world infant healthcare, is it crucial to understand, to take into account and to address these contextual factors, when researching and caring for children presenting with HIVE.

EPIDEMIOLOGY

HIVE is the most common primary HIV-related CNS complication in children. Reported prevalence in historical cohorts of untreated children has ranged from 20% to 60% (Epstein et al. 1986; Blanche et al. 1989; Lobato et al. 1995; Englund et al. 1996; Chase et al. 2000; Bruck et al. 2001; Foster et al. 2006; Tahan et al. 2006). This severe neurological complication may present before the development of significant immunosuppression but, when present in an HIV-infected child, HIVE constitutes an AIDS-defining condition (see Box 5.1).

Before the advent of combination antiretroviral therapy (cART) regimens, HIVE was relatively common amongst HIV-infected children, and even more so in children with advanced disease (Epstein et al. 1986; Lobato et al. 1995). In one of the earliest accounts, 20 (55%) of 36 HIV-infected children undergoing clinical surveillance in the USA between 1981 and 1985, developed progressive HIVE. A further eight HIV-infected children developed a static form of encephalopathy (Epstein et al. 1986). However, a much larger, multi-site USA study investigating 1811 cases of perinatal HIV infection occurring between 1988 and 1992, found HIVE was the fourth most common AIDS-defining condition, affecting 23% of children with AIDS and 9.8% of all HIV-infected children (Lobato et al. 1995). The incidence of HIVE thus varies significantly in terms of the sample size, time period, setting, and clinical status of the cohort involved, and these are therefore factors to be considered when interpreting study data.

> **Box 5.1 Centers for Disease Control and Prevention (CDC): HIV encephalopathy criteria for classification**
>
> According to the CDC, encephalopathy must include criteria in at least one of the following areas for at least 2 months in the absence of a concurrent illness:
>
> - Loss of, or failure to attain, developmental milestones, or loss of intellectual ability, verified by a standard developmental scale or by neuropsychological testing.
> - Impaired brain growth, or acquired microcephaly, evident by head circumference measurements or brain atrophy shown on computed tomography or magnetic resonance imaging; serial imaging is required for children less than 2 years of age.
> - Acquired symmetric motor deficits, including two or more of the following: paresis, pathological reflexes, ataxia, or gait disturbance.

Access to cART has Revolutionised the Treatment of HIV

Access to cART has been shown to substantially reduce HIVE incidence. Seminal work by Patel et al., investigating the year-to-year incidence of HIVE amongst children enrolled in a large prospective cohort between 1993 and 2007 (Patel et al. 2009), found that after a peak of more than 20 cases of HIVE per 1000 person-years in 1995, new cases declined by approximately 10-fold over the subsequent years as cART coverage improved. Thereafter, the incidence of HIVE appeared to remain stable at less than three cases per 1000 person-years with more than 90% cART coverage from approximately 2003 to 2006 (the end of the study period). Significantly, Patel et al. (2009) found a 50% reduction in cases of HIVE when comparing children prescribed cART versus single-drug ART regimens, further emphasising the importance of a combination therapy approach. Moreover, it was demonstrated that cART regimens with a higher central nervous system penetration (CNSP) score conferred a greater reduction in the risk of HIVE than those with a lower CNSP score (Patel et al. 2009).

Data from more recent cohorts such as the large CHER (Children with HIV Early Antiretroviral Therapy) trial, showed that early initiation of cART led to better short-term neurodevelopmental outcomes in infants compared to those where treatment was deferred. This study highlighted the critical need for early access to cART for both brain health and development in early life (Laughton et al. 2012). Further, HIV-infected school-aged children with early initiation of cART from the same CHER trial had similar neurocognitive developmental trajectories to those without infection, although it was noted that all cART-treated children remained at risk for cognitive deficits across early school ages (van Wyhe et al. 2021).

Setting-related Challenges Affect Uptake and Outcomes in sub-Saharan Africa

Although some studies from the 2000s support a low prevalence of HIVE (Chiriboga et al. 2005; Mbaye et al. 2005), other studies continued to report a relatively high rate of between 18% (Hamid et al. 2008) and 33% (Govender et al. 2011) respectively. The reasons for this are likely to be multifactorial, including setting-related challenges such as access to the expertise to make a HIVE diagnosis and cART distribution challenges.

At a Red Cross War Memorial Children's Hospital satellite clinic in Cape Town, one-third of HIV-infected children born between 2006 and 2007 presented with HIVE. Of these, only 55% were found to be receiving ART (Govender et al. 2011). A subsequent case series reported that 87 of the 145 (60%)

HIV-infected children who were seen at this clinic were diagnosed with HIVE at a different clinic within the same hospital system between 2008 and 2012 (Donald et al. 2015). These findings raise concerns that in many high-burden communities, general medical services may lack the capacity to provide the necessary neurological screening to identify children at risk of developing HIVE, and those cases of HIVE that are diagnosed may represent only the most severe presentations (Donald et al. 2015).

Further Research Required to Understand HIVE in Under-resourced Settings

In summary, the transition from the pre-ART era to the cART era has produced a substantial reduction in the prevalence of HIVE. The full-blown version of this condition has become uncommon in well-resourced settings able to provide comprehensive cART coverage (Chiriboga et al. 2005; Shanbhag et al. 2005; Patel et al. 2009). However, current understanding of HIVE epidemiology is based primarily on large cohort studies from the USA, a relatively high-resource, low-burden setting. Much less is known about HIVE epidemiology in high-burden, low-resource settings where provision of cART was, or still is, suboptimal. New studies investigating the prevalence of HIVE (particularly the milder forms of the condition) in high-burden, low-resource settings would provide insight and awareness of the current burden in this context.

Since the introduction of cART in the mid-1990s, mortality of HIV-infected children has steadily dropped as they increasingly survive their early, high-risk years and are successfully transferred into adult care (Koekkoek et al. 2008; Banks et al. 2015). cART increases CD4 counts, decreases HIV RNA levels and, in turn, reduces the AIDS-related consequences (Egger et al. 2002; Cole et al. 2003). As a result of these gains, greater numbers of children are surviving but, of course, they live with HIV as a chronic condition, to a varying degree. The timing of cART initiation, compartmentalisation, and the neurotoxic effects of the drugs all play a significant role in the severity and complexity of neurological outcomes in children with HIVE (Whitehead, Potterton, and Coovadia 2014). Although cART reduces the viral load and inflammatory markers, it has limited ability to reverse CNS injury brought about by HIV. Where a child has been exposed to the virus even for only a short period of time – for example, where ARTs have been administered early – or for those first infected in the perinatal window, the fact that foetal life occurred in an altered inflammatory and immune environment, puts the child at risk of the more subtle CNS effects (see Chapter 15), including learning difficulties, developmental delays, and executive function problems. Children with vertically-acquired HIV who do not have access to cART, or who started treatment later in life, remain at risk of developing CNS sequelae (Abubakar et al. 2008; Baillieu and Potterton 2008; Hilburn, Potterton, and Stewart 2010; Govender et al. 2011; Devendra et al. 2013; Banks et al. 2015).

PATHOGENESIS AND AETIOLOGY OF HIVE

HIV has been shown to enter the CNS compartment within days or weeks of infection. The virus acts through both direct and indirect mechanisms, resulting in a spectrum of CNS and peripheral nervous system (PNS) sequelae, of which HIVE is the primary paediatric manifestation. In children, the majority of whom are infected through vertical transmission, the disease process can start as early as during the antenatal period. The virus may directly infect the microglia, astrocytes, oligodendroglia, and cells of the monocyte-macrophage lineage in the brain. Prominent reservoirs of HIV are the microglial cells; once infected, they secrete chemokines which escalate recruitment of HIV-infected monocytes, in turn secreting tumour necrosis factor alpha and nitric oxide. Thus neuronal function is impaired even where neurons themselves are not infected by the virus. The virus infiltrates the immature developing brain, putting the child at risk of a number of neurological outcomes, including neuronal dysfunction, neural cell death, and altered neurogenesis. Studies using quantitative brain magnetic resonance imaging (MRI) are enhancing our understanding of the neurobiological effects of HIV on developing brains in the clinical context. Ackermann and colleagues (2014), using structural MRI, reported abnormal white matter signals in many of the brains of very young HIV-infected children (mean age: 31.4 months), all of whom had been initiated on cART before they were 3 months old. This suggests that the virus infiltrates the CNS at an extremely early stage of infection (Ackermann et al. 2014).

HIV Subtypes and Clades: Clade C, the Most Common and the Most Neurotropic

HIV type 1 (HIV-1) virus strain is classified into four groups: M, N, O, and P. Of these, group M is the major group causing the global epidemic. Within the M group, there are at least nine other subtypes, differing in CNS macrophage trophic properties, brain virulence, CNS penetrance in cART treatment drug categories, and subsequent HIVE risk and prevalence (Boivin et al. 2010; Bangirana et al. 2017; Ruiseñor-Escudero et al. 2018).

M group subtypes are categorised as A, B, C, D, F, G, H, J, and K (Hemelaar 2012). Of these, subtypes A, C, and D are predominant in East, South, West, and Central Africa (Geretti 2006), with certain subtypes being associated with a greater risk of transmission or disease progression than others, although published data on this point demonstrate inconsistent findings across studies and contexts (Pant Pai, Shivkumar, and Cajas 2012). Nearly 50% of all people living with HIV globally have subtype (or clade) C (Sturdevant et al. 2012; Gartner et al. 2020). Clade C is not only the most prevalent subtype in Africa, the region with the highest incidence of HIV worldwide, but it has also been noted to be the most neurotropic HIV-1 virus strain.

Clinical and Laboratory Predictors of HIVE in HIV-infected Children

Studies have identified HIV-related risk factors associated with HIVE. These include maternal and child immune status, high cerebrospinal fluid and plasma viral load, high circulating monocytes, timing of infection, route of transmission, and availability of early treatment (Msellati et al. 1993; Le Doaré, Bland, and Newell 2012). Regarding the latter, a study by Laughton et al. (2012) revealed that children who had early initiation of cART, had better locomotor and general scores at the median age of 11 months compared to their counterparts who deferred treatment. Likewise, Patel et al. (2009) found that a cART regimen with a high CNSP score is associated with a significantly lower hazard score. There is also evidence that cART may arrest the course of progressive HIVE, improving neurological outcomes in some children, including brain growth and cognitive function (Pizzo et al. 1988; Brouwers et al. 1990; DeCarli et al. 1991; Chiriboga et al. 2005). These improvements are correlated with a decrease in the HIV viral load measured in the cerebrospinal fluid, although the magnitude of change in CNS viral load does not directly predict the magnitude of change in neurological outcomes (DeCarli et al. 1991; McCoig et al. 2002).

The ongoing CHER study aims to determine whether early clinical indicators, including both infant and maternal health, are predictive of later health and neurodevelopmental outcomes. This includes whether HIV and cART exposure affect infant neurodevelopment, and whether the duration of in utero cART exposure affects outcomes. Notwithstanding this work, a definitive clinical or imaging predictor has yet to be identified.

For infected children who are on cART treatment and whose viral loads are undetectable, understanding the pathway that leads to a variation in CNS presentation between different individuals is especially important. Postulated pathways include viral suppression and associated improved immunologic function, as well as via indirect mechanisms (Zink et al. 1999; Willen 2006; Heaton et al. 2011). Finally, and most crucially, despite progress being made to identify risk factors associated with the manifestation of HIVE, it remains unclear what factors cause the onset of HIVE. Encouragingly, mechanisms for how cART acts to mitigate the risk of CNS effects from HIV infection are being established, and advances are being made in establishing clinical and laboratory predictors of CNS outcomes in HIV-infected children.

The Role of Indirect Factors on HIVE Presentation

Beyond these direct effects, the manifestation of HIV in a child is affected by the interplay between cytotoxic viral effects, immune-mediated inflammatory response, secondary neurological conditions, adverse effects of cART as well as variable entry and effectiveness of individual cART agents in the CNS (Bass et al. 2017). In discussing HIVE in low- and middle-income countries (LMICs), and especially in the sub-Saharan African region, adverse environmental factors remain highly relevant. The challenge is to understand the extent to which neurodevelopmental risk is due to HIV as a proximal (direct) cause, or due to more distal causes such as psychosocial risk factors, including caregiving, poor nutrition, and micronutrient deficiencies (mothers living with HIV in a subsistence agricultural or resource-constrained urban setting) (Boivin et al. 2016). This has become yet more challenging in the era of COVID pandemic lockdowns and related socioeconomic challenges.

Major Gaps Remain in Our Understanding of the Different Clades

Data on HIVE have primarily originated from the Americas and now more recently in Africa. Considering the paucity of information from other major regions impacted by HIV, there are still major gaps in our understanding of different clades and their specific mode of action and effects on the developing child (see Box 5.2 describing the Nurturing Care Framework).

Box 5.2 The Nurturing Care Framework for Early Childhood Development

To reach their full potential, children need the five inter-related and indivisible components of nurturing care: good health, adequate nutrition, safety and security, responsive caregiving, and opportunities for learning.

The Nurturing Care Framework for Early Childhood Development is aimed at helping children SURVIVE and THRIVE to TRANSFORM health and human potential. It builds on evidence of how child development unfolds and of the effective policies and interventions that can improve early childhood development. The framework was developed by the World Health Organization, UNICEF, and the World Bank Group, in collaboration with the Partnership for Maternal, Newborn & Child Health, the Early Childhood Development Action Network, and many other partners, to provide a roadmap for ensuring attainment of the Sustainable Development Goals and survive, thrive, and transform goals of the Global Strategy on Women's, Children's and Adolescents' Health. Launched alongside the 71st World Health Assembly in May 2018, it outlines why efforts to improve health and well-being must begin in the earliest years, from pregnancy to age 3 years; the major threats to early childhood development; how nurturing care protects young children from the worst effects of adversity and promotes physical, emotional, and cognitive development; and what families and caregivers need in order to provide nurturing care for young children.

More information is available at: https://nurturing-care.org/about/what-is-the-nurturing-care-framework/

RANGE IN SEVERITY OF HIVE AND ITS CLINICAL MANIFESTATIONS

Range in Severity of HIVE

Paediatric HIVE was first described in the mid-1980s (Belman et al. 1985; Epstein et al. 1985; Epstein et al. 1986). This was followed in 1994 by the standardised Centers for Disease Control and Prevention criteria (CDC 1994). Children with HIVE must meet one of the following criteria for at least 2 months in the absence of concurrent illness: (1) failure to attain, plateau, or loss of developmental milestones or loss of intellectual ability, (2) impaired brain growth, or acquired microcephaly, and/or (3) acquired symmetric motor deficit, which clinically manifests as paresis, pathological reflexes or gait disturbances (CDC 1994).

NEURODEVELOPMENTAL DELAY

Neurodevelopmental delay is the most typical sign of HIVE, and it can vary in both severity and presentation. The severity of encephalopathy can present in either a static or a progressive (plateau or sub-acute) pattern (Brouwers et al. 1990; Hilburn, Potterton, and Stewart 2010).

STATIC ENCEPHALOPATHY

Children with static encephalopathy will present with delays in their neurodevelopment but will not experience neurological deterioration over time, so they will still attain their motor milestones. As presented in Figure 5.1 (Brouwers et al. 1990), there is linear mental growth. However, this is slower when compared to typical neurocognitive development trajectories, resulting in a gap between chronological age and developmental age over time. This form of HIVE is the most commonly seen presentation in the cART era.

PLATEAU ENCEPHALOPATHY

Children with plateau encephalopathy will show linear neurological development during the first few months of life. This progression is slower when compared to children with typical neurological development. After the first few months of growth, children begin to deteriorate neurologically, losing their previously acquired skills and resulting in both motor and cognitive impairments. These children do not progress in their development, but may not show deterioration for lengthy periods of time (Hilburn, Potterton, and Stewart 2010).

SUBACUTE PROGRESSIVE ENCEPHALOPATHY

During the first few months of life, children with subacute progressive encephalopathy develop in the same manner as a typically developing child, but then show a sudden deterioration in their neurological abilities, resulting in the loss of previously-obtained motor milestones. Mentally, these children are initially only slightly behind their typically developing peers but they suddenly regress, displaying a rapid deterioration in mental age as they lose their previously obtained cognitive and motor milestones. These children may remain relatively stable for extended time periods before a new loss is appreciated.

CLINICAL MANIFESTATIONS

The presentation of paediatric HIVE is extremely variable. The neurodevelopmental complications in children with HIV involve delays in both gross and fine motor control. In the more severe forms of HIVE, the onset of both walking and talking may be delayed until after the child is 2 years old. Affected

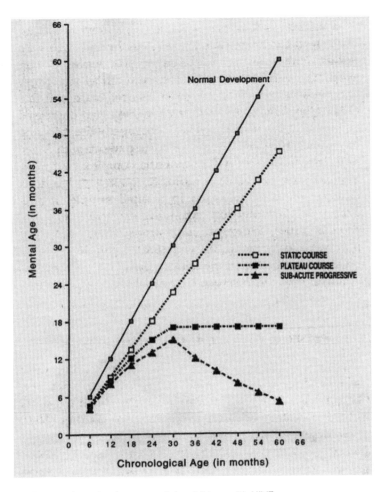

Figure 5.1 Natural history trajectories (conceptual) for children with HIVE.
Source: Reproduced from Brouwers P, Walters P, and Civitello L. Central nervous system manifestations and assessment. In: PA Pizzo PA, Wilfert CM, editors, *Pediatric AIDS. 3rd Edition.* Baltimore, MD: Williams & Williams, 1998: 293–308. With kind permission of the authors and publishers.

children often have difficulty with both hearing and language. Language impairment in these children is classified as primary or concurrent, and may occur with or without cognitive and/or hearing impairment (Rice et al. 2012). Common speech-language deficits include loss of speech–language milestones, and poor language development with the progression of the infection (Baillieu and Potterton 2008). The language domain has been found to be at risk even when HIV-infected children are compared to those exposed but not infected. Further, amongst children who are HIV-exposed but not infected compared to unexposed peers, risk for poor language development in early life also appears important, arguing for the role of inflammatory and immune dysregulation in the aetiological pathway to these impairments (see Chapter 16). Further, neurocognitive impairment has also been frequently described, often additionally resulting in behavioural problems and difficulties coping with school to the point of needing to repeat grades due to poor performance (Van Rie et al. 2007; Abubakar et al. 2008; Hilburn, Potterton, and Stewart 2010; Le Doaré, Bland, and Newell 2012; Laughton et al. 2013; Donald et al. 2015).

Impaired Brain Growth

Another cardinal sign of HIVE is decreased brain growth, measured by a child having a smaller head circumference compared to typically developing children. Microcephaly is diagnosed when the child's head circumference is more than two standard deviations below the 50th percentile circumference for their age reflected on World Health Organization (WHO 2016) growth charts (Figure 5.2). Microcephaly was reported in 48% to 69% of the cases described in HIVE cohorts (Chiriboga et al.

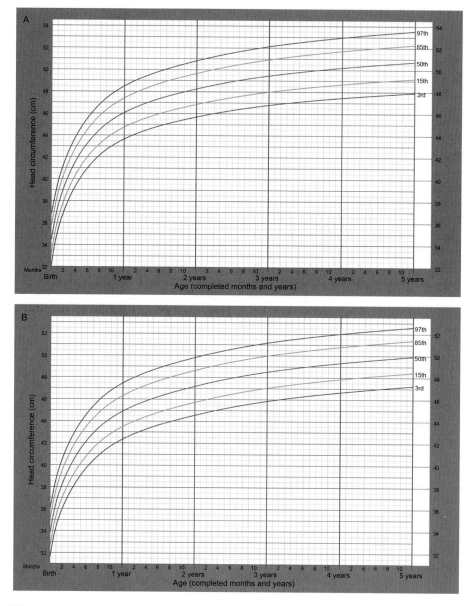

Figure 5.2   WHO head circumference-for-age charts – from birth until 5 years – for boys (A) and girls (B) (WHO 2016).

2005; Donald et al. 2015) and is often associated with impaired development in other anthropometric measures, such as weight and height (Donald et al. 2015).

Motor Deficits

Motor deficits often present as bilateral lower limb spasticity and other gait disturbances (Epstein et al. 1986), similar to the clinical presentation observed in children with cerebral palsy (CP). In more severe HIVE presentations, children show spasticity in both lower extremities, which is recognised as bilateral lower limb spasticity or diparesis (Epstein et al. 1986). This motor impairment was described in about 54% and 63% of the HIVE study cohorts reported by Chiriboga et al. (2005) and Donald et al. (2015) respectively. Due to hypertonicity in the child's legs, such children generally present with an abnormal posture and an atypical walking pattern. They often require an assistive device, like crutches or a walker, to ambulate successfully (Figures 5.3a and 5.3b).

The gait pattern of children with HIVE is recognised as a tip-toe, scissor-like gait, often observed in bilateral lower limb spasticity. Langerak et al. (2014) reported in their three-dimensional gait-study, that this walking pattern differs from the typical CP gait (jump, crouch, true or apparent equinus gait), although the functional gait impairment in the severest cases was very similar to their peers with a diagnosis of CP (Rodda et al. 2004). About two-thirds of their study cohort walked with mild limitations, and one-third showed some of the typical CP characteristics while ambulating, including the equinus ankle and stiff knee (Wren, Rethlefsen, and Kay 2005). It was concluded that, based on both gait analyses and physical examinations, children with HIVE and bilateral lower limb spasticity who walked with an impaired gait pattern, had greater involvement of the distal muscle groups than the children with CP (Langerak et al. 2014).

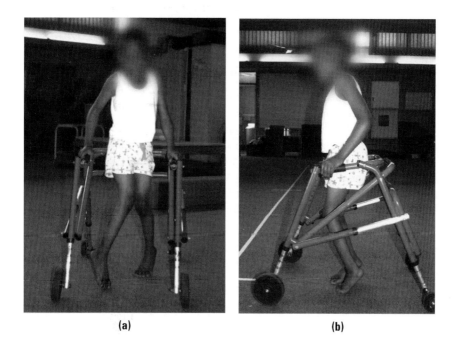

(a)   (b)

Figure 5.3 A child with HIVE and bilateral lower limb spasticity.

In addition to the data supporting impaired lower limb function in children with HIVE and bilateral lower limb spasticity, Mann et al. (2016) also reported impaired fine motor control in the upper limb function of these children. Mann et al. (2016) also observed that the upper limb motor performance and limitations among the participants were not correlated with severity of functional impairment in the lower limbs.

Comorbidities

Children with HIVE often present with other comorbidities, including other symptoms of CNS dysfunction as well as other organ systems, reflecting the systemic nature of the HIV infection. Conditions that are particularly frequently associated with HIVE, include seizures, ear diseases, behavioural problems (Donald et al. 2015), cardiomyopathy (Epstein et al. 1986; Lobato et al. 1995; Cooper et al. 1998), hepatosplenomegaly and lymphadenopathy (Hamid et al. 2008).

THE DIAGNOSTIC PATHWAY FOR INVESTIGATING AND REFERRING PAEDIATRIC HIVE CASES

As discussed earlier, diagnosis of HIVE at the milder end of the disease spectrum is often missed in clinics with high patient loads. Furthermore, children with severe HIVE are often misdiagnosed: for example, bilateral lower limb spasticity is often treated as CP, while those presenting with secondary abnormalities, such as epilepsy, might be misdiagnosed with other medical conditions (Langerak et al. 2014). A child with HIVE requires specialised care, including cART for the HIV infection itself. Ideally, a multidisciplinary team should be engaged to assist in the diagnosis of HIVE where confounding symptoms are present, before initiating comorbidity treatments and interventions.

Investigating the possibility of paediatric HIVE should begin with excluding other causes of motor and cognitive decline. Relevant comorbid conditions – which may contribute to the clinical picture, management of disease, and timely decision-making – must be identified before HIVE-related specific care can be initiated. Investigations should utilise an approach that incorporates an understanding of both the medical condition and the situational context:

- If cognitive impairment develops in an HIV-infected child who is receiving ART, check for both viral load and adherence to the current medication regime.
- If a child's previously achieved milestones are regressing, or if an older child develops new educational or behaviour problems, and there is no obvious explanation for either, the child should be referred for further evaluation, even if the HIV infection is well managed.
- Possible contributing treatable conditions should be screened through routine history-taking, frequent examination, and ordering relevant diagnostic tests (Table 5.1).
- Exclude indirect complications of HIV infections. These include opportunistic CNS infections (including tuberculous meningitis or cytomegalovirus infection), or intrauterine exposure to teratogens.

Refer for assessment by a specialist paediatrician (or developmental paediatrician) for:

- Neuroimaging.
- A psychologist for cognitive testing and for neuropsychological battery.
- Electroencephalography, if there is a concern for seizures.
- Occupational therapy and audiology, for assessment of hearing and language development as well as potential speech therapy.
- Audiometry, if there is a delay in language development.

Table 5.1	Management of HIV-infected children at primary, secondary, and tertiary care.
Primary	– Document milestones, measure head circumference at birth, enrolment and 6 monthly thereafter.
	– Monitor growth and nutrition.
	– Actively investigate and manage treatable conditions, e.g. chronic middle ear infection, epilepsy, iron deficiency anaemia.
	– Review copies of school reports, refer educational support if possible.
	– Monitor side effects of medication, e.g. sleep disturbances.
	– Refer to secondary level if complicated epilepsy, positive diagnosis of HIVE, or if HIV-associated neurocognitive disorder, attention problems, or behavioural problems are suspected.
Secondary	– Paediatricians, psychiatrists, physiotherapists, occupational therapists, and speech therapists at secondary level *must be made available to all primary healthcare workers for up-referral as necessary.*
	– Strengthen links between educators (teacher or learning support professional at the school) and health professionals in order to provide education goals which are realistic and which will ensure the child achieves their maximum potential.
	– Screening by specialists to decide if tertiary intervention required and to manage some of the more complex general medical problems.
Tertiary	– Assessment by specialist paediatrician (or developmental paediatrician).
	– Refer for neuroimaging.
	– Refer psychologist for cognitive testing and/or neuropsychological battery (if indicated).
	– Refer electroencephalography if indicated.
	– Refer occupational therapy, audiology, assessment, speech therapy.
	– Referral for audiometry when language delay is present.

Source: Reproduced from Nassen et al. (2014) with kind permission of the Southern African HIV Clinicians Society and the publishers.

Neuroimaging remains the most useful diagnostic tool in assessing a child with HIVE. Neuroimaging findings in children with HIVE, from some of the earliest radiological descriptions of this disorder, revealed some key characteristics, which included generalised atrophy, basal ganglia calcification, and ventriculomegaly (Kieck and Andronikou 2004; Tucker et al. 2004). Although these are the most frequently reported neuroimaging findings in HIVE overall, on an individual level they appear to be relatively uncommon amongst children with HIVE, especially in the cART era. Other less specific findings from MRI studies of children meeting the clinical criteria for HIVE diagnosis, included microstructural changes to white matter in some children. These studies suggest that structural and microstructural changes secondary to HIVE are visible on brain imaging, and that the likelihood of identifying these changes is related to the severity of HIVE (Donald et al. 2015; Ackerman et al. 2016). Thus, neuroanatomical changes in HIV-infected children may reveal indicators of disease progression which are visible on neuroimaging (see Chapter 4).

MANAGEMENT AND PROGNOSIS

HIV

Children with HIVE typically have a significantly higher HIV-1 viral load than those not infected with HIV (Chiriboga et al. 2005), and have a higher viral load in the first year of life when compared to

HIV-infected children without HIVE (Cooper et al. 1998). HIV should be clinically controlled by cART, as described by the WHO guidelines (WHO 2010). In addition to decreasing HIVE incidence rates (Patel et al. 2009), cART improves both survival rates (Patel et al. 2009) and childhood development outcomes (Foster et al. 2006; Laughton et al. 2013). Access to cART is thought to reduce a mother's viral load, so that, even if vertical HIV transmission occurs, her child benefits from lower exposure to viral load. Further, early initiation of ART in children can reduce the CNS reservoir of HIV, allowing the child to achieve viral suppression at an earlier age, resulting in improved long-term neurological outcomes (Crowell 2018; Laughton et al. 2019).

In a recently reported clinical cohort, the specific diagnosis of HIVE was seldom recognised in general medical or paediatric services, even in its most severe forms (Donald et al. 2015). Possible explanations for this include environments where heavy service load makes it challenging to perform a full neurological examination due to time constraints. Specialist paediatric services (particularly specialised paediatric neurology services) are particularly under-represented across many LMICs. This is especially true in sub-Saharan Africa, where the major burden of HIV infection in children resides (Donald et al. 2014). Thus, the milder forms of HIVE may be overlooked in these overburdened healthcare systems. Therefore, despite the successful roll-out of ART, HIVE remains an important and frequently undiagnosed clinical problem.

Comorbidities and Secondary Abnormalities

It is imperative that comorbidities of HIVE, such as seizures, attention-deficit/hyperactivity disorder, and cardiovascular problems, are addressed by healthcare professionals. Children with HIVE need to be cared for by both infectious disease and neurodevelopmental specialists. They also require a multidisciplinary team approach including other clinicians, psychologists, social workers, teachers, and allied health professionals (Nassen et al. 2014).

Children with motor deficits like bilateral lower limb spasticity, or other abnormalities, such as joint and bony deformities, need specialised care (Langerak et al. 2014). However, it is still not clear if the aetiology of HIVE-associated bilateral lower limb spasticity is the same as or similar to CP-associated bilateral lower limb spasticity. Bilateral lower limb spasticity in CP is static and these children can be referred to orthopaedics or neurosurgery for interventions to improve function. It is unclear whether HIVE-associated bilateral lower limb spasticity is similarly stable or if it is progressive, with evidence suggesting that it varies per child. Mann et al. (2015) found that children with unresolved tone abnormalities were likely to have presented with more severe disease at an earlier age, and reported resolution of lower limb spasticity in 13 out of 19 children who had previously been diagnosed with HIVE. However, it is as yet unclear why lower limb tone abnormalities resolve in some children and not in others, making decisions regarding which children should receive surgical interventions for their conditions a challenging task.

Identification and Management of Other Indirect Factors

Factors unrelated to HIVE can also influence the well-being of a child diagnosed with HIVE. These include environmental and socioeconomic factors, nutrition, and opportunistic infections (e.g. tuberculous meningitis), as well as exposure to alcohol, or other harmful substances. In Table 5.2, Nassen et al. (2014) set out a range of conditions, their diagnosis, potential effect on cognition, and management. These factors should be considered, recognised, and managed alongside HIVE in the patient.

Table 5.2 Medical conditions that may impact on cognition.

Condition	Diagnosis	Potential effect on cognition	Management
Iron deficiency anaemia	History and full blood count	Attention problems	Iron supplements
Nasal obstruction	History, sleep studies	Learning difficulties and attention problems	Nasal spray Referral to ear, nose, and throat specialist
Chronic middle ear infection	History and examination	Decreased hearing resulting in learning difficulties	Audiology Referral to ear, nose, and throat specialist
Visual impairment	History and examination (e.g. use of Snellens chart for older children and small items such as edible 100's and 1000's for young children)	Visuomotor problems as well as difficulty managing in the classroom	Refer optometrist/ ophthalmologist as appropriate
Malnutrition	Growth charts	Specific learning difficulties and attention problems	Referral to dietician Medical follow-up Refer to nutrition supplementation programme
Efavirenz side effects	Sleep history and co-lateral from teacher. May sleep at school. High EFV level	Decreased concentration and focus. Poor memory	Detailed history Consider lower dose (discuss with specialist)
Emotional problems	History and behaviour check lists	Cognitive problems, attention problems, poor scholastic performance	Refer to psychiatric service

Source: Reproduced from Nassen et al. (2014) with kind permission of the Southern African HIV Clinicians Society and the publishers.

THE IMPACT OF ANTIRETROVIRAL THERAPY ON NEUROLOGICAL OUTCOMES

Poor HIVE Prognosis in the pre-cART Era

In the pre-cART era, a diagnosis of progressive HIVE was considered to be a poor prognostic sign for future health (Epstein et al. 1986), with reports of severe morbidity and high mortality amongst affected children (Belman et al. 1985; Epstein et al. 1986; Lobato et al. 1995). Median survival time in children with HIVE from the point of diagnosis ranged from 8 to 22 months in different cohorts. Children with HIVE were also shown to have a significantly greater risk of dying within the study period when compared to those without a HIVE diagnosis (Epstein et al. 1986; Lobato et al. 1995; Cooper et al. 1998; Tardieu et al. 2000; Patel et al. 2009). For example, the Women and Infants Transmission Study reported a mortality rate of 41% among children with HIVE, compared to 12.5% amongst the total cohort of HIV-infected children (Cooper et al. 1998). This trend was observed even when comparing HIVE to other AIDS-defining conditions. A large, multi-site study in the USA reported a median survival time of 22 months among children with HIVE and 36 months among children with other AIDS-defining conditions when estimated from the point of diagnosis (Lobato et al. 1995). While most of these data are historical in the context of advanced, Western economies, there are areas in the world where reliable access to cART remains limited and hence remains a relevant factor to consider.

cART Has Dramatically Improved the Outlook for Children with HIVE

The advent of cART dramatically altered the outlook for children with a HIVE diagnosis. Access to cART has been reported to halve the risk of death among children with HIVE when compared to non-cART regimens (Patel et al. 2009). There is also preliminary evidence that, in some cases, cART may improve the motor deficits that are part of a HIVE diagnosis. For example, one study reported that only 7 out of 10 children, in whom increased lower limb tone formed part of the initial HIVE diagnosis, continued to present with hypertonia at follow-up assessments (Chiriboga et al. 2005). In a different report, lower limb tone abnormalities appeared to have resolved in 13 out of 19 children with HIVE. These children were recorded as having increased lower limb tone at a previous assessment (Mann et al. 2015). It has been noted that improvements in cognitive function and head size tend to occur before any improvements in motor function (Chiriboga et al. 2005). However, little is known about the progression of motor deficits in children with HIVE, or why these deficits appear to resolve in some cases but not in others. While cART regimens have been shown to arrest the progression of HIV and to improve neurological outcomes for affected children, these children are still likely to experience greater cognitive and functional impairment when compared to HIV-infected children with no previous HIVE diagnosis, and thus often require additional care (Cysique et al. 2009; Cysique, Waters, and Brew 2011). Less is known about the specific pharmacodynamics of cART in the brain and which particular agents are most effective at reducing risk for neurocognitive impairment (Smurzynski et al. 2011; Caniglia et al. 2014; Ellis et al. 2014). Further studies into the long-term prognosis of cART-treated paediatric HIVE is fast becoming a possibility, as effective treatment with cART is allowing these patients to grow into adolescence and adulthood.

Notwithstanding cART, Children with HIVE Have Worse Brain Development Outcomes

Although cART may significantly improve neurological outcomes in children with a history of HIVE, long-term prognosis is less favourable than in HIV-infected children without HIVE. Children with a history of HIVE had a significantly higher rate of residual neurological abnormalities, as well as a higher rate of placement at special needs schools, when compared to HIV-infected children with no previous HIVE diagnosis (Chiriboga et al. 2005). Those with a history of HIVE also experience significant limitations in daily living when compared to typically developing, uninfected children. For example, children with HIVE and bilateral lower limb spasticity showed significantly lower scores for the 'Daily Activities', 'Mobility', and 'Social/Cognitive' domains of the Paediatric Evaluation of Disability Inventory, when compared to a control group of typically developing children (Mann et al. 2016). All children with HIVE were receiving cART, according to the latest National Guidelines of the South African Department of Health, yet some individual participants had scores more than two standard deviations below the instrument norms (Mann et al. 2016).

Looking Forward

Worldwide, more than 25% of children under 5 years of age are physically and/or cognitively stunted, unable to realise their full potential. To what extent is healthy brain and cognitive development influenced by the prevalence of the HIV-1 virus, or by other environmental and economic factors in our vulnerable populations? Research has sought to address some of these fundamental questions by longitudinally mapping brain and cognitive growth across the early years of life in association with infant nutrition, parent–child interaction, substance exposure, prevalent infections, and general environmental stress.

Performed in low-resource settings, where there is a paucity of information and where children are at highest risk of poor developmental and cognitive outcomes, results from this research are aimed at quantifying the relative impact of these modifiable factors on infant brain growth and cognition, clarifying the time-period over which their influence is greatest, and determining their potential impact in ameliorating childhood cognitive stunting. In particular, research on the impact of prevalent risk factors, and on the development of the brain in the very early weeks and months of life, is contributing to our understanding of the effects of adverse exposures at this vulnerable and critical time point. New advances in technology are improving our ability to measure brain structures and to correlate these data with executive function. In particular, the development of low-field MRI allows for the more practical and less invasive imaging work to be conducted in LMIC settings.

Recent work has included looking at overlapping risk factors for children in these contexts. This includes the emerging concern about adolescents and their vulnerability to additional risk factors, such as substance abuse, that may result in poor outcomes. This work has particular significance for developing approaches to support these vulnerable populations in countries where HIV is prevalent. However, it also speaks to the emerging recognition of the importance of taking into account the additive effects of multiple risk factors often found in these populations.

REFERENCES

Abubakar A, Van Baar A, Van de Vijver FJ, Holding P, Newton CR (2008) Paediatric HIV and neurodevelopment in sub-Saharan Africa: A systematic review. *Tropical Medicine & International Health: TM & IH*, 13(7): 880–887.

Ackermann C, Andronikou SF, Laughton BF et al. (2014) White matter signal abnormalities in children with suspected HIV-related neurologic disease on early combination antiretroviral therapy. *Pediatric Infectious Disease Journal*, August; 33(8): e207–212. doi: 10.1097/inf.0000000000000288.

Baillieu N, Potterton J (2008) The extent of delay of language, motor, and cognitive development in HIV-positive infants. *Journal of Neurologic Physical Therapy: JNPT*, 32(3): 118–121. https://doi.org/10.1097/NPT.0b013e3181846232.

Bangirana P, Ruel TD, Boivin MJ et al. (2017) Absence of neurocognitive disadvantage associated with paediatric HIV subtype A infection in children on antiretroviral therapy. *Journal of the International AIDS Society*, 20(2): e25015. https://doi.org/10.1002/jia2.25015.

Banks LM, Zuurmond M, Ferrand R, Kuper H (2015) The relationship between HIV and prevalence of disabilities in sub-Saharan Africa: Systematic review (FA). *Tropical Medicine & International Health: TM & IH*, 20(4): 411–429. https://doi.org/10.1111/tmi.12449.

Bass JK, Opoka R, Familiar I et al. (2017) Randomized controlled trial of caregiver training for HIV-infected child neurodevelopment and caregiver well being. *AIDS (London, England)*, 31(13): 1877–1883. https://doi.org/10.1097/QAD.0000000000001563.

Belman AL, Ultmann MH, Horoupian D et al. (1985) Neurological complications in infants and children with acquired immune deficiency syndrome. *Annals of Neurology*, 18(5): 560–566.

Blanche S, Rouzioux C, Moscato ML et al. (1989) A prospective study of infants born to women seropositive for human immunodeficiency virus type 1. HIV infection in newborns French collaborative study group. *The New England Journal of Medicine*, 320(25): 1643–1648.

Boivin MJ, Ruel TD, Boal HE et al. (2010) HIV-subtype A is associated with poorer neuropsychological performance compared with subtype D in antiretroviral therapy-naive Ugandan children. *AIDS (London, England)*, 24(8): 1163–1170. https://doi.org/10.1097/qad.0b013e3283389dcc.

Boivin MJ, Ruiseñor-Escudero H, Familiar-Lopez I (2016) CNS impact of perinatal HIV infection and early treatment: The need for behavioral rehabilitative interventions along with medical treatment and care. *Current HIV/AIDS Reports*, 13(6): 318–327. https://doi.org/10.1007/s11904-016-0342-8.

Brouwers P, Moss H, Wolters P et al. (1990) Effect of continuous-infusion zidovudine therapy on neuropsychologic functioning in children with symptomatic human immunodeficiency virus infection. *The Journal of Pediatrics*, 117(6): 980–985.

Bruck I, Tahan TT, Cruz CR et al. (2001) Developmental milestones of vertically HIV infected and seroreverters children: Follow up of 83 children. *Arquivos De Neuro-Psiquiatria*, 59(3-B): 691–695.

Caniglia EC, Cain LE, Justice A et al. (2014) Antiretroviral penetration into the CNS and incidence of AIDS-defining neurologic conditions. *Neurology*, 83(2): 134–141.

CDC (1994) CDC: 1994 revised classification system for HIV infection in children less than 13 years of age. *CDC*, 443(RR12): 1–10.

Chase C, Ware J, Hittelman J et al. (2000) Early cognitive and motor development among infants born to women infected with human immunodeficiency virus. Women and Infants Transmission Study Group. *Pediatrics*, 106(2): E25.

Chiriboga CA, Fleishman S, Champion S, Gaye-Robinson L, Abrams EJ (2005) Incidence and prevalence of HIV encephalopathy in children with HIV infection receiving highly active anti-retroviral therapy (HAART). *The Journal of Pediatrics*, 146(3): 402–407.

Cole SR, Hernán MA, Robins JM et al. (2003) Effect of highly active antiretroviral therapy on time to acquired immunodeficiency syndrome or death using marginal structural models. *American Journal of Epidemiology*, 158(7): 687–694. https://doi.org/10.1093/aje/kwg206.

Cooper ER, Hanson C, Diaz C et al. (1998) Encephalopathy and progression of human immunodeficiency virus disease in a cohort of children with perinatally acquired human immunodeficiency virus infection. Women and Infants Transmission Study Group. *The Journal of Pediatrics*, 132(5): 808–812.

Crowell CS, Huo Y, Tassiopoulos K et al. (2015) Early viral suppression improves neurocognitive outcomes in HIV-infected children. *AIDS (London, England)*, 29(3): 295–304.

Cysique LA, Vaida F, Letendre S et al. (2009) Dynamics of cognitive change in impaired HIV-positive patients initiating antiretroviral therapy. *Neurology*, 73(5): 342–348.

Cysique LA, Waters EK, Brew BJ (2011) Central nervous system antiretroviral efficacy in HIV infection: A qualitative and quantitative review and implications for future research. *BMC Neurology*, 11(1): 1.

DeCarli C, Fugate L, Falloon J et al. (1991) Brain growth and cognitive improvement in children with human immunodeficiency virus-induced encephalopathy after 6 months of continuous infusion zidovudine therapy. *Journal of Acquired Immune Deficiency Syndromes*, 4(6): 585–592.

Devendra A, Makawa A, Kazembe PN, Calles NR, Kuper H (2013) HIV and childhood disability: A case-controlled study at a paediatric antiretroviral therapy centre in Lilongwe, Malawi. *PloS One*, 8(12): e84024. https://doi.org/10.1371/journal.pone.0084024.

Donald KA, Samia P, Kakooza A et al. (2014) Cerebral palsy in Africa: Where are we? *Journal of Child Neurology*, 30(8): 963–971. doi: 10.1177/0883073814549245.

Donald KA, Walker KG, Kilborn T et al. (2015) HIV encephalopathy: Pediatric case series description and insights from the clinic coalface. *AIDS Research and Therapy*, 12(1): 2. doi: 10.1186/s12981-014-0042-7.

Egger M, May M, Chêne G et al. (2002) Prognosis of HIV-1-infected patients starting highly active antiretroviral therapy: A collaborative analysis of prospective studies. *Lancet (London, England)*, 360(9327): 119–129. https://doi.org/10.1016/s0140-6736(02)09411-4.

Ellis RJ, Letendre S, Vaida F et al. (2014) Randomized trial of central nervous system-targeted antiretrovirals for HIV-associated neurocognitive disorder. *Clinical Infectious Diseases: An Official Publication of the Infectious Diseases Society of America*, 58(7): 1015–1022.

Englund JA, Baker CJ, Raskino C et al. (1996) Clinical and laboratory characteristics of a large cohort of symptomatic, human immunodeficiency virus-infected infants and children. AIDS clinical trials group protocol 152 study team. *The Pediatric Infectious Disease Journal*, 15(11): 1025–1036.

Epstein LG, Sharer LR, Joshi VV, Fojas MM, Koenigsberger MR, Oleske JM (1985) Progressive encephalopathy in children with acquired immune deficiency syndrome. *Annals of Neurology*, 17(5): 488–496.

Epstein LG, Sharer LR, Oleske JM et al. (1986) Neurologic manifestations of human immunodeficiency virus infection in children. *Pediatrics*, 78(4): 678–687.

Foster CJ, Biggs RL, Melvin D, Walters MD, Tudor-Williams G, Lyall EG (2006) Neurodevelopmental outcomes in children with HIV infection under 3 years of age. *Developmental Medicine and Child Neurology*, 48(8): 677–682.

Gartner MJ, Roche M, Churchill MJ, Gorry PR, Flynn JK (2020) Understanding the mechanisms driving the spread of subtype C HIV-1. *EBioMedicine*, 53: 102682. https://doi.org/10.1016/j.ebiom.2020.102682.

Geretti AM (2006) HIV-1 subtypes: Epidemiology and significance for HIV management. *Current Opinion in Infectious Diseases*, 19(1): 1–7. doi: 10.1097/01.qco.0000200293.45532.68.

Govender R, Eley B, Walker K, Petersen R, Wilmshurst JM (2011) Neurologic and neurobehavioral sequelae in children with human immunodeficiency virus (HIV-1) infection. *Journal of Child Neurology*, 26(11): 1355–1364.

Hamid MZ, Aziz NA, Zulkifli ZS, Norlijah O, Azhar RK (2008) Clinical features and risk factors for HIV encephalopathy in children. *The Southeast Asian Journal of Tropical Medicine and Public Health*, 39(2): 266–272.

Heaton RK, Franklin DR, Ellis RJ et al. (2011) HIV-associated neurocognitive disorders before and during the era of combination antiretroviral therapy: Differences in rates, nature, and predictors. *Journal of Neurovirology*, 17(1): 3–16.

Hemelaar J (2012) The origin and diversity of the HIV-1 pandemic. *Trends in Molecular Medicine*, 18(3): 182–192. https://doi.org/10.1016/j.molmed.2011.12.001.

Hilburn N, Potterton J, Stewart A (2010) Paediatric HIV encephalopathy in sub-Saharan Africa. *Physical Therapy Reviews*, 15(5): 410–417.

Kieck JR, Andronikou S (2004) Usefulness of neuro-imaging for the diagnosis of HIV encephalopathy in children. *South African Medical Journal = Suid-Afrikaanse Tydskrif Vir Geneeskunde*, 94(8): 628–630.

Koekkoek S, de Sonneville L, Wolfs TF, Licht R, Geelen S (2008) Neurocognitive function profile in HIV-infected school-age children. *European Journal of Paediatric Neurology: EJPN: Official Journal of the European Paediatric Neurology Society*, 12(4): 290–297. doi: 10.1016/j.ejpn.2007.09.002.

Langerak NG, du Toit J, Burger M, Cotton MF, Springer PE, Laughton B (2014) Spastic diplegia in children with HIV encephalopathy: First description of gait and physical status. *Developmental Medicine & Child Neurology*, 56(7): 686–694.

Laughton B, Cornell M, Grove D et al. (2012) Early antiretroviral therapy improves neurodevelopmental outcomes in infants. *AIDS (London, England)*, 26(13): 1685–1690. https://doi.org/10.1097/QAD.0b013e328355d0ce.

Laughton B, Cornell M, Boivin M, Van Rie A (2013) Neurodevelopment in perinatally HIV-infected children: A concern for adolescence. *Journal of the International AIDS Society*, 16(1): 18603. https://doi.org/10.7448/IAS.16.1.18603.

Laughton B, Naidoo S, Dobbels E et al. (2019) Neurodevelopment at 11 months after starting antiretroviral therapy within 3 weeks of life. *Southern African Journal of HIV Medicine*, 20(1): 1008. https://doi.org/10.4102/sajhivmed.v20i1.1008.

Le Doaré K, Bland R, Newell M (2012) Neurodevelopment in children born to HIV-infected mothers by infection and treatment status. *Pediatrics*, 130(5): e1326–e1344.

Lobato MN, Caldwell MB, Ng P, Oxtoby MJ (1995) Encephalopathy in children with perinatally acquired human immunodeficiency virus infection. Pediatric spectrum of disease clinical consortium. *The Journal of Pediatrics*, 126(5 Pt 1): 710–715.

Mann TN, Donald KA, Walker KG, Langerak NG (2015) Resolved lower limb muscle tone abnormalities in children with HIV encephalopathy receiving standard antiretroviral therapy. *AIDS Research and Therapy*, 12(1): 1.

Mann TN, Donald KA, Laughton B, Lamberts RP, Langerak NG (2016) HIV encephalopathy with bilateral lower limb spasticity: Upper limb motor function and level of activity and participation. *Developmental Medicine & Child Neurology*, 59(4): 412–419. doi: 10.1111/dmcn.13236.

Mbaye AD, Sy HS, Gueye ND et al. (2005) Aspects épidémiologiques et cliniques de l'infection à VIH de l'enfant au centre hospitalier national d'enfants Albert-Royer à dakar. *Archives De Pédiatrie*, 12(4): 404–409.

McCoig C, Castrejon MM, Castano E et al. (2002) Effect of combination antiretroviral therapy on cerebrospinal fluid HIV RNA, HIV resistance, and clinical manifestations of encephalopathy. *The Journal of Pediatrics*, 141(1): 36–44.

Msellati P, Lepage P, Hitimana D-G, Goethem C, Van de Perre P, Dabis F (1993) Neurodevelopmental testing of children born to human immunodeficiency virus type 1 seropositive and seronegative mothers: A prospective cohort study in Kigali, Rwanda. *Pediatrics*, 92(6): 843–848. doi.org/10.1542/peds.92.6.843.

Nassen R, Donald K, Walker K et al. (2014) Management of mental health disorders and central nervous system sequelae in HIV-positive children and adolescents. *Southern African Journal of HIV Medicine*, 15(3): 81–96.

Pant Pai N, Shivkumar S, Cajas JM (2012) Does genetic diversity of HIV-1 non-B subtypes differentially impact disease progression in treatment-naive HIV-1-infected individuals? A systematic review of evidence: 1996–2010. *Journal of Acquired Immune Deficiency Syndromes (1999)*, 59(4): 382–388. https://doi.org/10.1097/QAI.0b013e31824a0628.

Patel K, Ming X, Williams PL et al (2009) Impact of HAART and CNS-penetrating antiretroviral regimens on HIV encephalopathy among perinatally infected children and adolescents. *AIDS*, 23(14): 1893–1901.

Pizzo PA, Eddy J, Falloon J et al. (1988) Effect of continuous intravenous infusion of zidovudine (AZT) in children with symptomatic HIV infection. *The New England Journal of Medicine*, 319(14): 889–896.

Rice ML, Buchanan AL, Siberry GK et al. (2012) Language impairment in children perinatally infected with HIV compared to children who were HIV-exposed and uninfected. *Journal of Developmental and Behavioral Pediatrics: JDBP*, 33(2): 112–123. https://doi.org/10.1097/DBP.0b013e318241ed23.

Rodda JM, Graham HK, Carson L, Galea MP, Wolfe R (2004) Sagittal gait patterns in spastic diplegia. *The Journal of Bone and Joint Surgery. British Volume*, 86(2): 251–258.

Ruiseñor-Escudero H, Sikorskii A, Familiar-Lopez I et al. (2018) Neurodevelopmental outcomes in preschool children living with HIV-1 subtypes A and D in Uganda. *The Pediatric Infectious Disease Journal*, 37(12): e298–e303. https://doi.org/10.1097/INF.0000000000002097.

Shanbhag MC, Rutstein RM, Zaoutis T, Zhao H, Chao D, Radcliffe J (2005) Neurocognitive functioning in pediatric human immunodeficiency virus infection: Effects of combined therapy. *Archives of Pediatrics & Adolescent Medicine*, 159(7): 651–656.

Smurzynski M, Wu K, Letendre S et al. (2011) Effects of central nervous system antiretroviral penetration on cognitive functioning in the ALLRT cohort. *AIDS (London, England)*, 25(3): 357–365.

Sturdevant CB, Dow A, Jabara CB et al. (2012) Central nervous system compartmentalization of HIV-1 subtype C variants early and late in infection in young children. *PLoS Pathogens*, 8(12): e1003094. https://doi.org/10.1371/journal.ppat.1003094.

Tahan TT, Bruck I, Burger M, Cruz CR (2006) Neurological profile and neurodevelopment of 88 children infected with HIV and 84 seroreverter children followed from 1995 to 2002. *The Brazilian Journal of Infectious Diseases: An Official Publication of the Brazilian Society of Infectious Diseases*, 10(5): 322–326.

Tardieu M, Le Chenadec J, Persoz A, Meyer L, Blanche S, Mayaux MJ (2000) HIV-1-related encephalopathy in infants compared with children and adults. French pediatric HIV infection study and the SEROCO group. *Neurology*, 54(5): 1089–1095.

Tucker KA, Robertson KR, Lin W et al. (2004) Neuroimaging in human immunodeficiency virus infection. *Journal of Neuroimmunology*, 157(1–2): 153–162.

Van Rie A, Harrington PR, Dow A, Robertson K (2007) Neurologic and neurodevelopmental manifestations of pediatric HIV/AIDS: A global perspective. *European Journal of Paediatric Neurology: EJPN: Official Journal of the European Paediatric Neurology Society*, 11(1): 1–9.

van Wyhe KS, Laughton B, Cotton MF et al. (2021) Cognitive outcomes at ages seven and nine years in South African children from the children with HIV early antiretroviral (CHER) trial: A longitudinal investigation. *Journal of the International AIDS Society*, 24(7): e25734. https://doi.org/10.1002/jia2.25734.

Whitehead N, Potterton J, Coovadia A (2014) The neurodevelopment of HIV-infected infants on HAART compared to HIV-exposed but uninfected infants. *AIDS Care*, 26(4): 497–504. https://doi.org/10.1080/09540121.2013.841828.

WHO (2010) *Antiretroviral therapy of HIV infection in infants and children: Towards universal access: Recommendations for a Public Health Approach – 2010 revision*. World Health Organization. Available at https://apps.who.int/iris/handle/10665/164255.

WHO (2016) Child Growth Standards. Head circumference-for-age: Birth to 5 years. World Health Organization. Retrieved November 2016, from http://www.who.int/childgrowth/standards/hc_for_age/en/.

Willen EJ (2006) Neurocognitive outcomes in pediatric HIV. *Ment Retard Dev Disabil Res Rev*, 12(3): 223–228. doi: 10.1002/mrdd.20112.

Wren TA, Rethlefsen S, Kay RM (2005) Prevalence of specific gait abnormalities in children with cerebral palsy: Influence of cerebral palsy subtype, age, and previous surgery. *Journal of Pediatric Orthopaedics*, 25(1): 79–83.

Zink WE, Zheng J, Persidsky Y, Poluektova L, Gendelman HE (1999) The neuropathogenesis of HIV-1 infection. *FEMS Immunology and Medical Microbiology*, 26(3–4): 233–241.

Seizures and Epilepsy in Children Living with HIV

Pauline Samia, Subira Anzaya, and Jo M Wilmshurst

INTRODUCTION

People with epilepsy have recurring, unprovoked seizures caused by abnormalities in neuronal structure and function. Human immunodeficiency virus (HIV) infection and commonly associated infectious, vascular, or other disease processes, cause changes to brain structure and function which predispose HIV-infected individuals to epilepsy. HIV is an emerging cause of epilepsy worldwide and especially in sub-Saharan Africa. This chapter discusses common causes of epilepsy in paediatric patients infected with HIV, including HIV encephalopathy (HIVE), progressive multifocal leukoencephalopathy opportunistic infections, and vasculopathy. This chapter outlines the pathogenesis, clinical features, and management of these conditions and discusses the acute and long-term management of seizures in these patients.

CAUSES OF SEIZURES AND EPILEPSY IN PAEDIATRIC PATIENTS WITH HIV

Epilepsy is a brain disorder characterised by 'recurrent' and 'unpredictable' seizures (Fisher et al. 2005, 2014). A seizure is an electrical event occurring in the brain during which there is synchronous or excessive discharging of many neurons (D'Cruz 2015). This excessive electrical activity is caused by a disturbance in the normal excitatory and inhibitory control of neuronal activity (Rho and Stafstrom 2006). In epilepsy, there are numerous causes of an imbalance in the excitatory-inhibitory control of neurons (Rho and Stafstrom 2006). In general, this imbalance is a result of abnormalities in the structure and function of neurons, which can arise during the development of the nervous system, following brain injury in postnatal life, or as the result of abnormal metabolism (Rho and Stafstrom 2006).

The definition of epilepsy is not restricted to an enduring predisposition to generate epileptic seizures, but extends to include the neurobiological, cognitive, psychological, and social consequences of the disease (Fisher et al. 2005, 2014). This is because epilepsy is a disease that has a marked impact not just on the physical, but also on the cognitive, social, and psychological domains of an individual's life (D'Cruz 2015).

Approximately 50% to 90% of untreated children infected with HIV will develop neurological complications of the disease, which include seizures and epilepsy. Seizures are the presenting clinical symptoms in 3% to 17% of cases of HIV infection (Pascual-Sedano et al. 1999). Treatment with antiretroviral therapy (ART) either prevents or delays the onset of neurological disease, especially epilepsy (Bale 2006; Bearden et al. 2015). Unfortunately, in sub-Saharan Africa, many children infected with HIV are not being treated with ART and between 6% and 14% of HIV-infected children have epilepsy, with late diagnosis of HIV being positively linked to higher rates of epilepsy in children (Govender et al. 2011; Samia et al. 2013; Donald et al. 2014; Michaelis et al. 2020).

There are various causes of epilepsy and new-onset seizures in HIV-infected children, including direct HIV toxicity, opportunistic infections, stroke due to HIV-associated vasculopathy, HIV-associated malignancy, metabolic abnormalities related to multi-organ dysfunction, as well as the side effects of multiple medications (Visudtibhan, Visudhiphan, and Chiemchanya 1999; Narayan, Samuels, and Barrow 2002; Benjamin et al. 2012; Bearden et al. 2015; Moog, Kakooza-Mwesige, and Tan 2017). All these conditions produce neuronal damage and dysfunction which predisposes these patients to recurrent seizures (Mintz 1996; Donald et al. 2014). The pathogenesis of neuronal injury and death, as well as the clinical features and management of some of these conditions, is described in this chapter.

There is a paucity of existing information on the subject of epilepsy in paediatric patients with HIV. As such, the three most commonly reported causes of epilepsy in paediatric HIV patients in Africa are reviewed in this chapter.

HIV ENCEPHALOPATHY

Pathogenesis

According to a study by Bearden et al. (2015), direct HIV toxicity may be the most common cause of epilepsy in an African context. Damage to and subsequent dysfunction of neurons and oligodendrocytes potentially occurs following exposure to the neurotoxic cytokines produced by HIV-infected glial and immune cells (Atwood et al. 1993; Mintz 1996; Bale 2006). These toxins lead to overstimulation of the neurons resulting in the production of free radicals, which contributes to hypersynchronisation and seizure generation. In one study, in approximately one-fifth of patients there was no other identified cause for new-onset seizures apart from HIV infection (Holtzman, Kaku, and So 1989).

ART has been found to be effective in reducing viral load and improving the neurological and cognitive function of children with HIVE (Mintz 1996; Bale 2006). Seizures can develop in children following the initiation of ART in children as part of an immune reconstitution inflammatory syndrome. In these situations, the antiretroviral agent in question should be discontinued temporarily and the inflammatory condition managed appropriately (e.g. with corticosteroids) (Orikiiriza et al. 2010; Link-Gelles et al. 2014).

OPPORTUNISTIC INFECTIONS

In the African context, infections of the central nervous system (CNS) may account for one-third of all the cases of epilepsy in children with HIV (Bearden et al. 2015). These can be viral, bacterial, or parasitic in nature.

Viral Infections

PATHOGENESIS

Viral infections produce neurological disease by directly infecting neurones or neuroglia; or by generating an immune response that impairs normal neuronal function, thereby predisposing the child to new-onset seizures (Bale 2006). Cytomegalovirus (CMV) infections are considered the most common viral infections involving the CNS in paediatric patients with HIV in resource-poor settings (Donald et al. 2014). Like CMV, herpes simplex virus (HSV) is another member of the herpes virus family that has been identified in HIV-infected paediatric patients with seizures in the context of encephalitis (Mintz 1996; Misra and Kalita 1998). HSV lyses neuronal cells, destroying them, and it can also cause intracerebral haemorrhage (Bale 2006). Other viruses that are also associated with seizures in children with HIV are the John Cunningham virus and the measles virus. The John Cunningham virus infects and destroys myelin-forming oligodendrocytes, resulting in demyelination and neurological dysfunction that is characteristic of progressive multifocal leukoencephalopathy (Bale 2006). The measles virus directly invades the neurons, causing neuronal degeneration which can produce seizures in HIV-infected children in the context of encephalitis (Koppel et al. 1996; Poon, Tchertkoff, and Win 1998; Bale 2006). Severely immunocompromised children can develop a form of measles encephalitis known as measles body inclusion encephalitis (MIBE), also known as subacute measles encephalitis (SME), which usually occurs 9 months following exposure to the measles virus (Hardie et al. 2013). Infection with a mutant measles virus in the context of defective cell-medicated immunity due to HIV results in an early-onset, 'fulminant' form of subacute sclerosing panencephalitis (SSPE), which is a disorder that ordinarily occurs in immunocompetent hosts several years after infection with the measles virus (Dasopoulou and Covanis 2004; Muthusamy et al. 2015; Maurya et al. 2016).

Clinical Features

Viral encephalitis tends to present with non-specific features such as headache and vomiting, as well as other more systemic features including skin rash, enlargement of the parotid gland, lymphadenopathy, and hepatosplenomegaly (Bale 2006). Seizures are a common presentation in paediatric patients with encephalitis, affecting 15% to 60% of these children (Bale 2006). Seizures may be focal or generalised; however, focal seizures should raise concern of herpes simplex encephalitis (Bale 2006). In immuno-compromised children, SME occurs 1 to 7 months after measles infection and is associated with altered mental status and seizures, which may be either focal or generalised. Epilepsia partialis continua is a typical presentation of SME (Bale 2006). SSPE presents with progressive cognitive and behavioural impairment, as well as atonic seizures and myoclonic jerks in the trunk, limbs, and face (Kija et al. 2015; Muthusamy et al. 2015; Maurya et al. 2016).

Treatment and Management

Seizures commonly occur in paediatric patients with viral encephalitis and, in the acute phase, lorazepam can be used to provide seizure control (Bale 2006). Following acute management, patients should be maintained on suitable antiseizure medications (ASMs) (Samia et al. 2013; Donald 2014). For seizures in patients who have SSPE without HIV, carbamazepine is the preferred therapy (Kija et al. 2015). In this setting this agent does not exacerbate the myoclonus but is instead the optimal agent to control the movements. Despite the cross reactivity with ARTs and carbamazepine, the benefits of seizure control on the quality of life for the child support carbamazepine use as long as there are careful adjustments and monitoring of ART dosages. Without careful monitoring there is risk of carbamazepine toxicity and ART failure.

HSV and varicella-zoster virus (VZV) encephalitis should be treated with acyclovir, which should be started as soon as HSV infection is suspected (Bale 2006). Even when treatment with acyclovir is initiated early, 40% of neonates or children will develop long-term neurological sequelae, including epilepsy (which may be partial or generalised), intellectual disability, and language and motor limitations (Bale 2006). CMV infections are effectively treated with ganciclovir or foscarnet (Bale 2006). Ribavirin can be used to treat patients with SME but the outcome of this condition is often poor. Coinfection with HIV, HSV, Epstein–Barr virus, and CMV has been reported in the oral cavities of children with HIV, particularly those with high viral loads (Grando et al. 2005). Where epilepsy is part of the sequelae of HSV infection, adequate seizure control with broad spectrum ASMs such as valproic acid and levetirac-etam would be recommended.

Bacterial Infections

PATHOGENESIS

Bacteria-driven inflammation in the blood vessels results in the development of occlusive thrombi and, subsequently, neuronal damage (Taüber and Schaad 2006). The sequelae of toxic bacterial products stim-ulate an immune response and the subsequent production of cytokines, which can also be neurotoxic (Misra and Kalita 1998; Taüber and Schaad 2006). Common causes of bacterial meningitis in this pop-ulation include: *streptococcus pneumoniae, haemophilus influenzae,* and *mycobacterium tuberculosis* (Madhi et al. 2001; Donald et al. 2015).

HIV predisposes patients to the development of tuberculosis (TB) and, whilst both HIV and TB are major global health concerns, the burden of HIV-TB coinfection is highest in sub-Saharan Africa (Tarekegne et al. 2016).

Clinical Features

Bacterial meningitis is a common cause of neurological disability in paediatric patients with HIV and can manifest with acute convulsive seizures, which can be focal or generalised (van Toorn et al. 2012; Donald et al. 2014). Focal seizures are an indication of permanent brain damage and hence of future neurological deficits (Taüber and Schaad 2006). Epilepsy is more than three times more common in children following bacterial meningitis in comparison to a population similar in age without this history (Taüber and Schaad 2006).

Treatment and Management

In the acute phase, patients with seizures should be provided with adequate airway, ventilation, and car-diovascular support; as well as ASM therapy (Taüber and Schaad 2006). There is no antiepileptic therapy that is 'specific' to the management of seizures in bacterial meningitis. Phenobarbital, fosphenytoin, diazepam, and lorazepam, individually or in combination, have been used to provide seizure control in the acute phase (Taüber and Schaad 2006). Epilepsy is a common consequence of TB meningitis, as with other forms of bacterial meningitis. In HIV-positive children with epilepsy, ASM-use combined with ongoing anti-TB therapy requires close monitoring and judicious use of requisite agents due to the possibility of drug–drug interactions (Taüber and Schaad 2006; Samia et al. 2013).

Fungal Infections

PATHOGENESIS

Cryptococcus neoformans is a ubiquitous fungus that most commonly infects immunocompromised hosts (Glaser, Lewis, and Schuster 2006; Kellinghaus et al. 2008). It invades and replicates in brain tissue causing necrosis (Lee, Dickson, and Casadevall 1996; Klock, Cerski, and Goldani 2009).

Clinical Features

Cryptococcal central nervous system (CNS) infections in children with HIV can present with seizures (Gumbo et al. 2002; Glaser, Lewis, and Schuster 2006). Cryptococcal meningoencephalitis in HIV-infected patients also commonly presents with fever, headache, photophobia, meningitis, and altered mental status (Gumbo et al. 2002; Glaser, Lewis, and Schuster 2006). Focal deficits may also occur, although this is less common (Glaser, Lewis, and Schuster 2006).

In addition to meningoencephalitis, cryptococcal infection can result in the formation of granulomas and brain abscesses. This may lead to increased intracranial pressure as well as focal neurological deficits (e.g. hemiparesis) and seizures (Glaser, Lewis, and Schuster 2006).

Treatment and Management

Cryptococcal meningitis in patients with HIV should initially be treated with amphotericin B and flucy-tosine, with oral fluconazole being an alternative for amphotericin B (Glaser, Lewis, and Schuster 2006).

Parasitic Infections

TOXOPLASMOSIS

Pathogenesis

Toxoplasma gondii has been associated with causing epilepsy in children with HIV (Bearden et al. 2015). Necrosis and formation of cysts are some of the ways in which a toxoplasma gondii infection destroys the nervous system (Glaser, Lewis, and Schuster 2006).

Clinical Features

Infants with HIV will often present with toxoplasmosis between 3 and 4 months of age, with signs and symptoms similar to those of HIV-negative paediatric patients with congenital toxoplasmosis (Glaser, Lewis, and Schuster 2006). These include vomiting, hydrocephalus (as indicated by a tense and bulging fontanelle), a high-pitched cry, and opisthotonos (Glaser, Lewis, and Schuster 2006). Epilepsy is one of the long-term consequences of toxoplasma infection of the CNS (Glaser, Lewis, and Schuster 2006).

MALARIA

In children age 6 months or older, malaria is associated with acute seizures and is also a significant cause of status epilepticus (Idro et al. 2008).

Plasmodium vivax occurs more commonly in Asia while *Plasmodium falciparum* is more prevalent in Africa. Both *P. vivax* and *P. falciparum* can cause seizures (Singhi 2011; Ssenkusu et al. 2016).

Clinical Features

Children hospitalised with *P. falciparum* malaria may present with seizures (Singhi 2011). Seizures can occur in patients with uncomplicated malaria as well as in those with the most severe form of malaria – cerebral malaria, a comatose state due to *P. falciparum* malaria infection (Singhi 2011). Seizures may occur in the acute febrile phase; however, in up to 50% of cases, seizures occur in the afebrile phase of the illness (Singhi 2011). Seizures are focal in nature and may or may not become generalised. Some patients may have subtle or even purely electrographic seizures (Singhi 2011). Status epilepticus can occur in one-third of paediatric patients with malaria (Singhi 2011). Following malaria infection, 10% of children will subsequently develop epilepsy (Singhi 2011).

Treatment and Management

Seizures occurring in the context of *P. falciparum* malaria infections may be refractory to readily available antiseizure medications such as diazepam and midazolam (Mpimbaza et al. 2009). Hypoglycaemia and cerebral malaria may be independent predictors of persistent and recurrent seizures in spite of these medications (Mpimbaza et al. 2009).

VASCULOPATHY AND STROKE

Vasculopathy and subsequent stroke are uncommon occurrences in HIV-infected children such that between 1.2% and 2.6% of HIV-infected children develop stroke. Stroke may present with seizures with eventual development of epilepsy resulting from associated gliosis. (Philippet et al. 1994). Prevalence of cerebrovascular disease in HIV-infected children is underestimated because of limited neuroimaging in low- and middle-income countries, unidentified cerebrovascular events without overt motor manifestations, and mislabelling as HIVE for non-motor manifestations such as behavioural and cognitive difficulties (Hammond et al. 2016).

Clinical Features

Stroke, often presents overtly with hemiparesis, focal seizures, aphasia, and reduced responsiveness and this may be the first presentation for a child with HIV infection (Philippet et al. 1994).

Treatment and Management

Basic management would involve normalising body temperature, blood glucose, and oxygen levels; controlling blood pressure; correcting dehydration, coagulopathies, and anaemia; and avoidance of micro- and macronutrient deficiencies (Philippet et al. 1994). Inclusion of prophylactic ASM at commencement of acute care for stroke in children helps reduce the risk of new-onset seizures with accompanying increased metabolic demands on a brain already compromised by inadequate vascular function. In the setting of cerebrovascular disease, occurrence of seizures can be extremely detrimental to the clinical course of the child, which makes the neurological damage from the stroke more severe.

Following the treatment of coexisting opportunistic infections, initiation of ART may improve outcomes of vascular disease.

LONG-TERM ANTISEIZURE MEDICATION

Evidence to support the optimal ASM interventions in paediatric patients with HIV is scarce, with most studies focusing on the management of epilepsy in HIV-infected adults.

Paediatric patients with HIV are at higher risk of developing epilepsy than the uninfected paediatric population (Mintz 1996). Between 7.6% and 14% of HIV-infected children will develop epilepsy, which requires the initiation of long-term ASM (Mintz 1996; Wilmshurst et al. 2006; Samia et al. 2013; Donald et al. 2014).

In addition to seizure control, ASMs are useful for treating other neurological and psychiatric comorbidities in patients with HIV, such as neuropathic pain and anxiety (Kellinghaus et al. 2008; Birbeck et al. 2012).

More patients with HIV will be on long-term ART, as the intervention is becoming more available even in poorer regions of the world such as sub-Saharan Africa (Birbeck et al. 2012). Furthermore, the World Health Organization (WHO) recommends that all HIV-infected children who are younger than 10 years of age and all adolescents (defined as 10–19 years) with HIV be commenced on ART regardless of WHO clinical stage or the CD4 cell count (WHO 2016).

There are no reviews describing the interactions between ASMs and antiretroviral medications in children (WHO 2015). However, according to studies in adults, there is great potential for 'complex' and 'extensive' interactions between ASMs and ARTs (Birbeck et al. 2012). Some of these relate to the cytochrome P450 system, whereby the older generation ASMs (i.e. phenytoin, phenobarbital, and carbamazepine), which tend to be more readily available in low- and low-middle-income countries, induce the P450 enzymes (Birbeck et al. 2012; Samia et al. 2013). This results in increased metabolism and in decreased serum levels of several antiretroviral drugs, including non-nucleoside reverse transcriptase inhibitors and protease inhibitors (Birbeck et al. 2012). Lowered ART levels favour HIV replication and the development of resistance and, hence, more rapid progression of the disease (Garg 1999; Kellinghaus et al. 2008; Satishchandra and Sinha 2008; Yacoob et al. 2011).

Gastrointestinal malabsorption (which occurs in patients with HIV) and certain ARTs can also lower the levels of ASMs, resulting in poor seizure control (Satishchandra and Sinha 2008; Birbeck et al. 2012).

ASMs that are more protein-bound may cause toxicity in HIV-infected patients since patients with HIV tend to have lower levels of serum albumin (Satishchandra and Sinha 2008). In addition, patients with HIV can have elevated gammaglobulin levels, which may predispose them to hypersensitivity reactions following the initiation of ASM (Satishchandra and Sinha 2008). For example, the use of lamotrigine in patients may result in greater risk of a skin rash, which can range in severity from milder to life-threatening forms (Messenheimer 1998).

According to studies in adults, newer drugs such as levetiracetam, topiramate, and pregabalin, which do not induce cytochrome P450 enzymes, should be used in HIV patients with seizures (Satishchandra and Sinha 2008; Ruiz-Giménez et al. 2010). Levetiracetam does not have any of the documented interactions with ARV medications as can occur with carbamazepine and, overall, has a better side-effect profile than phenobarbital. Levetiracetam would be more effective than phenytoin, especially for long-term use for children with HIV. Unlike other more recently developed ASMs gaining popularity in high-income countries (HICs), levetiracetam has undergone clinical trials in the paediatric African context and has been deemed safe and effective (Birbeck et al. 2019).

A South African paediatric study described viral suppression in children on ASMs and ART; although patient numbers were small, viral suppression was maintained in patients taking sodium valproate or lamotrigine or a combination of sodium valproate and topiramate (Samia et al. 2013).

Carbamazepine is highly effective in controlling seizures in children with SSPE. The occurrence of SSPE in the context of HIV is rare, and, although carbamazepine is not usually recommended for patients on ART, children with SSPE and HIV may still experience good seizure control on carbamazepine use. However, careful monitoring of viral titres and carbamazepine drug levels may be indicated (Kija et al. 2015; Maurya et al. 2016).

According to adult-based studies and evidence-based guidelines from the American Academy of Neurology (AAN) and the International League Against Epilepsy, phenytoin may decrease the drug levels of protease inhibitors lopinavir and ritonavir, and about a '30%' increase in the dose of these ARVs may be required to counteract the effects of phenytoin. The levels of zidovudine, an NRTI, may be increased in the presence of valproic acid and, hence, the dose of zidovudine may need to be decreased when taken in the context of valproic acid. On the other hand, when administered with valproic acid, the dose of efavirenz, a nucleoside reverse transcriptase inhibitor, may not need to be changed. Protease inhibitors ritonavir and atazanavir may decrease the levels of lamotrigine and, hence, a '50%' increase in the dosage of this ASM is recommended (Birbeck et al. 2012). Fewer interactions have been reported with the use of newer antiretroviral medications when used with ASMs. With ART being commenced in young children at HIV diagnosis, this observation provides the possibility to achieve better outcomes for children with the dual diagnosis of HIV and epilepsy (Zaporojan et al. 2018).

CONCLUSION

Epilepsy is the tendency to have recurrent seizures due to abnormalities in neuronal structure or function (Fisher et al. 2005; Rho and Stafstrom 2006; David 2016). HIV infection is highly prevalent in sub-Saharan Africa and HIV infection itself, as well as HIV-associated infections or disorders, can result in the subsequent development of epilepsy, brain injury, and death (Mintz 1996; Taüber and Schaad 2006; Donald et al. 2014; Bearden et al. 2015).

A significant proportion of children with HIV – between 7.6% and 14% – will develop epilepsy. HIV encephalopathy, opportunistic infections, and stroke are common neurological conditions associated with epilepsy in these children (Visudtibhan, Visudhiphan, and Chiemchanya 1999; deVeber 2006; Govender et al. 2011; Donald et al. 2014). ART should be initiated as early as possible to improve immune, neurological, and cognitive function; additionally, any associated infections should be treated appropriately (Bale 2006). Long-term management of seizures using ASMs is also necessary (Garg 1999; Kellinghaus et al. 2008; Satishchandra and Sinha 2008; Birbeck et al. 2012).

However, there are several complex and unwanted interactions between antiretroviral medications and ASMs, particularly with respect to the older generation of ASMs (i.e. phenytoin, phenobarbital, and carbamazepine) (Birbeck et al. 2012). Additionally, patients with HIV have other systemic problems – such as hypoalbuminemia or gastrointestinal dysfunction – that may result in toxic levels or, in contrast, decreased absorption of ASMs (Satishchandra and Sinha 2008; Birbeck et al. 2012).

Newer ASMs with fewer such interactions, such as levetiracetam, topiramate, and pregabalin should be utilised where possible (Satishchandra and Sinha 2008; Wilmshurst et al. 2015). Where older-generation ASMs are in use, the dose of particular ART should be appropriately adjusted to maintain adequate serum levels and viral suppression (Satishchandra and Sinha 2008). On the other hand, particular ART may alter the serum concentration of certain ASMs leading to poor seizure control, or certain ASMs may result in altered ART levels. In these cases, the dosages of either the ART or ASM would need to be adjusted accordingly (Satishchandra and Sinha 2008).

In conclusion, accurate diagnosis of seizure-associated neurological conditions, as well as appropriate general and seizure-specific management of these conditions, is vital to the effective therapeutic management of seizures and epilepsy in HIV-infected children.

REFERENCES

Atwood WJ, Berger JR, Kaderman R, Tornatore CS, Major EO (1993) Human immunodeficiency virus type 1 infection of the brain. *Clin Microbiol Rev*, 6: 339–366.

Bale JF (2006) Viral infections of the nervous system. In: Swaiman K, Ashwal S, and Ferriero D, editors, *Pediatric Neurology: Principles and Practice*. Philadelphia: Mosby Elsevier, pp. 1595–1630.

Bearden D, Steenhoff AP, Dlugos DJ et al. (2015) Early antiretroviral therapy is protective against epilepsy in children with human immunodeficiency virus infection in Botswana. *J Acquir Immune Defic Syndr*, 69: 193–199. doi: 10.1097/QAI.0000000000000563.

Benjamin LA, Bryer A, Emsley HC, Khoo S, Solomon T, Connor MD (2012) HIV infection and stroke: Current perspectives and future directions. *Lancet Neurol*, 11: 878–890. doi: 10.1016/S1474-4422(12)70205-3.

Birbeck GL, French JA, Perucca E et al. (2012) Antiepileptic drug selection for people with HIV/AIDS: Evidence-based guidelines from the ILAE and AAN. *Epilepsia*, 53: 207–214. doi: 10.1111/j.1528-1167.2011.03335.x.

Birbeck GL, Herman ST, Capparelli EV et al. (2019) A clinical trial of enteral Levetiracetam for acute seizures in pediatric cerebral malaria. *BMC Pediatrics*, 19 (1): 399. doi: 10.1186/s12887-019-1766-2.

Dasopoulou M, Covanis A (2004) Subacute sclerosing panencephalitis after intrauterine infection. *Acta Paediatr*, 93: 1251–1253.

David K (2016) Epilepsy and seizures [Online]. Available at: http://emedicine.medscape.com/article/1184846-overview [accessed 28 December 2016].

D'Cruz O (2015) Outcome-centered antiepileptic therapy: Rate, rhythm and relief: Implementing AAN epilepsy quality measures in clinical practice. *Epilepsy Behav*, 53: 108–111. doi: 10.1016/j.yebeh.2015.09.021.

deVeber GA (2006) Cerebrovascular disease. In: Swaiman K, Ashwal S, and Ferriero D, editors, *Pediatric Neurology: Principles and Practice*. Philadelphia: Mosby Elsevier, 1759–1802.

Donald KA, Hoare J, Eley B, Wilmshurst JM (2014) Neurologic complications of pediatric human immunodeficiency virus: Implications for clinical practice and management challenges in the African setting. *Semin Pediatr Neurol*, 21: 3–11. doi: 10.1016/j.spen.2014.01.004.

Donald KA, Walker KG, Kilborn T et al. (2015) HIV encephalopathy: Pediatric case series description and insights from the clinic coalface. *AIDS Res Ther*, 12: 2. doi: 10.1186/s12981-014-0042-7.

Fisher RS, van Emde Boas W, Blume W et al. (2005) Epileptic seizures and epilepsy: Definitions proposed by the international league against epilepsy (ILAE) and the international bureau for epilepsy (IBE). *Epilepsia*, 46: 470–472.

Fisher RS, Acevedo C, Arzimanoglou A et al. (2014) ILAE official report: A practical clinical definition of epilepsy. *Epilepsia*, 55: 475–482. doi: 10.1111/epi.12550.

Garg RK (1999) HIV infection and seizures. *Postgrad Med J*, 75: 387–390.

Glaser CA, Lewis PF, Schuster FL (2006) Fungal, rickettsial and parasitic diseases of the nervous system. In: Swaiman K, Ashwal S, and Ferriero D, editors, *Pediatric Neurology: Principles and Practice*. Philadelphia: Mosby Elsevier, pp. 1631–1683.

Govender R, Eley B, Walker K, Petersen R, Wilmshurst JM (2011) Neurologic and neurobehavioral sequelae in children with human immunodeficiency virus (HIV-1) infection. *J Child Neuro*, 26: 1355–1364. doi: 10.1177/0883073811405203.

Grando LJ, Machado DC, Spitzer S et al. (2005) Viral coinfection in the oral cavity of HIV-infected children: Relation among HIV viral load, CD4+T lymphocyte count and detection of EBV, CMV and HSV. *Brazilian Oral Research, Sociedade Brasileira de Pesquisa Odontológica – SBPqO*. 19(3): 228–234.

Gumbo T, Kadzirange G, Mielke J, Gangaidzo IT, Hakim JG (2002) Cryptococcus neoformans meningoencephalitis in African children with acquired immunodeficiency syndrome. *Pediatr Infect Dis J*, 21: 54–56.

Hammond CK, Eley B, Wieselthaler N, Ndondo A, Wilmshurst JM (2016) Cerebrovascular disease in children with HIV-1 infection. *Dev Med Child Neurol*, 58: 452–460. doi: 10.1111/dmcn.13080. Epub 2016 Feb 18. Review.

Hardie DR, Albertyn C, Heckmann JM, Smuts HE (2013) Molecular characterisation of virus in the brains of patients with measles inclusion body encephalitis (MIBE). *Virol J*, 10: 283. doi: 10.1186/1743-422X-10-283.

Holtzman DM, Kaku DA, So YT (1989) New-onset seizures with human immunodeficiency virus infection: Causation and clinical features in 100 cases. *Am J Med*, 87: 173–177.

Idro R, Gwer S, Kahindi M et al. (2008) The incidence, aetiology and outcome of acute seizures in children admitted to a rural Kenyan district hospital. *BMC Pediatr*, 8: 5. doi: 10.1186/1471-2431-8-5.

Kellinghaus C, Engbring C, Kovac S et al. (2008) Frequency of seizures and epilepsy in neurological HIV-infected patients. *Seizure*, 17: 27–33.

Kija E, Ndondo A, Spittal G, Hardie DR, Eley B, Wilmshurst JM (2015) Subacute sclerosing panencephalitis in South African children following the measles outbreak between 2009 and 2011. *S Afr Med J*, 105: 713–718. doi: 10.7196/SAMJnew.7788.

Klock C, Cerski M, Goldani LZ (2009) Histopathological aspects of neurocryptococcosis in HIV-infected patients: Autopsy report of 45 patients. *Int J Surg Pathol*, 17: 444–448. doi: 10.1177/1066896908320550.

Koppel BS, Poon TP, Khandji A, Pavlakis SG, Pedley TA (1996) Subacute sclerosing panencephalitis and acquired immunodeficiency syndrome: Role of electroencephalography and magnetic resonance imaging. *J Neuroimaging*, 6: 122–125.

Lee SC, Dickson DW, Casadevall A (1996) Pathology of cryptococcal meningoencephalitis: Analysis of 27 patients with pathogenetic implications. *Hum Pathol*, 27: 839–847.

Link-Gelles R, Moultrie H, Sawry S, Murdoch D, Van Rie (2014) Tuberculosis immune reconstitution inflammatory syndrome in children initiating antiretroviral therapy for HIV infection: A systematic literature review. *Pediatr Infect Dis J*, 33: 499–503. doi: 10.1097/INF.0000000000000142.

Madhi SA, Madhi A, Petersen K, Khoosal M, Klugman KP (2001) Impact of human immunodeficiency virus type 1 infection on the epidemiology and outcome of bacterial meningitis in South African children. *Int J Infect Dis*, 5: 119–125.

Maurya PK, Thakkar MD, Kulshreshtha D, Singh AK, Thacker AK (2016) Subacute sclerosing panencephalitis in a child with human immunodeficiency virus co-infection. *Clin Med Res*, 14: 156–158. doi: 10.3121/cmr.2016.1331.

Messenheimer JA (1998) Rash in adult and pediatric patients treated with lamotrigine. *Can J Neurol Sci*, 25: S14–S18.

Michaelis IA, Nielsen M, Carty C, Wolff M, Sabin CA, Lambert JS (2020) Late diagnosis of human immunodeficiency virus infection is linked to higher rates of epilepsy in children in the Eastern Cape of South Africa. *Southern African Journal of HIV Medicine*, 21(1): 1–6.

Mintz M (1996) Neurological and developmental problems in pediatric HIV infection. *J Nutr*, 126: 2663S–2673S.

Misra UK, Kalita J (1998) Neurophysiological studies in herpes simplex encephalitis. *Electromyogr Clin Neurophysiol*, 38: 177–182.

Moog CJ, Kakooza-Mwesige MA, Tan CT (2017) Epilepsy in the tropics: Emerging etiologies. *Seizure*, 44: 108–112. doi: 10.1016/j.seizure.2016.11.032.

Mpimbaza A, Staedke SG, Ndeezi G, Byarugaba J, Rosenthal PJ (2009) Predictors of anti-convulsant treatment failure in children presenting with malaria and prolonged seizures in Kampala, Uganda. *Malar J*, 8: 145. doi: 10.1186/1475-2875-8-145.

Muthusamy K, Yoganathan S, Thomas MM, Alexander M, Verghese VP (2015) Subacute sclerosing panencephalitis in a child with human immunodeficiency virus (HIV) infection on antiretroviral therapy. *Ann Indian Acad Neurol*, 18: 96–98. doi: 10.4103/0972-2327.144299.

Narayan P, Samuels OB, Barrow DL (2002) Stroke and pediatric human immunodeficiency virus infection. Case report and review of the literature. *Pediatr Neurosurg*, 37: 158–163.

Orikiiriza J, Bakeera-Kitaka S, Musiime V, Mworozi EA, Mugyenyi P, Boulware DR (2010) The clinical pattern, prevalence, and factors associated with immune reconstitution inflammatory syndrome in Ugandan children. *AIDS*, 24: 2009–2017. doi: 10.1097/QAD.0b013e32833b260a.

Pascual-Sedano B, Iranzo A, Marti-Fàbregas J, Domingo P, Escartin A, Fuster M, Barrio JL, Sambeat MA (1999) Prospective study of new-onset seizures in patients with human immunodeficiency virus infection: etiologic and clinical aspects. *Arch Neurol*, 56(5): 609–612. doi: 10.1001/archneur.56.5.609.

Philippet P, Blanche S, Sebag G, Rodesch G, Griscelli C, Tardieu M (1994) Stroke and cerebral infarcts in children infected with human immunodeficiency virus. *Arch Pediatr Adolesc Med*, 148: 965–970.

Poon TP, Tchertkoff V, Win H (1998) Subacute measles encephalitis with AIDS diagnosed by fine needle aspiration biopsy. A case report. *Acta Cytol*, 42: 729–733.

Rho JM, Stafstrom CE (2006) Neurophysiology of epilepsy. In: Swaiman K, Ashwal S, Ferriero D, editors, *Pediatric Neurology: Principles and Practice*. Philadelphia: Mosby Elsevier, pp. 991–1008.

Ruiz-Giménez J, Sánchez-Alvarez JC, Cañadillas-Hidalgo F, Serrano-Castro PJ, Andalusian Epilepsy Society (2010) Antiepileptic treatment in patients with epilepsy and other comorbidities. *Seizure*, 19: 375–382. doi: 10.1016/j.seizure.2010.05.008.

Samia P, Petersen R, Walker KG, Eley B, Wilmshurst JM (2013) Prevalence of seizures in children infected with human immunodeficiency virus. *J Child Neurol*, 28: 297–302. doi: 10.1177/0883073812446161.

Satishchandra P, Sinha S (2008) Seizures in HIV-seropositive individuals: NIMHANS experience and review. *Epilepsia*, 49: 33–41. doi: 10.1111/j.1528-1167.2008.01754.x.

Singhi P (2011) Infectious causes of seizures and epilepsy in the developing world. *Dev Med Child Neurol*, 53: 600–609. doi: 10.1111/j.1469-8749.2011.03928.x.

Ssenkusu JM, Hodges JS, Opoka RO et al. (2016) Long-term behavioural problems in children with severe malaria. *Pediatrics*, 138(5): e20161965.

Tarekegne D, Jemal M, Atanaw T et al. (2016) Prevalence of human immunodeficiency virus infection in a cohort of tuberculosis patients at Metema Hospital, Northwest Ethiopia: A 3 years retrospective study. *BMC Res Notes*, 9: 192. doi: 10.1186/s13104-016-2004-8.

Taüber MG, Schaad UB (2006) Bacterial infections of the nervous system. In Swaiman K, Ashwal S, Ferriero D, editors, *Pediatric Neurology: Principles and Practice*, Philadelphia: Mosby Elsevier, pp. 1571–1594.

van Toorn R, Rabie H, Dramowski A, Schoeman JF (2012) Neurological manifestations of TB-IRIS: A report of 4 children. *Eur J Paediatr Neurol*, 16: 676–682. doi: 10.1016/j.ejpn.2012.04.005.

Visudtibhan A, Visudhiphan P, Chiemchanya S (1999) Stroke and seizures as the presenting signs of pediatric HIV infection. *Pediatr Neurol*, 20: 53–56.

WHO (2015) Anti-epileptic medications for adults and children with HIV [Online]. Available at: http://www.who.int/mental_health/mhgap/evidence/epilepsy/q14/en/ [accessed 15 March 2017].

WHO (2016) Consolidated guidelines on the use of antiretroviral drugs for treating and preventing HIV infection: Summary of recommendations [Online]. Available at: http://www.who.int/entity/hiv/pub/arv/summary-recommendations.pdf [accessed 21 March 2017].

Wilmshurst JM, Burgess J, Hartley P, Eley B (2006) Specific neurologic complications of human immunodeficiency virus type 1 (HIV-1) infection in children. *J Child Neurol*, 21: 788–794.

Wilmshurst JM, Burman R, Gaillard WD, Cross JH (2015) Treatment of infants with epilepsy: Common practices around the world. *Epilepsia*, 56(7): 1033–1046.

Yacoob Y, Bhigjee AI, Moodley P, Parboosing R (2011) Sodium valproate and highly active antiretroviral therapy in HIV-positive patients who develop new-onset seizures. *Seizure*, 20: 80–82. doi: 10.1016/j.seizure.2010.09.009.

Zaporojan L, McNamara PH, Williams JA, Bergin C, Redmond J, Doherty CP (2018) Seizures in HIV: The case for special consideration. *Epilepsy Behav Case Rep*, 10: 38–43.

Neuroinfections in Children Infected with HIV

Brian Eley, Babatunde O Ogunbosi, Ebrahim Banderker, and Charles K Hammond

INTRODUCTION

According to the joint United Nations Programme on HIV/AIDS (UNAIDS), at the end of 2019 the total number of children less than 15 years of age living with human immunodeficiency virus (HIV) infection was 1.8 million, of whom 1.62 million (90.0%) were living in sub-Saharan Africa (SSA) and 140 000 (7.8%) in Asia and the Pacific region (UNAIDS 2020). A highly effective global prevention of mother-to-child transmission (PMTCT) intervention strategy has resulted in a decrease in the annual number of incident (new) HIV infections among children, from more than 500 000 in 2000 to 150 000 in 2019 (UNAIDS 2020). Combination antiretroviral therapy (cART) when administered to HIV-infected children suppresses HIV replication, reverses HIV-induced immune deficiency that developed before cART initiation, prevents the progression of immune deficiency, reverses existing coinfection, and lowers the risk of acquiring new coinfections. At the end of 2019, the global cART coverage of children less than 15 years of age was only 53% (UNAIDS 2020). Thus, many HIV-infected children, particularly in low- and middle-income countries (LMICs), are at risk of developing a wide spectrum of coinfections. These include coinfections of the central nervous system (CNS) and the peripheral nervous system, collectively referred to in this chapter as neuroinfections.

The clinical progression of HIV infection has been divided into four stages by the World Health Organization (WHO 2010). Coinfections are common manifestations of paediatric HIV infection, and they occur throughout the four disease stages. Stage four, the most advanced stage of HIV infection, includes several neuroinfections, most notably recurrent acute bacterial infection such as bacterial meningitis, tuberculous meningitis (TBM), cytomegalovirus (CMV) infection, cerebral toxoplasmosis, and cryptococcal meningitis (WHO 2010). Neuroinfections can affect between 8% and 34% of HIV-infected children (Donald et al. 2014). The risk of acquiring coinfections is influenced by the severity of the immune deficiency, regularity of cART administration, administration of antimicrobial preventive therapy, and response to routinely administered childhood vaccines. Social variables that are prevalent in the LMICs where most HIV-infected children reside, such as overcrowding, nutritional status, and exposure to air pollution, also affect the risk of acquiring coinfections (Eley and Nuttall 2007).

IMMUNE DEFICIENCY IN HIV INFECTION

Chronic HIV infection causes profound immune dysfunction, resulting in characteristic clinical manifestations, including predisposition to infections caused by a range of pathogenic and opportunistic microorganisms. Thus, both adaptive and innate immunity are affected. Immune dysfunction results from direct HIV effects after the virus enters specific immune cells, notably CD4+ T-lymphocytes (CD4 cells). Immune dysfunction also occurs when virions or specific viral glycoproteins act on uninfected cells of the immune system, as well as when chronic immune activation arises from both the HIV infection and the host's response to the infection (McMichael and Rowland-Jones 2001; Doitsh et al. 2014; Roider, Muenchhoff, and Goulder 2016).

The major immunological disturbances in HIV infection are progressive attrition and dysfunction of the CD4+ T-lymphocytes. The immunological hallmark of HIV infection is CD4+ T-lymphocytopaenia. The rate of progression of HIV infection varies according to age, being more rapid in infants and young children when compared to adults. Several direct and indirect mechanisms have been proposed to explain the destruction of CD4+ T-lymphocytes in HIV infection (Pantaleo, Graziosi, and Fauci 1993; Badley et al. 2000; Eley 2003; Swanstrom and Coffin 2012; Doitsh et al. 2014). Recent research has shown that HIV-induced caspase-3-mediated apoptosis and caspase-1-mediated pyroptosis, which is triggered by abortive viral infection and chronic immune activation, are the mechanisms responsible for most CD4+ T-lymphocyte attrition. In fact, caspase-1-mediated pyroptosis is responsible for more than 95% of CD4+ T-lymphocyte death (Doitsh et al. 2014). Over and above the quantitative CD4+ T-lymphocyte loss, viable, circulating naïve and memory CD4+ T-lymphocytes show evidence of dysfunction, including a depressed response to soluble antigens and mitogens, defective interleukin receptor expression, and impaired activation (Meyaard et al. 1994). CD8+ T-lymphocyte-mediated viral clearance is also impaired in HIV infection. This has been attributed, in part, to both virus escape from CD8+ T-lymphocyte recognition and to CD8+ T-lymphocyte dysfunction (McMichael and Rowland-Jones 2001; Jones and Walker 2016).

Although B-lymphocytes are not infected by HIV, several defects in humoral immunity occur during HIV infection, including non-specific activation of B-lymphocytes resulting in characteristic polyclonal hypergammaglobulinaemia. Other humoral immunity deficits include loss of memory B-lymphocytes, attenuated immunoglobulin production in response to both new and recall antigens including vaccines, and loss of specific antibody responses previously gained during routine childhood immunisations (Titanji et al. 2006; Pensieroso et al. 2009; Cagigi et al. 2012).

HIV infection also compromises innate immunity. HIV affects the function of monocytes, macrophages, and neutrophils. Disturbances include decreased phagocytosis affecting monocytes/macrophages, and altered chemotaxis and cytokine production affecting both cell types. Along with cell-mediated immune deficiencies, phagocytic dysfunction can contribute to poor granuloma formation seen in HIV infection, and hence prevent containment of important pathogens such as *Mycobacterium tuberculosis* (Pugliese et al. 2005). Natural killer (NK) cells are critical antiviral effectors of the innate immune system, being responsible for an early antigen-independent cytolytic response against infected cells. However, they also play a critical role in the adaptive immune response through antibody-mediated cellular cytotoxicity and antigen-mediated immunological memory. During HIV infection, NK lytic activity and cytokine production are impaired (Ansari et al. 2015; Scully and Alter 2016).

HIV also causes generalised activation of the innate and adaptive immune systems. Generalised immune activation is now considered a central feature of the immunopathogenesis of HIV infection, leading to CD4+ T-lymphocyte depletion through activation-induced cell death from apoptosis and pyroptosis of bystander cells (Doitsh et al. 2014). Therefore, immune activation drives progression to advanced HIV infection, or AIDS, and risk of coinfections. Even though cART-mediated suppression of HIV replication reduces immune activation significantly, immune activation pathways remain abnormal during antiretroviral therapy. Chronic HIV infection, gastrointestinal bacterial translocation, and coinfections such as CMV infection likely contribute to the persistence of immune activation during therapy (Roider, Muenchhoff, and Gouder 2016; Utay and Hunt 2016).

The net effect of HIV-mediated immune deficiency is to compromise both adaptive and innate immunity and predispose HIV-infected children to a wide range of viral, bacterial, fungal, and parasitic coinfections, including a similar spectrum of neuroinfections.

EFFECT OF cART ON IMMUNE FUNCTION

Following the initiation of cART, immunological reconstitution in HIV-infected children occurs mainly via the naïve T-lymphocyte compartment. Although both thymic activity and peripheral T-lymphocyte proliferation are involved in immunological reconstitution, thymic output is the major source of CD4+ T-lymphocyte repopulation. Recovery of the naïve T-lymphocytes is more rapid if cART is started at a young age and is better in children with larger thymuses (Gibb et al. 2000; De Rossi et al. 2002; Ometto et al. 2002). This response differs from immunological reconstitution in adults, where thymic function is compromised (Haynes et al. 1999; Eley 2003).

In HIV-infected children, cART restores the T-lymphocyte receptor Vβ repertoire of naïve T-lymphocytes because of thymic activity (Yin et al. 2009). Thymic output increases significantly with time on cART (Sandgaard et al. 2014). In children, cART significantly reduces the concentration of activated CD4+ and CD8+ T-lymphocytes and promotes the reconstitution of both IL-7Rα-expressing CD8+ T-lymphocytes and resting memory B-lymphocytes (Rainwater-Lovett et al. 2014a, 2014b). The immunological reconstitution to specific microorganisms (pathogen-specific immunity) has also been documented after cART initiation. In one such study using a functional whole blood in vitro assay for evaluating antimycobacterial immunity, significant containment of mycobacterial replication was demonstrated within a few months of commencing cART in HIV-infected children residing in Cape Town, a high tuberculosis (TB) endemic setting (Kampmann et al. 2004, 2006).

Children who initiate cART when they have low CD4+ cell counts and those at a relatively older age are less likely to achieve normal CD4+ cell counts. Furthermore, HIV-infected children with low CD4+ counts who commence cART at a younger age experience better long-term immunological reconstitution than older children (Lewis et al. 2012; Picat et al. 2013). In one study of 933 children aged 5 years or older, CD4+ counts remained less than 500 cells/μL in 8% of patients, 2 years after achieving virological suppression (Krogstad et al. 2015). Another study of 507 children tracked on cART for a median of 7 years showed that 22% failed to achieve a CD4+ percentage of at least 25%. An age of greater than 7 years and a CD4+ percentage of less than less than 5% before cART initiation was associated with poor immunological reconstitution (Collins et al. 2013).

Commencement of early cART during infancy preserves the existing memory T- and B-lymphocyte compartment. Consequently, protective antibody titres induced by routine childhood immunisation are maintained (Pensieroso et al. 2009). Early cART also results in immunological reconstitution of the naïve T-lymphocyte compartment involving both CD4+ and CD8+ naïve T-lymphocytes (Azzoni et al. 2015).

An important consequence of cART is the development of immune reconstitution inflammatory syndrome (IRIS). This occurs in approximately 20% of HIV-infected children (Smith et al. 2009). Two forms of IRIS have been described: paradoxical IRIS, in which there is new or worsening manifestations of a previously diagnosed and treated coinfection, and unmasking IRIS, in which a new coinfection manifests. After the initiation of cART, there is marked suppression of viral replication and restoration of pathogen-specific immunity. Without normal immunological homeostatic controls, an exaggerated inflammatory response can be induced by an existing infection. The exuberant inflammatory response can be induced by both viable and non-viable antigens, causing clinical deterioration. These IRIS events usually occur within the first 3 months of cART. IRIS may be triggered by several neuroinfections including TBM, cryptococcal meningitis, and progressive multifocal leukoencephalopathy (PML). This results in varying degrees of neurological deterioration, including progression to death in a subset of patients (Nuttall et al. 2004; van Toorn et al. 2012; Bahr et al. 2013).

IMPACT OF cART ON THE RISK OF INFECTION

A recent systematic review and meta-analysis compared the incidence and prevalence of 14 opportunistic infections in cART-naïve and cART-treated HIV-infected children less than 18 years of age and who were residing in LMICs (B-Lajoie et al. 2016). The 14 infections included cryptococcal meningitis, cerebral toxoplasmosis, extrapulmonary TB, and bacterial infections like bacterial meningitis. Data from 35 incidence studies involving more than 23 000 children were analysed. A significant reduction in incidence risk was documented after cART initiation in most opportunistic infections. The greatest effect of cART on incidence risk was for cerebral toxoplasmosis, *Cryptosporidium* diarrhoea, and extrapulmonary TB. The incidence risk of extrapulmonary TB, which included TBM cases, declined from 7.26% in cART-naïve children to 1.12% in children receiving cART, an 85% reduction in risk. Furthermore, after cART initiation, the incidence risk declined to less than 1.5% for some of the infections evaluated, including cryptococcal meningitis, cerebral toxoplasmosis, bacterial meningitis, and extrapulmonary TB. Data from 60 prevalence studies involving more than 36 000 children were evaluated and significant reduction in prevalence was only documented for *Cryptosporidium* diarrhoea and bacteraemia, not for any of the neuroinfectious organisms evaluated (B-Lajoie et al. 2016).

THE SPECTRUM OF NEUROINFECTIONS

More than two decades after the effectiveness of cART was first demonstrated, HIV-infected children and adults continue to be at risk for a wide spectrum of neuroinfections. Several factors contribute to this status quo, including inadequate cART coverage, suboptimal adherence, unplanned treatment interruptions, and viral resistance to antiretroviral agents. Some neuroinfections were rare before the emergence of the HIV pandemic but have since been shown to be more common in HIV-infected individuals. These include cryptococcal meningitis, cerebral toxoplasmosis, and PML (Bowen et al. 2016).

The spectrum of neuroinfections (Table 7.1) in HIV-infected individuals varies according to age and geographical region. In SSA, TBM, cryptococcal meningitis, CMV infection, and malaria are common, whereas in Asia and the Pacific region, cryptococcal meningitis, cerebral toxoplasmosis, TBM, and Japanese encephalitis B are the most prevalent infections (Tan et al. 2012). Acute bacterial meningitis and tuberculous meningitis (TBM) are the most reported neuroinfections in HIV-infected children who live in LMICs. Cryptococcal meningitis and PML are less common in HIV-infected children than in HIV-infected adults (Meiring et al. 2012; Wilmshurst et al. 2018). Presumed viral meningitis is not easily confirmed in LMICs because of limited access to cerebrospinal fluid (CSF) molecular screening. Thus, viral meningitis is under-studied in HIV-infected children who live in LMICs. CMV encephalitis coinfection is likely under-reported in HIV-infected children because of diagnostic constraints.

Table 7.1   CNS infections in HIV-infected children.

CNS infection	Spectrum of microorganisms
Acute bacterial meningitis	Frequently caused by *Streptococcus pneumoniae*, *Haemophilus influenzae* type B, non-typhoid *Salmonella enterica*, and *Neissaria meningitidis*.
	Less frequent causes: Gram-negative organisms e.g. *Klebsiella pneumoniae*, *Escherichia coli*, *Pseudomonas species*, multi-drug resistant bacterial infection.
	Unusual pathogens include *Treponema pallidum*, *Bartonella* species, *Listeria monocytogenes*, and *Nocardia asteroides* complex.
Tuberculous meningitis	Mainly caused by *Mycobacterium tuberculosis*; rarely caused by atypical mycobacteria and *Mycobacterium bovis* Bacille Calmette-Guérin (BCG).
Fungal infections	Frequently caused by *Cryptococcus neoformans*.
	Less frequent causes: *Cryptococcus gatti*, *Candida* species, *Aspergillus fumigatus*, Zygomycetes infection.
Viral neuroinfections	John Cunningham virus causing progressive multifocal leukoencephalopathy.
	Herpes simplex viruses 1 and 2, varicella zoster virus, cytomegalovirus, Japanese encephalitis virus.
	Common causes of viral meningitis, e.g. enteroviruses and parechoviruses.
	Measles virus-induced complications.
Parasitic neuro-infections	Cerebral malaria: *Plasmodium falciparum*. Less frequently by *Plasmodium vivax* especially outside sub-Saharan Africa. Rarely by *Plasmodium ovale* or *Plasmodium malariae*.
	Cerebral toxoplasmosis: *Toxoplasma gondii*.
	Trypanosomiasis: *Trypanosoma brucei gambiense*, *Trypanosoma brucei rhodesiense*, *Trypanosoma cruzi*.
	Neurocysticercosis: *Taenia solium*.
	Neuroschistosomiasis: Cerebral infection, often by *Schistosoma japonicum*. Spinal infections often by *Schistosoma mansoni* and *Schistosoma haematobium*.
	Other causes: *Echinococcus granulosus*, *Entamoeba histolytica*, *Leishmania* species, *Microsporidium* species.
Virus-induced neoplasms	Epstein–Barr virus induced non-Hodgkin lymphoma and herpes simplex virus-8 causing Kaposi sarcoma.

Cerebral malaria and other CNS parasitic diseases can coinfect HIV-infected children in SSA (Mallewa and Wilmshurst 2014). Less frequently encountered neuroinfections in HIV-infected children include cerebral toxoplasmosis and herpes simplex virus encephalitis. Rarely, CNS infection may be caused by atypical mycobacteria, *Treponema pallidum*, *Bartonella* species, *Listeria monocytogenes*, and *Nocardia asteroides* complex (Wilmshurst, Eley, and Brew 2014; Wilmshurst et al. 2018).

Neuroinfections may have devastating consequences, contributing appreciably to morbidity and mortality. In HIV-infected adults, cryptococcal meningitis is responsible for 15% to 20% of deaths attributed to HIV-associated opportunistic infections, and the case-fatality rate of TBM may exceed 50% (Kwan and Ernst 2011; Bowen et al. 2016). The incidence and prevalence of neurological morbidity following neuroinfections have not been estimated in HIV-infected children who live in LMICs but they are likely not insignificant. At an individual patient level, neurological morbidity may be severe and complex, due to the combined effects of the HIV infection and one or more neuroinfections acting together or sequentially on the developing nervous system (Wilmshurst et al. 2006).

Acute Bacterial Meningitis

Bacterial meningitis is an important cause of morbidity and mortality worldwide. The common bacteria causing childhood meningitis are *Streptococcus pneumoniae*, *Haemophilus influenzae* type B (Hib), and *Neissaria meningitidis*. Before widespread use of protein-conjugate vaccines to prevent severe bacterial infection, mortality rates associated with pneumococcal, Hib, and meningococcal meningitis in SSA were 45%, 29%, and 8% respectively (Peltola 2001). Global introduction of pneumococcal and Hib protein-conjugate vaccines is currently progressing. Most countries in SSA administer these vaccines as part of their childhood immunisation programmes, and they are consequentially benefiting from a substantially reduced meningitis risk. A systematic review and meta-analysis concluded that approximately 75% of bacterial meningitis deaths can be prevented through routine administration of these vaccines (Davis, Feikin, and Johnson 2013). In 2010, mass immunisation with a meningococcal serogroup A protein-conjugate vaccine began in 26 countries in the African meningitis belt, targeting individuals between 1 and 29 years old. However, these mass immunisation campaigns are currently being superseded by routine immunisation during childhood. At the end of 2020, all countries within the African meningitis belt had introduced the vaccine through campaigns, and 15 countries had introduced it in their routine childhood immunisation programmes. These initiatives are further reducing the bacterial meningitis risk in SSA (WHO 2019).

Bacterial meningitis is more prevalent in HIV-infected children than in HIV-infected adults, especially in unvaccinated children. Frequently cultured bacteria include *S. pneumoniae*, Hib, non-typhoid *Salmonella enterica* (NTS), and *N. meningitidis*. Generally, the clinical presentation of bacterial meningitis is similar in HIV-infected and uninfected children (Madhi et al. 2001; Molyneux et al. 2003). However, impaired consciousness is significantly more common in HIV-infected children (Madhi et al. 2001). Bacterial meningitis causes significantly higher mortality in HIV-infected children than in uninfected children. Pneumococcal meningitis is associated with poorer outcomes, including neurological sequalae and death, in HIV-infected children compared to uninfected children (Madhi et al. 2001; Molyneux et al. 2003). A risk factor analysis showed that HIV infection increases the odds of death from bacterial meningitis by 165% (McCormick et al. 2013). Furthermore, HIV-infected children are at a higher risk of recurrent meningitis than uninfected children are, and *S. pneumoniae* and NTS are the main causes of recurrent meningitis in HIV-infected children in SSA (Molyneux et al. 2003).

Management should include both laboratory workup for specific bacterial pathogens and appropriate antibiotic treatment. The duration of antibiotic therapy has not been optimised for bacterial meningitis in HIV-infected children. A randomised trial showed that it is safe to treat clinically stable, uninfected children aged 2 months to 12 years with bacterial meningitis caused by *S. pneumoniae*, Hib, or *N. meningitidis* with 5 days of parenteral ceftriaxone (Molyneux et al. 2011). However, a more conservative approach should be adopted in HIV-infected children. For *N. meningitides*, the duration of antibiotic therapy should be 7 days; for *H. influenzae*, 7 to 10 days; for *S. pneumoniae*, 10 to 14 days; and for Gram-negative bacilli, 21 days (McMullan et al. 2016). There is insufficient evidence to direct clinical practice with regard to using restricted versus maintenance fluid therapy in children with bacterial meningitis (Maconochie and Bhaumik 2016). In high-income countries, corticosteroids lower the risk of neurological sequelae and deafness. However, in LMICs, glucocorticosteroids have not been shown to have a beneficial effect in children with acute bacterial meningitis (Molyneux et al. 2002; Brouwer et al. 2015). Immunisation and long-term trimethoprim-sulfamethoxazole (co-trimoxazole) prophylaxis are important interventions for preventing invasive bacterial infections, including meningitis, in HIV-infected children (Davis, Feikin, and Johnson 2013; Bwakura-Dangarembizi et al. 2014).

Tuberculous Meningitis

HIV-infected individuals are at an increased risk for all forms of extrapulmonary TB including TBM. TBM in HIV-infected children is particularly common in settings where both TB and HIV infection are highly endemic, such as in southern Africa. The clinical presentation and CSF findings of TBM in children, both with and without HIV infection, are similar (van der Weert et al. 2006). Significantly more HIV-infected children with TBM have radiographic evidence of pulmonary TB than uninfected children do. However, typical neuroimaging features of TBM, such as basal meningeal enhancement and hydrocephalus (as shown in Figure 7.1), can be blunted or absent in HIV-infected children. Cerebral infarcts are reported to be more common in HIV-infected adults with TBM, but the prevalence of infarction in HIV-infected and uninfected children with TBM is not dissimilar (Schutte 2001; van der Weert et al. 2006). A low threshold for TBM diagnostic considerations is necessary in HIV-infected children. Furthermore, some screening tests for TB, such as the tuberculin skin tests and chest radiographs,

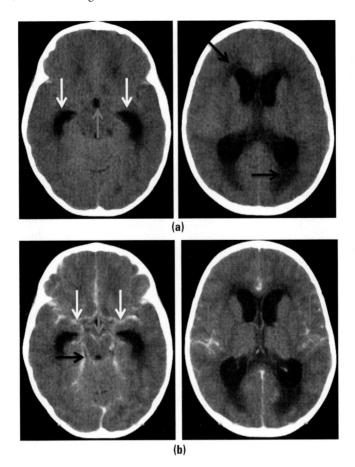

Figure 7.1 Tuberculous meningitis. **(a)** Uncontrasted CT brain scan image: Obstructive hydrocephalus as evidenced by bilateral temporal horn prominence (white arrows), rounding of the third ventricle (upward central arrow, left-hand image) and transependymal fluid shift (black arrows, right-hand image). **(b)** Contrast-enhanced CT brain scan image: Extensive basal meningeal enhancement within the middle cerebral artery cisterns (white arrows, left-hand image), interpeduncular (red arrow) and ambient wing (black arrow) cisterns. Also note extensive leptomeningeal enhancement (arrows, right-hand image).

should be interpreted with caution, as the results may not be as definitive as in immunocompetent children (Lancella et al. 2016). A recent study showed that the pathology of TBM in both HIV-infected and uninfected children is not confined to the brain, but that spinal pathology, commonly arachnoiditis and tuberculomata, occur in approximately 75% of HIV-infected and uninfected children (Rohlwink et al. 2016).

There are also challenges in the management of HIV-TBM coinfection. The optimal anti-TB drug regimen and duration of therapy have not been adequately researched. Current treatment recommendations are based on observational studies. The WHO recommends a 12-month anti-TB regimen for TBM, comprising a 2-month 4-drug intensive phase (isoniazid, rifampicin, pyrazinamide, and ethambutol) followed by a 10-month, 2-drug maintenance phase (isoniazid and rifampicin) (WHO 2014). A South African prospective non-randomised study showed that a 4-drug intensified regimen (isoniazid, rifampicin, pyrazinamide, and ethionamide) administered for 9 months to HIV-infected children or for 6 months to uninfected children resulted in a satisfactory outcome in 80% of patients, low mortality of 3.8% and no difference in outcome between the two groups (van Toorn et al. 2014). This regimen is being used in some parts of South Africa. Glucocorticosteroids reduce the mortality risk in uninfected individuals with TBM by approximately 25% (Prasad, Singh, and Ryan 2016). Although glucocorticosteroid therapy has not been demonstrated to be beneficial in HIV-infected children and adults with TBM, it is used in both HIV-infected and uninfected patients with TBM (van Toorn and Solomons 2014; Wasserman and Meintjes 2014).

In antiretroviral-naïve HIV-infected patients in whom TBM is diagnosed, anti-TB drug treatment should be commenced as soon as is possible, and the initiation of cART can be delayed by 4 through 8 weeks. The delay in cART initiation is supported by a randomised trial showing that immediate cART initiation is associated with significantly more severe adverse events (Torok et al. 2011). Significant drug interactions may also complicate the management of TBM. Rifampicin induces the metabolism of lopinavir, a protease inhibitor, resulting in a marked reduction in its concentration. When rifampicin-containing anti-TB treatment is administered together with the lopinavir/ritonavir coformulation in HIV-infected children, additional ritonavir should be administered to prevent subtherapeutic lopinavir concentration with resultant viral escape and development of lopinavir resistance (Ren et al. 2008). Doubling the dose of lopinavir/ritonavir coformulation does not overcome the effect of rifampicin on the metabolism of lopinavir in young children. Thus, this practice is discouraged in children (McIlleron et al. 2011).

With regards to the non-nucleoside reverse transcriptase inhibitors, reduced nevirapine concentration occurs when administered concomitantly with rifampicin-containing anti-TB treatment. To partially overcome this effect, the nevirapine lead-in dosing should be omitted, and patients commenced on twice daily dosing (Cohen et al. 2008). Furthermore, the WHO recommends that when nevirapine is used with rifampicin in HIV-infected children the dose be increased to 200mg/m^2 twice daily (WHO 2010).

The effect of rifampicin on efavirenz concentration is complex because of the interaction with hepatic metabolic pathways. Mid-dosing concentration of efavirenz usually decreases marginally when efavirenz is coadministered with rifampicin. Thus, efavirenz dose modification is not required (Ren et al. 2009; McIlleron et al. 2013). However, rifampicin administration may, on occasion, cause a paradoxical elevation in plasma efavirenz concentration as a result of *CYP2B6* loss of function polymorphisms (Gengiah et al. 2012; Bertrand et al. 2014; Dooley et al. 2015). Isoniazid coadministration with efavirenz usually causes a mild, insignificant decrease in efavirenz mid-dosing plasma concentration. Isoniazid may also increase efavirenz concentration by inhibiting *CYP2A6*, an important pathway for metabolising efavirenz in individuals who are *CYP2B6* slow metabolisers. Isoniazid is usually metabolised by the enzyme NAT2. Loss-of-function polymorphisms in NAT2 cause increased isoniazid exposure, increasing the risk of *CYP2A6* pathway inhibition. Furthermore, individuals with slow metaboliser phenotypes for both *CYP2B6* and *NAT2* genes have been shown to have markedly elevated efavirenz concentrations when cotreated with rifampicin and isoniazid-containing anti-TB treatment (Bertrand et al. 2014; Luetkemeyer et al. 2015).

An additional treatment consideration is the development of paradoxical, or unmasking, TBM-IRIS events during the first few months of cART. This may aggravate neurological dysfunction or disability caused by TBM and can even cause mortality (van Toorn et al. 2012; Bahr et al. 2013; Kalk et al. 2013). Risk factors for paradoxical TBM-IRIS in adult patients include evidence of disseminated TB, such as the presence of abnormalities on chest radiograph, higher CSF neutrophil count, and a CSF cytokine profile characterised by high tumour necrosis factor-α and low interferon-γ concentrations (Marais et al. 2013).

Cryptococcal Meningitis

Cryptococcal meningitis, a fungal infection, is usually caused by *Cryptococcus neoformans* and occasionally by *Cryptococcus gatti*. Cryptococcal meningitis is less common in the paediatric population than in adult patients. In a laboratory-based study in South Africa that analysed more than 16 000 incident cases of cryptococcosis, the risk was 1 in per 100 000 population for children less than 15 years old and 19 per 100 000 population in adults, and 47 per 100 000 population in HIV-infected children less than 15 years old and 120 per 100 000 population in adults. Amongst HIV-infected children, a peak risk of 517 cases per 100 000 persons was documented in children aged 10 to 14 years, confirming that in HIV-infected children cryptococcal meningitis is a disease that predominantly affects older children (Meiring et al. 2012). Although cryptococcal meningitis has a worldwide distribution, the highest burden of the disease and the highest case-fatality rate occurs in SSA (Park et al. 2009).

Cryptococcal meningitis is a subacute meningoencephalitis. It can present with subtle, non-specific symptoms, such as a headache or fever. This disease typically evolves over days to weeks before symptom presentation. At presentation, fever and headache are dominant features but the typical signs of meningism may be absent. Thus, a high index of clinical suspicion is required by the attending clinician (Siberry et al. 2013). CSF analysis will reveal typical changes, including pleocytosis, high protein concentration, and increased CSF pressure. The diagnosis is confirmed either by cryptococcal antigen, lateral flow assay, or India ink test examination of CSF (WHO 2011). The few paediatric reports of cryptococcal meningitis in HIV-infected children in SSA have shown that HIV-infected children can present with either acute, fulminating meningitis, or in the more classic, subacute manner (Gumbo et al. 2002; Nyazika et al. 2016).

Treatment of cryptococcal meningitis in children is based on intervention trials in adult patients. During the 2-week induction phase, combination therapy is recommended. A phase-III randomised controlled trial showed that amphotericin B plus flucytosine is associated with better survival when compared to the combination of amphotericin B and fluconazole (Day et al. 2013). Flucytosine is not readily available in SSA because of its high cost, so the combination of amphotericin B and fluconazole is frequently used during induction (WHO 2011; Govender and Dlamini 2014). The induction phase is followed by consolidation treatment of fluconazole monotherapy for 8 weeks. After completion of consolidation treatment, the patient is maintained on fluconazole mono-prophylaxis until there is sufficient immunological reconstitution (WHO 2011). During cryptococcal meningitis, an elevated CSF pressure is experienced by 50% to 75% of patients. Serial lumbar punctures are used to relieve intracranial pressure and consequently improve survival significantly (Bowen et al. 2016). If relapse episodes occur, the induction phase of antifungal therapy is extended to 4 to 8 weeks (WHO 2011). The timing of cART initiation was addressed in a clinical trial conducted in HIV-infected adults with cryptococcal meningitis. The results showed that 6-month mortality was significantly higher when cART was started within 2 weeks of starting cryptococcal induction therapy, compared to the deferment of cART initiation for 5 weeks (Boulware et al. 2014). Thus, cART is generally started 4 to 6 weeks after commencing antifungal therapy, irrespective of the degree of immunosuppression (Govender and Dlamini 2014).

Because cryptococcal meningitis is associated with high mortality even with appropriate therapy, two approaches have been used to prevent the development of this infection in HIV-infected adults. Primary antifungal prophylaxis can be considered in patients with a CD4 count of less than 100 cells/μL if there is anticipated delay in the start of cART. Alternatively, serum or plasma can be screened for cryptococcal antigen in patients with a CD4+ count of less than 100 cells/μL to identify patients with subclinical systemic cryptococcal infection prior to the development of meningitis. Subclinical cryptococcal infection can then be treated with fluconazole. The latter approach is recommended by the WHO and has been implemented in some countries (WHO 2011; Govender and Dlamini 2014). However, prevention therapy is currently not recommended for children (WHO 2011).

Viral Neuroinfections

A diverse spectrum of viruses can enter the CNS, causing acute and chronic neurological disorders. Virus-induced CNS diseases are influenced by routes of viral entry, viral tropism, and immune responses. In the immunocompetent host, CNS immune reactions limit the spread of the virus to contain the infection. In the HIV-infected immunocompromised child, this mechanism may be ineffective, leading to severe disease (Swanson and McGavern 2015).

PROGRESSIVE MULTIFOCAL LEUKOENCEPHALOPATHY

PML, which is caused by a neurotropic human polyomavirus, the John Cunningham virus, is rare in HIV-infected children. Fewer than 25 cases have been reported in the published literature (Nuttall et al. 2004; Shah and Chudgar 2005; Wilmshurst et al. 2006; Schwenk et al. 2014). The typical findings on MRI scans are symmetrical white-matter T2-hyperintense, T1-hypointense lesions without oedema, most common in the frontal and parieto-occipital regions (Schwenk et al. 2014). Definitive diagnosis of PML requires the detection of John Cunningham virus DNA in the CSF or in tissue obtained at brain biopsy (Wilmshurst, Eley, and Brew 2014). Although there are no effective antiviral drugs for this infection, administration of cART improves survival significantly (Schwenk et al. 2014). Glucocorticosteroid therapy may reverse the effects of PML-IRIS (Nuttall et al. 2004).

HERPES SIMPLEX VIRUSES (HSV-1 AND HSV-2)

Herpes simplex viruses (HSV-1 and HSV-2) cause meningitis and encephalitis in children. HSV initially infects keratinocytes, migrates to peripheral sensory neurons, and finally moves to the CNS. HSV-1 has also been thought to reach the CNS via olfactory sensory neurons whose dendrites are directly exposed to airways in the nose. HSV-1 establishes latency in the trigeminal ganglia following primary infection, and CNS infections can result from either the primary infection or reactivation of the latent virus. The virus has tropism for both the meninges and the cortical parenchyma, leading to meningitis and encephalitis respectively. The virus can also lead to meningoencephalitis when both the meninges and the cortical parenchyma are infected. Common symptoms of HSV meningitis include fever, headache, and neck stiffness (Swanson and McGavern 2015).

The mechanisms that drive HSV encephalitis remain unknown but histological analysis reveals perivascular inflammatory infiltrates, HSV-infected neurons, and engulfment of neurons by microglia

(Swanson and McGavern 2015). Some studies implicate a protective role for the immune system, as individuals with immunosuppression are more susceptible to HSV encephalitis (Bradford et al. 2009). Children with HSV encephalitis or meningoencephalitis present with fever, headache, altered personality, focal or generalised seizures, altered cognition, and disturbed consciousness (Whitley 2014). CSF examination shows pleocytosis and proteinosis, and polymerase chain reaction (PCR) detection of HSV DNA in the CSF confirms the diagnosis (Whitley 2014). HSV infection in both immunocompetent and HIV-infected persons is treated with acyclovir for 14 to 21 days. If untreated, there is a high fatality rate. Long-term neurological complications include seizures, developmental delay, and cognitive, memory, personality, and behavioural impairments (John et al. 2015).

Varicella-zoster Virus

Varicella-zoster virus (VZV) causes chicken pox as a primary infection, and it remains dormant in the cranial and dorsal root ganglia with the potential for reactivation as shingles (zoster) (Eshleman, Shahzad, and Cohrs 2011). Neurological complications occur with both the primary infection and with reactivation, especially in the immunocompromised host. Reactivated VZV can cause a wide variety of neurological disease. In many cases, subclinical meningeal irritation can occur, but HIV-infected persons may present with acute and severe meningoencephalitis, vasculitis, ventriculitis, severe necrotising myelitis, postherpetic neuralgia, and leukoencephalopathy (Annunziato and Gershon 1998; Corti 2000). Reactivation of the primary infection leading to neurological disease, without the classic herpes zoster exanthema, has been reported, confirming the ability of the latent virus to travel directly to the CNS without the classic skin involvement (Echevarria et al. 1994; Ibrahim et al. 2015). Fever, headache, nausea, vomiting, and signs of meningeal irritation are commonly seen but patients may present with papilloedema, sixth nerve palsies, diplopia, and elevated CSF opening pressures (Ibrahim et al. 2015). A positive VZV PCR in the CSF establishes this diagnosis. Treatment is intravenous acyclovir for 14 to 21 days (Corti 2000). Neurological sequelae include stroke, chronic pain, and major depression (John et al. 2015).

Cytomegalovirus Infection

CMV infection is common during childhood. In SSA, where HIV infection abounds, the burden of CMV disease has not been completely defined because of limited access to CMV diagnostics (Bates and Brantsaeter 2016). However, a recent study showed that maternal HIV infection was associated with high congenital CMV prevalence (Mwaanza et al. 2014). Although CMV infection may be acquired in utero or throughout childhood, research suggests that most children from SSA are infected with CMV during early infancy, irrespective of their HIV status (Bates and Brantsaeter 2016).

HIV infection tends to progress more rapidly in children coinfected with CMV (Siberry et al. 2013). Before cART was available, CMV end-organ disease was common in HIV-infected adults, particularly in those with a very low CD4 cell count of less than 50 cells/µL (Brantsaeter et al. 2002). In HIV-infected adults, the spectrum of neurological diseases includes encephalitis, retinitis, radiculitis, and myelitis (Bowen et al. 2016). End-organ disease of the nervous system has also been documented in HIV-infected children, CMV retinitis being the most frequent severe manifestation (Marriage et al. 1996; Zaknun et al. 1997; Siberry et al. 2013). After the introduction of cART, CMV disease has become relatively uncommon in HIV-infected children and adults (Gona et al. 2006; Slyker 2016).

Neurodevelopmental and hearing outcomes of symptomatic congenital CMV infection are improved with valganciclovir administered for 6 months (Kimberlin et al. 2015). Antiviral therapy should be considered for HIV-infected children with congenital infection (Siberry et al. 2013). CMV retinitis and other neurological manifestations should also be treated with anti-CMV agents. Combination therapy with ganciclovir and foscarnet is recommended for retinitis if ganciclovir monotherapy fails. Because of poor penetration into the CNS, combined therapy with ganciclovir and foscarnet is preferred for acquired CMV neurological disease (Siberry et al. 2013). Unfortunately, antiviral therapy is not widely available for treating CMV disease in HIV-infected children living in LMICs (Bates and Brantsaeter 2016).

JAPANESE ENCEPHALITIS VIRUS

Japanese encephalitis virus is transmitted between vertebrate animals by the *Culex* mosquito. Pigs act as reservoirs but do not exhibit symptoms (Kumar and Singh 2014). In humans, infection with Japanese encephalitis virus can be asymptomatic, or it can present as an acute undifferentiated febrile illness with an aseptic meningitis or encephalitis (Solomon 2003). The disease course starts with a prodrome of fever, headache, vomiting, and diarrhoea. This is followed, in hours to days, by severe neurological complications, notably delirium, seizures, axial rigidity, extrapyramidal signs, cranial nerve palsies, ataxia, focal deficits, paraplegia, and segmental sensory disturbances (Kumar and Singh 2014; John et al. 2015). Severe cases may be complicated by hyperventilation, raised intracranial pressure, and shock. In about a third of patients, death may occur in quick succession (Kumar and Singh 2014). In survivors, there is a gradual improvement over a period of weeks to a few months with sequelae, including polio-like lower motor neuron weakness (Kumar and Singh 2014).

CSF examination may be normal, or it may show mild to moderate pleocytosis with elevated protein but normal sugar. The mainstay for diagnosis is enzyme-linked immunosorbent assay (ELISA) in the CSF or serum, but PCR assays are now being employed. Neuroimaging reveals changes in the basal ganglia, thalamus, and the brainstem. Electrophysiological studies, including EEG and evoked potentials, are often abnormal (Kumar and Singh 2014). There is currently no definitive treatment, and management is supportive (Kumar and Singh 2014). Prevention is through vector control and immunisation. Among survivors, 30% to 50% have significant neurological, cognitive, or psychiatric sequelae (John et al. 2015).

COMPLICATIONS OF MEASLES

Children with vertically transmitted HIV infection have lower measles antibody titres due to inefficient transplacental transfer, rapid antibody decay, reduced response rates, and reduced immunologic memory following measles vaccination, making them susceptible to early measles infection with a more severe clinical course. In the severely immunocompromised child, there might not be a rash with a measles infection, and the mortality rate is higher than in immunocompetent children (Kaplan et al. 1992). The CNS complications of measles can occur within days or years of acute infection (Buchanan and Bonthius 2012).

Primary measles encephalitis occurs during active measles infection, with onset during the exanthem. The CSF has marked lymphocytic pleocytosis, mildly elevated protein, and normal glucose (Buchanan and Bonthius 2012). Treatment is largely supportive (Buchanan and Bonthius 2012).

Acute postinfectious measles encephalomyelitis, or measles-induced acute disseminated encephalomyelitis, is an immune-mediated demyelination disorder that occurs within weeks to months after the active infection or, rarely, after vaccination. It presents with motor and sensory deficits, ataxia, and mental status changes. The CSF shows mild to moderate lymphocytic pleocytosis, and MRI studies confirm disseminated white matter lesions in the brain and spinal cord (Buchanan and Bonthius 2012). Treatment includes high-dose intravenous glucocorticosteroid therapy, followed by an oral tapering course. Intravenous immunoglobulin and plasmapheresis are used in fulminant presentations (Pohl et al. 2016).

Measles inclusion body encephalitis affects immunocompromised children who, within the past year, have either been acutely infected with measles virus or vaccinated with a live-attenuated measles vaccine. It is caused by persistence of the infectious measles virus. HIV-infected children are at risk due to their immunodeficiency (Mustafa et al. 1993; Buchanan and Bonthius 2012). The presentation includes altered mental status, intractable focal seizures, focal motor deficits, cortical blindness, language or artic-ulation problems, and dysphagia (Mustafa et al. 1993; Buchanan and Bonthius 2012). Less frequently, patients present with autonomic manifestations (Buchanan and Bonthius 2012). There is no effective treatment, although prolonged intravenous ribavirin has achieved limited success (Mustafa et al. 1993; Freeman et al. 2004; Buchanan and Bonthius 2012).

Subacute sclerosing panencephalitis (SSPE) is a late complication of measles in children who are infected with the virus in early life; the earlier the age of measles infection, the greater the risk of devel-oping SSPE (Mekki et al. 2019). Mutations in the gene encoding the surface F protein, which enhances the fusion properties of the measles virus, promote invasion of neural cells. Persistent CNS infection precedes SSPE; however, the mechanisms by which the measles virus causes the disease remain unclear (Angius et al. 2019). SSPE typically presents 6 to 15 years after primary measles. In the early stages, patients present with behavioural problems and declining cognition. This is followed by motor dysfunc-tion, notably myoclonic jerks, dyskinesia, cerebellar ataxia, and, later, rigidity. Necrotising retinitis, optic neuritis, and cortical blindness can occur. With disease progression, patients lapse into a stupor, mutism, autonomic instability, and, eventually, death (Buchanan and Bonthius 2012; Griffin 2014; Mekki et al. 2019). In the antiretroviral-naïve HIV-infected child, this disease may manifest earlier with a more ful-minant and rapidly progressive course (Manesh et al. 2017). The diagnosis of SSPE is confirmed by the detection of high levels of measles-specific antibodies in the CSF and in the serum. Electroencephalogram shows characteristic periodic slow-wave complexes with burst αsuppression. Neuroimaging is typical for focal leukodystrophy and diffuse cortical atrophy (Buchanan and Bonthius 2012; Kija et al. 2015). Therapeutic agents have been used to slow down the progression of SSPE, the most common being a combination of Isoprinosine and interferon-α (Gascon and International Consortium on Subacute Sclerosing Panencephalitis 2003; Griffin 2014). Carbamazepine may decrease the myoclonic jerks in SSPE (Ravikumar and Crawford 2013).

NEUROLOGICAL ASSOCIATIONS OF COVID-19

Although predominantly a respiratory disease, neurological manifestations have been reported in chil-dren with SARS-CoV-2 infection, including encephalopathy, Guillain-Barré syndrome, headaches, brainstem and cerebellar signs, muscle weakness, and reduced reflexes. These manifestations are thought to either be from direct effects of the virus on the nervous system, para- or post-infectious immune-mediated disease, or neurological complications of the systemic COVID-19 infection (Abdel-Mannan et al. 2020; Ellul et al. 2020). There are suggestions that HIV-infected children might be at increased risk of SARS-CoV-2 infection or severe COVID-19, especially those with comorbidity, lower CD4 count, or high HIV RNA load. By contrast, HIV-associated immunosuppression might protect HIV-infected individuals from developing the cytokine storm observed in severe COVID-19 (Xu, Zhang, and Wang 2020). Further studies are required to explore these hypotheses.

Cerebral Malaria

HIV infection and malaria are leading causes of under-5 mortality globally. They share significant geo-graphical overlap, particularly in SSA. In 2019, about 229 million malaria episodes and about 409 000 malaria-related deaths occurred globally, with more than 93% of cases and 89% of deaths occurring in

SSA (WHO 2020). The most prevalent malarial species in SSA, *Plasmodium falciparum,* causes almost 99% of malaria deaths. Of these deaths, 67% occur in children less than 5 years old (WHO 2020). Cerebral malaria accounts for more than half of malaria-related deaths (Carme, Bouquety, and Plassart 1993). The WHO defines cerebral malaria as an unarousable coma, with asexual *P. falciparum* parasitaemia, and absence of other causes of coma (WHO 2000). HIV coinfection increases the frequency of malaria episodes and also increases the risk for severe malaria (Whitworth et al. 2000; Grimwade et al. 2003; Bronzan et al. 2007), especially in areas of unstable malaria transmission. HIV coinfection additionally increases with worsening immune suppression (Whitworth et al. 2000; Grimwade et al. 2004; Cohen et al. 2005; Korenromp et al. 2005). HIV coinfection is also associated with higher parasite load and poor parasite clearance, suggesting enhanced parasite replication in the HIV-infected, as well as a probable increased ability to transmit malaria (Bharti et al. 2012). Malaria, conversely, increases HIV replication, reduces CD4 cell counts, and promotes the spread of HIV infection (Kublin et al. 2005; Mermin, Lule, and Ekwaru 2006).

The effect of HIV infection on cerebral malaria presentation and outcome has been inconsistent, partially due to the challenges of cerebral malaria definition. Some have used the WHO definition of cerebral malaria, while others use a more stringent retinopathy positive cerebral malaria (RPCM), i.e. the WHO-defined cerebral malaria with patchy retinal whitening, vessel colour changes, or white-centred haemorrhages (Taylor et al. 2004). Also, up to 25% of children with RPCM have co-viral infections, which significantly impacts mortality (Mallewa et al. 2013). In children with WHO-defined cerebral malaria, HIV infection is a risk factor for cerebral malaria and malaria-related mortality, irrespective of the degree of immunosuppression. However, in those with RPCM, HIV coinfection was associated with a longer duration of time required to fully recover from a coma, but this does not appear to be associated with increased mortality (Hochman et al. 2015; Seydel et al. 2015; Mbale et al. 2016). The only consistent finding is that of patients with HIV coinfection being older children, and this is thought to be due to loss of malaria immunity with HIV disease progression (Tembo et al. 2014; Hochman et al. 2015; Mbale et al. 2016).

In children with RPCM, MRI findings include basal ganglia defects, increased cerebral volume, and white matter, pons, brainstem, and diffuse cortical changes (Potchen et al. 2012). Increased brain volume on MRI is directly related to mortality (Seydel et al. 2015). Differences between HIV-infected and uninfected children have not been delineated.

About 10% of children with cerebral malaria develop permanent neurological sequelae, including gross motor deficits, epilepsy, ataxia, visual, hearing, and speech impairments, and neurocognitive deficits (Roca-Feltrer, Carneiro, and Armstrong Schellenberg 2008). The effect of HIV coinfection on the spectrum and severity of neurodisabilities in cerebral malaria has not been studied.

In HIV-infected individuals, intravenous artesunate is a recommended drug for cerebral malaria, usually until consciousness is regained or until 7 days of use. This is followed by 3-day oral artemisinin-based combination therapy once oral intake is possible (WHO 2015). Alternatives include intramuscular artesunate, parenteral artemether, or quinine. Suspicion of cerebral malaria should prompt immediate treatment before diagnosis is confirmed, and other neuroinfections should be actively sought. Use of artesunate/amodiaquine is associated with increased risk of neutropenia in HIV coinfected individuals, especially those on zidovudine or cotrimoxazole prophylaxis (Gasasira et al. 2008). Efavirenz is also associated with higher risk of hepatotoxicity in patients on artesunate/amodiaquine combination (German et al. 2007).

Long-term cotrimoxazole prophylaxis in HIV-infected individuals reduces the incidence of malaria (Bwakura-Dangarembizi et al. 2014). Additional prophylaxis with sulfadoxine/pyrimethamine in HIV-infected pregnant females or infants on cotrimoxazole prophylaxis is not recommended (WHO 2015) Four doses of malaria vaccine RTS,S/AS01 reduces malaria episodes and severe malaria in children, and it has a good safety profile and immunogenicity in HIV-infected children on antiretroviral therapy and cotrimoxazole (Otieno et al. 2016).

Non-malarial Parasitic Neuroinfections

Besides cerebral malaria, parasitic neuroinfections of importance in HIV infection include cerebral toxoplasmosis, neurocysticercosis, neuroschistosomiasis, and both American and African forms of trypanosomiasis.

Cerebral Toxoplasmosis

The risk of cerebral toxoplasmosis is high in HIV-infected individuals who are seropositive for *Toxoplasma gondii*, especially in HIV-infected adults with CD4+ counts less than 100 cells/µL and who are not on antimicrobial prophylaxis (Belanger et al. 1999; Bowen et al. 2016). This risk is substantially reduced by administering cART (B-Lajoie et al. 2016). In HIV-infected children, toxoplasmosis is often due to reactivation of a latent infection (Mallewa and Wilmshurst 2014). Toxoplasmosis usually manifests with cerebral abscesses. Abscess formation may mimic a neoplasm. Less frequently, it causes diffuse encephalitis or chorioretinitis in HIV-infected individuals (Bowen et al. 2016).

Neurocysticercosis

Globally, neurocysticercosis is both the most common CNS parasitic infection and the most common cause of acquired epilepsy (Zhao et al. 2016). There are relatively few case reports of HIV-neurocysticercosis coinfection, even in regions such as SSA, where both HIV infection and *Taenia solium* infestation are highly prevalent (Figure 7.2) (Serpa et al. 2007; Anand et al. 2015; Schmidt et al. 2016). One matched cross-sectional study from northern Tanzania reported no significant differences between HIV-infected and uninfected individuals in the seroprevalence of *T. solium* and cysticercosis antibodies or in cysticercosis antigenaemia (Schmidt et al. 2016).

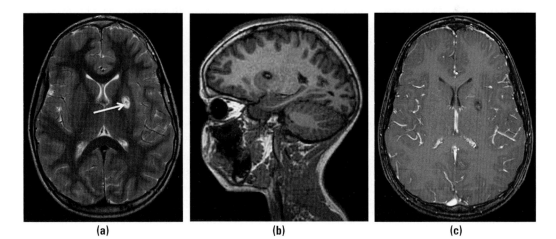

(a)   (b)   (c)

Figure 7.2   Colloidial vesticular stage of neurocysticercosis in a 3-year-old HIV-positive patient with focal seizures. **(a)** T2-weighted axial MRI scan: Ovoid cyst within the left lentiform nucleus containing a low signal eccentric scolex (white arrow) with a superior rim of subtle high signal inflammatory oedema. **(b)** T1-weighted sagittal MRI scan: High signal scolex within a cyst that returns signal isointense to that of CSF. **(c)** T1-weighted gadolinium enhanced axial MRI scan: Demonstrating superior rim enhancement.

Schistosomiasis

Schistosomiasis affects more than 200 million individuals, more than 90% of whom live in SSA. More than 60% of children in Africa have schistosome infections (Mutapi 2015). Neuroschistosomiasis, a severe form of this infection, affects less than 5% of patients with schistosomiasis (Ross et al. 2012). Both cerebral and spinal manifestations can occur as a result of egg deposition and granuloma formation. Cerebral schistosomiasis is more common with *Schistosoma japonicum* infection, and myelopathy is frequently caused by *S. mansoni* and *S. haematobium* (Ross et al. 2012). Schistosomiasis may impair cognition and short-term memory among children (Jukes et al. 2002). Few cases of neuroschistosomiasis have been described in HIV-infected individuals, so the effects of coinfections have not been elucidated (Mallewa and Wilmshurst 2014).

Trypanosomiasis

Human African trypanosomiasis is caused by *Trypanosoma brucei gambiense* in western and central Africa and *T. brucei rhodesiense* in eastern Africa. Stage two of this disease presents with CNS manifestations, including classic sleep disturbances (Walker, Kublin, and Zunt 2006). Limited research on HIV-infected individuals suggests that they are at a higher risk for treatment failure and poor outcome (Pepin et al. 1992). Chagas disease, caused by *T. cruzi*, is endemic in the Americas. In endemic countries 1.3% to 7.1% of HIV-infected individuals are chronically infected with *T. cruzi*. In the absence of cART, reactivation of Chagas disease occurs in 15% to 35% of coinfected patients (Corti 2000; Sartori et al. 2007; Perez-Molina 2014). Single or multiple space-occupying lesions or meningoencephalitis are common manifestations of reactivation disease in HIV-infected individuals (Perez-Molina 2014).

PREVENTION BY IMMUNISATION

Routine immunisation is one of the most important and effective public health interventions for preventing disease. Several vaccines used in national immunisation programmes provide substantial protection against neurological infections in HIV-infected children, including Hib, pneumococcal and meningococcal protein-conjugate vaccines, Bacille Calmette-Guérin live-attenuated vaccine, measles live-attenuated vaccine, and Japanese encephalitis inactivated and live-attenuated vaccines.

The efficacy of the RTS,S/AS01 malaria vaccine directed against *Plasmodium falciparum* in children who are 5 through 17 months old after a four-dose schedule, was 39.0% at 48 months (RTS and S Clinical Trials Partnership 2015). The WHO has recognised the public health potential of the RTS,S/AS01 vaccine and has recommended further evaluation of this vaccine before country-level introduction is considered. Pilot implementation studies are currently underway in Ghana, Kenya, and Malawi (WHO 2016). Besides the RTS,S/AS01 vaccine there are more than 30 other malarial vaccines in development (WHO 2016). Non-typhoid *Salmonella enterica* serovars are important causes of invasive bacterial infection, including meningitis in SSA. Although vaccines for the predominant NTS serovars, Typhimurium and Enteritidis, are under development, a multivalent vaccine that targets five through six serovars may ultimately be required to protect against most NTS disease (Tennant et al. 2016). New and safer vaccines against TB are in development or are being evaluated in human trials (Kaufmann 2014). There are currently no vaccines for most of the other neuroinfections that affect HIV-infected individuals, including cryptococcal meningitis, CMV encephalitis, HSV encephalitis, and PML.

Because HIV infection causes dysfunction of both T- and B-lymphocyte compartments, the effectiveness and sustainability of the immunological response after immunisation may be compromised (Cagigi et al. 2012). Intervention with cART, particularly when initiated during early infancy, is important for preserving existing immunity, reversing immunodeficiency and improving subsequent responses to immunisation (Pensieroso et al. 2009; Cagigi et al. 2012). Therefore, optimising cART administration is essential for maximising the effectiveness of current and future vaccines for the prevention of neuro-infections in HIV-infected children.

RESEARCH GAPS

Despite an ever-expanding body of information on paediatric HIV infection and its consequences, there are many gaps in our knowledge of the neuroinfections affecting HIV-infected children (Table 7.2).

Access to affordable and accurate rapid diagnostic tests, particularly point-of-care tests, and inexpensive neuroimaging modalities are major factors limiting our understanding of the epidemiology of neuroinfections, as well as the impact of HIV infection on the clinical presentation, neuroimaging features, and outcome of many neuroinfections. Several initiatives have been taken to overcome these diagnostic challenges (Yansouni et al. 2013). Inadequate diagnostic capacity also limits access to effective care, including existing antimicrobial therapies. Development of new classes of antimicrobial agents are needed to overcome adverse event profiles of existing therapies and to treat neuroinfections for which there are currently no effective therapies, including many viral infections. Supportive interventions such as fluid therapy, nutrition, and immunomodulatory agents, as well as the timing of cART, should be evaluated to improve the overall care and outcome of HIV-infected children with neuroinfections.

Table 7.2 Research priorities for the neuroinfections.

Research area	Important research foci
Pathogenesis	• Host response pathways in HIV-infected children with neuroinfections • The role of host response in disease containment, clinical manifestations, and neurodisability • Pathogen-specific factors producing neuroinfections in HIV-infected children • The role of the human microbiome in the pathogenesis of neuroinfections • Pathogenic differences between HIV-infected children, adolescents, and adults
Diagnosis	• Accurate and inexpensive point-of-care tests • Low-cost neuroimaging modalities • The role of innovative technologies in the design of new diagnostics • Improved diagnostics in the face of immunodeficiency, especially serological assays • Simple screening tools for identifying neurodisability and neurocognitive deficits
Epidemiology	• Incidence and distribution of neuroinfections among HIV-infected children • Determinants of mortality, neurodisability, and neurocognitive deficits
Disease presentation	• Impact of HIV infection on the clinical and neuroimaging manifestations of neuroinfections • Spectrum and severity of neurodisability
Treatment	• New and safer antimicrobial therapies • Optimisation of adjunctive therapies • Development of effective therapies that do not require intravenous administration • Appropriateness and timing of cART in HIV-infected children with neuroinfections
Prevention	• New, more effective and safer vaccines for preventing neuroinfections • Role of adjuvants in optimising vaccine responses in HIV-infected children • Ideal vaccine administration in relation to cART • Improved vector control programmes, including environment-friendly insecticide-based interventions

Improved preventative measures such as new vaccines and vector control programmes are also required (John et al. 2015). Anticipated improvements in the effectiveness of the global prevention of mother-to-child transmission intervention strategy and cART coverage among HIV-infected children should further reduce the size of the paediatric HIV epidemic and the burden of neuroinfections in HIV-infected children, resulting in fewer opportunities to research the interactions between paediatric HIV infection and a range of neuroinfections. Advancement in knowledge will thus depend on collaborative, multi-centre studies on children, and improvement in care will continue to rely on adult studies for the foreseeable future.

REFERENCES

Abdel-Mannan O, Eyre M, Löbel U et al. (2020) Neurologic and radiographic findings associated with COVID-19 infection in children. *JAMA Neurology*, 77(11): 1440–1445. doi: 10.1001/jamaneurol.2020.2687.

Anand KS, Wadhwa A, Garg J et al. (2015) HIV-associated neurocysticercosis. *J Int Assoc Provid AIDS Care*, 14(2): 120–122. doi: 10.1177/2325957414555232.

Angius F, Smuts H, Rybkina K et al. (2019) Analysis of a subacute sclerosing panencephalitis genotype B3 virus from the 2009–2010 South African measles epidemic shows that hyperfusogenic F proteins contribute to measles virus infection in the brain. *Journal of Virology*, 93(4): e01700–01718. doi: 10.1128/JVI.01700-18.

Annunziato P, Gershon A (1998) *Herpesvirus Infections in Children Infected with HIV*. Baltimore: Williams & Wilkins.

Ansari AW, Ahmad F, Meyer-Olson D et al. (2015) Natural killer cell heterogeneity: Cellular dysfunction and significance in HIV-1 immuno-pathogenesis. *Cell Mol Life Sci*, 72(16): 3037–3049. doi: 10.1007/s00018-015-1911-5.

Azzoni L, Barbour R, Papasavvas E et al. (2015) Early ART results in greater immune reconstitution benefits in HIV-infected infants: Working with data missingness in a longitudinal dataset. *PLoS One*, 10(12): e0145320. doi: 10.1371/journal.pone.0145320.

B-Lajoie M, Drouin O, Bartlett G et al. (2016) Incidence and prevalence of opportunistic and other infections and the impact of antiretroviral therapy among HIV-infected children in low- and middle-income countries: A systematic review and meta-analysis. *Clin Infect Dis*, 62(12): 1586–1594. doi: 10.1093/cid/ciw139.

Badley AD, Pilon AA, Landay A et al. (2000) Mechanisms of HIV-associated lymphocyte apoptosis. *Blood*, 96(9): 2951–2964. doi: 10.1182/blood.V96.9.2951.

Bahr N, Boulware DR, Marais S et al. (2013) Central nervous system immune reconstitution inflammatory syndrome. *Curr Infect Dis Rep*, 15(6): 583–593. doi: 10.1007/s11908-013-0378-5.

Bates M, Brantsaeter AB (2016) Human cytomegalovirus (CMV) in Africa: A neglected but important pathogen. *J Virus Erad*, 2(3): 136–142. doi: 10.1016/S2055-6640(20)30456-8.

Belanger F, Derouin F, Grangeot-Keros L et al. (1999) Incidence and risk factors of toxoplasmosis in a cohort of human immunodeficiency virus-infected patients: 1988–1995. HEMOCO and SEROCO Study Groups. *Clin Infect Dis*, 28(3): 575–581. doi: 10.1086/515147.

Bertrand J, Verstuyft C, Chou M et al. (2014) Dependence of efavirenz- and rifampicin-isoniazid-based antituberculosis treatment drug-drug interaction on CYP2B6 and NAT2 genetic polymorphisms: ANRS 12154 study in Cambodia. *J Infect Dis*, 209(3): 399–408. doi: 10.1093/infdis/jit466.

Bharti AR, Saravanan S, Madhavan V et al. (2012) Correlates of HIV and malaria co-infection in Southern India. *Malar J*, 11306. doi: 10.1186/1475-2875-11-306.

Boulware DR, Meya DB, Muzoora C et al. (2014) Timing of antiretroviral therapy after diagnosis of cryptococcal meningitis. *N Engl J Med* 370(26): 2487–2498. doi: 10.1056/NEJMoa1312884.

Bowen LN, Smith B, Reich D et al. (2016) HIV-associated opportunistic CNS infections: Pathophysiology, diagnosis and treatment. *Nat Rev Neurol*, 12(11): 662–674. doi: 10.1038/nrneurol.2016.149.

Bradford RD, Pettit AC, Wright PW et al. (2009) Herpes simplex encephalitis during treatment with tumor necrosis factor-alpha inhibitors. *Clin Infect Dis*, 49(6): 924–927. doi: 10.1086/605498.

Brantsaeter AB, Liestol K, Goplen AK et al. (2002) CMV disease in AIDS patients: Incidence of CMV disease and relation to survival in a population-based study from Oslo. *Scand J Infect Dis*, 34(1): 50–55. doi: 10.1080/00365540110076976.

Bronzan RN, Taylor TE, Mwenechanya J et al. (2007) Bacteremia in Malawian children with severe malaria: Prevalence, etiology, HIV coinfection, and outcome. *J Infect Dis*, 195(6): 895–904. doi: 10.1086/511437.

Brouwer MC, McIntyre P, Prasad K et al. (2015) Corticosteroids for acute bacterial meningitis. *Cochrane Database Syst Rev*, (9): CD004405. doi: 10.1002/14651858.CD004405.pub5.

Buchanan R, Bonthius DJ (2012) Measles virus and associated central nervous system sequelae. *Semin Pediatr Neurol*, 19(3): 107–114. doi: 10.1016/j.spen.2012.02.003.

Bwakura-Dangarembizi M, Kendall L, Bakeera-Kitaka S et al. (2014) A randomized trial of prolonged co-trimoxazole in HIV-infected children in Africa. *N Engl J Med*, 370(1): 41–53. doi: 10.1056/NEJMoa1214901.

Cagigi A, Cotugno N, Giaquinto C et al. (2012) Immune reconstitution and vaccination outcome in HIV-1 infected children: Present knowledge and future directions. *Hum Vaccin Immunother*, 8(12): 1784–1794. doi: 10.4161/hv.21827.

Carme B, Bouquety JC, Plassart H (1993) Mortality and sequelae due to cerebral malaria in African children in Brazzaville, Congo. *Am J Trop Med Hyg*, 48(2): 216–221. doi: 10.4269/ajtmh.1993.48.216.

Cohen C, Karstaedt A, Frean J et al. (2005) Increased prevalence of severe malaria in HIV-infected adults in South Africa. *Clin Infect Dis*, 41(11): 1631–1637. doi: 10.1086/498023.

Cohen K, van Cutsem G, Boulle A et al. (2008) Effect of rifampicin-based antitubercular therapy on nevirapine plasma concentrations in South African adults with HIV-associated tuberculosis. *J Antimicrob Chemother*, 61(2): 389–393. doi: 10.1093/jac/dkm484.

Collins I, Ngo-Giang-Huong N, Jourdain G et al. (2013) *Long-term immune response in HIV-infected children receiving highly active antiretroviral therapy in Thailand: Outcomes at 7 years.* In 7th IAS Conference on HIV Pathogenesis, Treatment and Prevention. Kuala Lumpur, Malaysia Abstract TUPE314. doi: 10.1097/COH.0000000000000027.

Corti M (2000) AIDS and Chagas' disease. *AIDS Patient Care STDS*, 14(11): 581–588. doi: 10.1089/10872910050193752.

Davis S, Feikin D, Johnson HL (2013) The effect of *Haemophilus influenzae* type B and pneumococcal conjugate vaccines on childhood meningitis mortality: A systematic review. *BMC Public Health*, 13(Suppl 3): S21. doi: 10.1186/1471-2458-13-S3-S21.

Day JN, Chau TT, Wolbers M et al. (2013) Combination antifungal therapy for cryptococcal meningitis. *N Engl J Med*, 368(14): 1291–1302. doi: 10.1056/NEJMoa1110404.

De Rossi A, Walker AS, Klein N et al. (2002) Increased thymic output after initiation of antiretroviral therapy in human immunodeficiency virus type 1-infected children in the Paediatric European Network for Treatment of AIDS (PENTA) 5 Trial. *J Infect Dis*, 186(3): 312–320. doi: 10.1086/341657.

Doitsh G, Galloway NL, Geng X et al. (2014) Cell death by pyroptosis drives CD4 T-cell depletion in HIV-1 infection. *Nature*, 505(7484): 509–514. doi: 10.1038/nature12940.

Donald KA, Hoare J, Eley B et al. (2014) Neurologic complications of pediatric human immunodeficiency virus: Implications for clinical practice and management challenges in the African setting. *Semin Pediatr Neurol*, 21(1): 3–11. doi: 10.1016/j.spen.2014.01.004.

Dooley KE, Denti P, Martinson N et al. (2015) Pharmacokinetics of efavirenz and treatment of HIV-1 among pregnant women with and without tuberculosis coinfection. *J Infect Dis*, 211(2): 197–205. doi: 10.1093/infdis/jiu429.

Echevarria JM, Casas I, Tenorio A et al. (1994) Detection of varicella-zoster virus-specific DNA sequences in cerebrospinal fluid from patients with acute aseptic meningitis and no cutaneous lesions. *J Med Virol*, 43(4): 331–335. doi: 10.1002/jmv.1890430403.

Eley B (2003) The immunology of HIV infection. *Current Allergy & Clinical Immunology*, 16(2): 40–46.

Eley B, Nuttall J (2007) Antiretroviral therapy for children: Challenges and opportunities. *Ann Trop Paediatr*, 27(1): 1–10. doi: 10.1179/146532807X170448.

Ellul MA, Benjamin L, Singh B et al. (2020) Neurological associations of COVID-19. *The Lancet Neurology*, 19(9): 767–783. doi: 10.1016/S1474-4422(20)30221-0.

Eshleman E, Shahzad A, Cohrs RJ (2011) Varicella zoster virus latency. *Future Virol*, 6(3): 341–355. doi: 10.2217/fvl.10.90.

Freeman AF, Jacobsohn DA, Shulman ST et al. (2004) A new complication of stem cell transplantation: Measles inclusion body encephalitis. *Pediatrics*, 114(5): e657–660. doi: 10.1542/peds.2004-0949.

Gasasira AF, Kamya MR, Achan J et al. (2008) High risk of neutropenia in HIV-infected children following treatment with artesunate plus amodiaquine for uncomplicated malaria in Uganda. *Clin Infect Dis*, 46(7): 985–991. doi: 10.1086/529192.

Gascon GG, International Consortium on Subacute Sclerosing Panencephalitis (2003) Randomized treatment study of inosiplex versus combined inosiplex and intraventricular interferon-alpha in subacute sclerosing panencephalitis (SSPE): International multicenter study. *J Child Neurol*, 18(12): 819–827. doi: 10.1177/088307380301801201.

Gengiah TN, Holford NH, Botha JH et al. (2012) The influence of tuberculosis treatment on efavirenz clearance in patients co-infected with HIV and tuberculosis. *Eur J Clin Pharmacol*, 68(5): 689–695. doi: 10.1007/s00228-011-1166-5.

German P, Greenhouse B, Coates C et al. (2007) Hepatotoxicity due to a drug interaction between amodiaquine plus artesunate and efavirenz. *Clin Infect Dis*, 44(6): 889–891. doi: 10.1086/511882.

Gibb DM, Newberry A, Klein N et al. (2000) Immune repopulation after HAART in previously untreated HIV-1-infected children. Paediatric European Network for Treatment of AIDS (PENTA) Steering Committee. *Lancet*, 355(9212): 1331–1332. doi: 10.1016/S0140-6736(00)02117-6.

Gona P, Van Dyke RB, Williams PL et al. (2006) Incidence of opportunistic and other infections in HIV-infected children in the HAART era. *JAMA*, 296(3): 292–300. doi: 10.1001/jama.296.3.292.

Govender NP, Dlamini S (2014) Management of HIV-associated cryptococcal disease in South Africa. *S Afr Med J*, 104(12): 896. doi: 10.7196/SAMJ.9070.

Griffin DE (2014) Measles virus and the nervous system. *Handbook of Clinical Neurology* 123577–123590. doi: 10.1016/B978-0-444-53488-0.00027-4.

Grimwade K, French N, Mbatha DD et al. (2003) Childhood malaria in a region of unstable transmission and high human immunodeficiency virus prevalence. *Pediatr Infect Dis J*, 22(12): 1057–1063. doi: 10.1097/01.inf.0000101188.95433.60.

Grimwade K, French N, Mbatha DD et al. (2004) HIV infection as a cofactor for severe falciparum malaria in adults living in a region of unstable malaria transmission in South Africa. *AIDS*, 18(3): 547–554.

Gumbo T, Kadzirange G, Mielke J et al. (2002) *Cryptococcus neoformans* meningoencephalitis in African children with acquired immunodeficiency syndrome. *Pediatr Infect Dis J*, 21(1): 54–56.

Haynes BF, Hale LP, Weinhold KJ et al. (1999) Analysis of the adult thymus in reconstitution of T lymphocytes in HIV-1 infection. *J Clin Invest*, 103(6): 921. doi: 10.1172/JCI5201.

Hochman SE, Madaline TF, Wassmer SC et al. (2015) Fatal pediatric cerebral malaria is associated with intravascular monocytes and platelets that are increased with HIV coinfection. *MBio*, 6(5): e01390–01315. doi: 10.1128/mBio.01390--15.

Ibrahim W, Elzouki AN, Husain A et al. (2015) Varicella zoster aseptic meningitis: Report of an atypical case and literature review. *Am J Case Rep*, 16594–597. doi: 10.12659/AJCR.894045.

John CC, Carabin H, Montano SM et al. (2015) Global research priorities for infections that affect the nervous system. *Nature*, 527(7578): S178–S186. doi: 10.1038/nature16033.

Jones RB, Walker BD (2016) HIV-specific CD8(+) T cells and HIV eradication. *J Clin Invest*, 126(2): 455–463. doi: 10.1172/JCI80566.

Jukes MC, Nokes CA, Alcock KJ et al. (2002) Heavy schistosomiasis associated with poor short-term memory and slower reaction times in Tanzanian schoolchildren. *Trop Med Int Health*, 7(2): 104–117. doi: 10.1046/j.1365-3156.2002.00843.x.

Kalk E, Technau K, Hendson W et al. (2013) Paradoxical Mycobacterium tuberculosis meningitis immune reconstitution inflammatory syndrome in an HIV-infected child. *Pediatr Infect Dis J*, 32(2): 157–162. doi: 10.1097/INF.0b013e31827031aa.

Kampmann B, Tena GN, Mzazi S et al. (2004) Novel human in vitro system for evaluating antimycobacterial vaccines. *Infect Immun*, 72(11): 6401–6407. doi: 10.1128/IAI.72.11.6401-6407.2004.

Kampmann B, Tena-Coki GN, Nicol MP et al. (2006) Reconstitution of antimycobacterial immune responses in HIV-infected children receiving HAART. *AIDS*, 20(7): 1011–1018. doi: 10.1097/01.aids.0000222073.45372.ce.

Kaplan LJ, Daum RS, Smaron M et al. (1992) Severe measles in immunocompromised patients. *JAMA*, 267(9): 1237–1241. doi: 10.1001/jama.1992.03480090085032.

Kaufmann SH (2014) Tuberculosis vaccine development at a divide. *Curr Opin Pulm Med*, 20(3): 294–300. doi: 10.1097/MCP.0000000000000041.

Kija E, Ndondo A, Spittal G et al. (2015) Subacute sclerosing panencephalitis in South African children following the measles outbreak between 2009 and 2011. *S Afr Med J*, 105(9): 713718. doi: 10.7196/SAMJNEW.7788.

Kimberlin DW, Jester PM, Sanchez PJ et al. (2015) Valganciclovir for symptomatic congenital cytomegalovirus disease. *N Engl J Med*, 372(10): 933–943. doi: 10.1056/NEJMoa1404599.

Korenromp EL, Williams BG, de Vlas SJ et al. (2005) Malaria attributable to the HIV-1 epidemic, sub-Saharan Africa. *Emerg Infect Dis*, 11(9): 1410–1419. doi: 10.3201/eid1109.050337.

Krogstad P, Patel K, Karalius B et al. (2015) Incomplete immune reconstitution despite virologic suppression in HIV-1 infected children and adolescents. *AIDS*, 29(6): 683–693. doi: 10.1097/QAD.0000000000000598.

Kublin JG, Patnaik P, Jere CS et al. (2005) Effect of Plasmodium falciparum malaria on concentration of HIV-1-RNA in the blood of adults in rural Malawi: A prospective cohort study. *Lancet*, 365(9455): 233–240. doi: 10.1016/S0140-6736(05)17743-5.

Kumar R, Singh RR (2014) Japanese encephalitis. In: Singhi P, Griffin DE, Newton CR, editors, *Central Nervous System Infections in Childhood* (International Review of Child Neurology Series). London: Mac Keith Press, pp. 126–135.

Kwan CK, Ernst JD (2011) HIV and tuberculosis: A deadly human syndemic. *Clin Microbiol Rev*, 24(2): 351–376. doi: 10.1128/CMR.00042-10.

Lancella L, Galli L, Chiappini E et al. (2016) Recommendations concerning the therapeutic approach to immunocompromised children with tuberculosis. *Clin Ther*, 38(1): 180–190. doi: 10.1016/j.clinthera.2015.10.012.

Lewis J, Walker AS, Castro H et al. (2012) Age and CD4 count at initiation of antiretroviral therapy in HIV-infected children: Effects on long-term T-cell reconstitution. *J Infect Dis*, 205(4): 548–556. doi: 10.1093/infdis/jir787.

Luetkemeyer AF, Rosenkranz SL, Lu D et al. (2015) Combined effect of CYP2B6 and NAT2 genotype on plasma efavirenz exposure during rifampin-based antituberculosis therapy in the STRIDE study. *Clin Infect Dis*, 60(12): 1860–1863. doi: 10.1093/cid/civ155.

Maconochie IK, Bhaumik S (2016) Fluid therapy for acute bacterial meningitis. *Cochrane Database Syst Rev*, 11CD004786. doi: 10.1002/14651858.CD004786.pub.5.

Madhi SA, Madhi A, Petersen K et al. (2001) Impact of human immunodeficiency virus type 1 infection on the epidemiology and outcome of bacterial meningitis in South African children. *Int J Infect Dis*, 5(3): 119–125. doi: 10.1016/S1201-9712(01)90085-2.

Mallewa M, Vallely P, Faragher B et al. (2013) Viral CNS infections in children from a malaria-endemic area of Malawi: A prospective cohort study. *Lancet Glob Health*, 1(3): e153–160. doi: 10.1016/S2214-109X(13)70060-3.

Mallewa M, Wilmshurst JM (2014) Overview of the effect and epidemiology of parasitic central nervous system infections in African children. *Semin Pediatr Neurol*, 21(1): 19–25. doi: 10.1016/j.spen.2014.02.003.

Manesh A, Moorthy M, Bandopadhyay R et al. (2017) HIV-associated sub-acute sclerosing panencephalitis – An emerging threat? *Int J STD & AIDS*, 28(9): 937–939. doi: 10.1177/0956462416687675.

Marais S, Meintjes G, Pepper DJ et al. (2013) Frequency, severity, and prediction of tuberculous meningitis immune reconstitution inflammatory syndrome. *Clin Infect Dis*, 56(3): 450–460. doi: 10.1093/cid/cis899.

Marriage SC, Booy R, Hermione Lyall EG et al. (1996) Cytomegalovirus myelitis in a child infected with human immunodeficiency virus type 1. *Pediatr Infect Dis J*, 15(6): 549–551.

Mbale EW, Moxon CA, Mukaka M et al. (2016) HIV coinfection influences the inflammatory response but not the outcome of cerebral malaria in Malawian children. *J Infect*, 73(3): 189–199. doi: 10.1016/j.jinf.2016.05.012.

McCormick DW, Wilson ML, Mankhambo L et al. (2013) Risk factors for death and severe sequelae in Malawian children with bacterial meningitis, 1997–2010. *Pediatr Infect Dis J*, 32(2): e54–e61. doi: 10.1097/INF.0b013e-31826faf5a.

McIlleron H, Ren Y, Nuttall J et al. (2011) Lopinavir exposure is insufficient in children given double doses of lopinavir/ritonavir during rifampicin-based treatment for tuberculosis. *Antivir Ther*, 16(3): 417–421. doi: 10.3851/IMP1757.

McIlleron HM, Schomaker M, Ren Y et al. (2013) Effects of rifampin-based antituberculosis therapy on plasma efavirenz concentrations in children vary by CYP2B6 genotype. *AIDS*, 27(12): 1933–1940. doi: 10.1097/qad.0b013e328360dbb4.

McMichael AJ, Rowland-Jones SL (2001) Cellular immune responses to HIV. *Nature*, 410(6831): 980–987. doi: 10.1038/35073658.

McMullan BJ, Andresen D, Blyth CC et al. (2016) Antibiotic duration and timing of the switch from intravenous to oral route for bacterial infections in children: Systematic review and guidelines. *Lancet Infect Dis* 16(8): e139–152. doi: 10.1016/S1473-3099(16)30024-X.

Meiring ST, Quan VC, Cohen C et al. (2012) A comparison of cases of paediatric-onset and adult-onset cryptococcosis detected through population-based surveillance, 2005–2007. *AIDS*, 26(18): 2307–2314. doi: 10.1097/QAD.0b013e3283570567.

Mekki M, Eley B, Hardie D et al. (2019) Subacute sclerosing panencephalitis: Clinical phenotype, epidemiology, and preventive interventions. *Developmental Medicine & Child Neurology*, 61(10): 1139–1144. doi: 10.1111/dmcn.14166.

Mermin J, Lule JR, Ekwaru JP (2006) Association between malaria and CD4 cell count decline among persons with HIV. *J Acquir Immune Defic Syndr*, 41(1): 129–130. doi: 10.1097/01.qai.0000179427.11789.a7.

Meyaard L, Otto SA, Hooibrink B et al. (1994) Quantitative analysis of CD4+ T cell function in the course of human immunodeficiency virus infection. Gradual decline of both naive and memory alloreactive T cells. *J Clin Invest*, 94(5): 1947–1952. doi: 10.1172/JCI117545.

Molyneux EM, Walsh AL, Forsyth H et al. (2002) Dexamethasone treatment in childhood bacterial meningitis in Malawi: A randomised controlled trial. *Lancet*, 360(9328): 211–218. doi: 10.1016/S0140-6736(02)09458-8.

Molyneux EM, Tembo M, Kayira K et al. (2003) The effect of HIV infection on paediatric bacterial meningitis in Blantyre, Malawi. *Arch Dis Child*, 88(12): 1112–1118. doi: 10.1136/adc.88.12.1112.

Molyneux E, Nizami SQ, Saha S et al. (2011) 5 versus 10 days of treatment with ceftriaxone for bacterial meningitis in children: A double-blind randomised equivalence study. *Lancet*, 377(9780): 1837–1845. doi: 10.1016/S0140-6736(11)60580-1.

Mustafa MM, Weitman SD, Winick NJ et al. (1993) Subacute measles encephalitis in the young immunocompromised host: Report of two cases diagnosed by polymerase chain reaction and treated with ribavirin and review of the literature. *Clin Infect Dis*, 16(5): 654–660. doi: 10.1093/clind/16.5.654.

Mutapi F (2015) Changing policy and practice in the control of pediatric schistosomiasis. *Pediatrics*, 135(3): 536–544. doi: 10.1542/peds.2014-3189.

Mwaanza N, Chilukutu L, Tembo J et al. (2014) High rates of congenital cytomegalovirus infection linked with maternal HIV infection among neonatal admissions at a large referral center in sub-Saharan Africa. *Clin Infect Dis*, 58(5): 728–735. doi: 10.1093/cid/cit766.

Nuttall JJ, Wilmshurst JM, Ndondo AP et al. (2004) Progressive multifocal leukoencephalopathy after initiation of highly active antiretroviral therapy in a child with advanced human immunodeficiency virus infection: A case of immune reconstitution inflammatory syndrome. *The Pediatric Infectious Disease Journal*, 23(7): 683–685. doi: 10.1097/01.inf.0000130954.41818.07.

Nyazika TK, Masanganise F, Hagen F et al. (2016) Cryptococcal meningitis presenting as a complication in HIV-infected children: A case series from sub-Saharan Africa. *Pediatr Infect Dis J*, 35(9): 979–980. doi: 10.1097/INF.0000000000001212.

Ometto L, De Forni D, Patiri F et al. (2002) Immune reconstitution in HIV-1-infected children on antiretroviral therapy: Role of thymic output and viral fitness. *AIDS*, 16(6): 839–849. doi: 10.1097/00002030-200204120-00003.

Otieno L, Oneko M, Otieno W et al. (2016) Safety and immunogenicity of RTS,S/AS01 malaria vaccine in infants and children with WHO stage 1 or 2 HIV disease: A randomised, double-blind, controlled trial. *Lancet Infect Dis*, 16(10): 1134–1144. doi: 10.1016/s1473-3099(16)30161-x.

Pantaleo G, Graziosi C, Fauci AS (1993) The immunopathogenesis of human immunodeficiency virus infection. *N Engl J Med*, 328(5): 327–335. doi: 10.1056/NEJM199302043280508.

Park BJ, Wannemuehler KA, Marston BJ et al. (2009) Estimation of the current global burden of cryptococcal meningitis among persons living with HIV/AIDS. *AIDS*, 23(4): 525–530. doi: 10.1097/QAD.0b013e328322ffac.

Peltola H (2001) Burden of meningitis and other severe bacterial infections of children in africa: Implications for prevention. *Clin Infect Dis*, 32(1): 64–75. doi: 10.1086/317534.

Pensieroso S, Cagigi A, Palma P et al. (2009) Timing of HAART defines the integrity of memory B cells and the longevity of humoral responses in HIV-1 vertically-infected children. *Proc Natl Acad Sci USA*, 106(19): 7939–7944. doi: 10.1073/pnas.0901702106.

Pepin J, Ethier L, Kazadi C et al. (1992) The impact of human immunodeficiency virus infection on the epidemiology and treatment of Trypanosoma brucei gambiense sleeping sickness in Nioki, Zaire. *Am J Trop Med Hyg*, 47(2): 133–140. doi: 10.4269/ajtmh.1992.47.133.

Perez-Molina JA (2014) Management of Trypanosoma cruzi coinfection in HIV-positive individuals outside endemic areas. *Curr Opin Infect Dis*, 27(1): 9–15. doi: 10.1097/QCO.0000000000000023.

Picat MQ, Lewis J, Musiime V et al. (2013) Predicting patterns of long-term CD4 reconstitution in HIV-infected children starting antiretroviral therapy in sub-Saharan Africa: A cohort-based modelling study. *PLoS Med*, 10(10): e1001542. doi: 10.1371/journal.pmed.1001542.

Pohl D, Alper G, Van Haren K et al. (2016) Acute disseminated encephalomyelitis: Updates on an inflammatory CNS syndrome. *Neurology*, 87(9 Suppl 2): S38–S45. doi: 10.1212/WNL.0000000000002825.

Potchen MJ, Kampondeni SD, Seydel KB et al. (2012) Acute brain MRI findings in 120 Malawian children with cerebral malaria: New insights into an ancient disease. *AJNR Am J Neuroradiol*, 33(9): 1740–1746. doi: 10.3174/ajnr.A3035.

Prasad K, Singh MB, Ryan H (2016) Corticosteroids for managing tuberculous meningitis. *Cochrane Database Syst Rev*, 4CD002244. doi: 10.1002/14651858.CD002244.pub4.

Pugliese A, Vidotto V, Beltramo T et al. (2005) Phagocytic activity in human immunodeficiency virus type 1 infection. *Clin Diagn Lab Immunol*, 12(8): 889–895. doi: 10.1128/CDLI.12.8.889-895.2005.

Rainwater-Lovett K, Nkamba H, Mubiana-Mbewe M et al. (2014a) Changes in cellular immune activation and memory T-cell subsets in HIV-infected Zambian children receiving HAART. *J Acquir Immune Defic Syndr*, 67(5): 455–462. doi: 10.1097/QAI.0000000000000342.

Rainwater-Lovett K, Nkamba HC, Mubiana-Mbewe M et al. (2014b) Antiretroviral therapy restores age-dependent loss of resting memory B cells in young HIV-infected Zambian children. *J Acquir Immune Defic Syndr*, 65(5): 505–509. doi: 10.1097/QAI.0000000000000074.

Ravikumar S, Crawford JR (2013) Role of carbamazepine in the symptomatic treatment of subacute sclerosing panencephalitis: A case report and review of the literature. *Case Rep Neurol Med*, 2013327647. doi: 10.1155/2013/327647.

Ren Y, Nuttall JJ, Egbers C et al. (2008) Effect of rifampicin on lopinavir pharmacokinetics in HIV-infected children with tuberculosis. *J Acquir Immune Defic Syndr*, 47(5): 566–569. doi: 10.1097/QAI.0b013e3181642257.

Ren Y, Nuttall JJ, Eley BS et al. (2009) Effect of rifampicin on efavirenz pharmacokinetics in HIV-infected children with tuberculosis. *J Acquir Immune Defic Syndr*, 50(5): 439–443. doi: 10.1097/QAI.0b013e31819c33a3.

Roca-Feltrer A, Carneiro I, Armstrong Schellenberg JR (2008) Estimates of the burden of malaria morbidity in Africa in children under the age of 5 years. *Trop Med Int Health*, 13(6): 771–783. doi: 10.1111/j.1365-3156.2008.02076.x.

Rohlwink UK, Kilborn T, Wieselthaler N et al. (2016) Imaging features of the brain, c erebral v essels and spine in pediatric tuberculous meningitis with associated hydrocephalus. *Pediatr Infect Dis J*, 35(10): e301–e310. doi: 10.1097/INF.0000000000001236.

Roider JM, Muenchhoff M, Goulder PJ (2016) Immune activation and paediatric HIV 1 disease outcome. *Curr Opin HIV AIDS*, 11(2): 146–155. doi: 10.1097/COH.0000000000000231.

Ross AG, McManus DP, Farrar J et al. (2012) Neuroschistosomiasis. *J Neurol*, 259(1): 22–32. doi: 10.1007/s00415-011-6133-7.

RTS S Clinical Trials Partnership (2015) Efficacy and safety of RTS,S/AS01 malaria vaccine with or without a booster dose in infants and children in Africa: Final results of a phase 3, individually randomised, controlled trial. *Lancet*, 386(9988): 31–45. doi: 10.1016/s0140-6736(15)60721-8.

Sandgaard KS, Lewis J, Adams S et al. (2014) Antiretroviral therapy increases thymic output in children with HIV. *AIDS*, 28(2): 209–214. doi: 10.1097/QAD.0000000000000063.

Sartori AM, Ibrahim KY, Nunes Westphalen EV et al. (2007) Manifestations of Chagas disease (American trypanosomiasis) in patients with HIV/AIDS. *Ann Trop Med Parasitol*, 101(1): 31–50. doi: 10.1179/136485907X154629.

Schmidt V, Kositz C, Herbinger KH et al. (2016) Association between *Taenia solium* infection and HIV/AIDS in northern Tanzania: A matched cross-sectional study. *Infect Dis Poverty*, 5(1): 111. doi: 10.1186/s40249-016-0209-7.

Schutte CM (2001) Clinical, cerebrospinal fluid and pathological findings and outcomes in HIV-positive and HIV-negative patients with tuberculous meningitis. *Infection* 29(4): 213–217. doi: 10.1007/s15010-001-1198-3.

Schwenk H, Ramirez-Avila L, Sheu SH et al. (2014) Progressive multifocal leukoencephalopathy in pediatric patients: Case report and literature review. *Pediatr Infect Dis J*, 33(4): e99–e105. doi: 10.1097/INF.0000000000000237.

Scully E, Alter G. (2016) NK cells in HIV disease. *Curr HIV/AIDS Rep*, 13(2): 85–94. doi: 10.1007/s11904-016-0310-3.

Serpa JA, Moran A, Goodman JC et al. (2007) Neurocysticercosis in the HIV era: a case report and review of the literature. *Am J Trop Med Hyg*, 77(1): 113–117. doi: 10.4269/ajtmh.2007.77.113.

Seydel KB, Kampondeni SD, Valim C et al. (2015) Brain swelling and death in children with cerebral malaria. *N Engl J Med*, 372(12): 1126–1137. doi: 10.1056/NEJMoa1400116.

Shah I, Chudgar P (2005) Progressive multifocal leukoencephalopathy (PML) presenting as intractable dystonia in an HIV-infected child. *J Trop Pediatr*, 51(6): 380–382. doi: 10.1093/tropej/fmi034.

Siberry GK, Abzug MJ, Nachman S et al. (2013) Guidelines for the prevention and treatment of opportunistic infections in HIV-exposed and HIV-infected children: Recommendations from the National Institutes of Health, Centers for Disease Control and Prevention, the HIV Medicine Association of the Infectious Diseases Society of America, the Pediatric Infectious Diseases Society, and the American Academy of Pediatrics. *Pediatr Infect Dis J*, 32(Suppl) 2i–KK4. doi: 10.1097/01.inf.0000437856.09540.11.

Slyker JA (2016) Cytomegalovirus and paediatric HIV infection. *J Virus Erad*, 2(4): 208–214. doi: 10.1016/S2055-6640(20)30873-6.

Smith K, Kuhn L, Coovadia A et al. (2009) Immune reconstitution inflammatory syndrome among HIV-infected South African infants initiating antiretroviral therapy. *AIDS*, 23(9): 1097–1107. doi: 10.1097/QAD.0b013e32832afefc.

Solomon T (2003) Recent advances in Japanese encephalitis. *J Neurovirol*, 9(2): 274–283. doi: 10.1080/13550280390194037.

Swanson PA 2nd, McGavern DB (2015) Viral diseases of the central nervous system. *Curr Opin Virol*, April, 11: 44–54. doi: 10.1016/j.coviro.2014.12.009.

Swanstrom R, Coffin J (2012) HIV-1 pathogenesis: The virus. *Cold Spring Harb Perspect Med*, 2(12): a007443. doi: 10.1101/cshperspect.a007443.

Tan IL, Smith BR, von Geldern G et al. (2012) HIV-associated opportunistic infections of the CNS. *Lancet Neurol*, 11(7): 605–617. doi: 10.1016/S1474-4422(12)70098-4.

Taylor TE, Fu WJ, Carr RA et al. (2004) Differentiating the pathologies of cerebral malaria by postmortem parasite counts. *Nat Med*, 10(2): 143–145. doi: 10.1038/nm986.

Tembo DL, Nyoni B, Murikoli RV et al. (2014) Differential PfEMP1 expression is associated with cerebral malaria pathology. *PLoS Pathog*, 10(12): e1004537. doi: 10.1371/journal.ppat.1004537.

Tennant SM, MacLennan CA, Simon R et al. (2016) Nontyphoidal salmonella disease: Current status of vaccine research and development. *Vaccine*, 34(26): 2907–2910. doi: 10.1016/j.vaccine.2016.03.072.

Titanji K, De Milito A, Cagigi A et al. (2006) Loss of memory B cells impairs maintenance of long-term serologic memory during HIV-1 infection. *Blood*, 108(5): 1580–1587. doi: 10.1182/blood-2005-11-013383.

Torok ME, Yen NT, Chau TT et al. (2011) Timing of initiation of antiretroviral therapy in human immunodeficiency virus (HIV)-associated tuberculous meningitis. *Clin Infect Dis*, 52(11): 1374–1383. doi: 10.1093/cid/cir230.

UNAIDS (2020) Fact sheet: World AIDS day 2020. https://www.unaids.org/sites/default/files/media_asset/UNAIDS_FactSheet_en.pdf [accessed 25 January 2021].

Utay NS, Hunt PW (2016) Role of immune activation in progression to AIDS. *Curr Opin HIV AIDS*, 11(2): 131–137. doi: 10.1097/COH.0000000000000242.

van der Weert EM, Hartgers NM, Schaaf HS et al. (2006) Comparison of diagnostic criteria of tuberculous meningitis in human immunodeficiency virus-infected and uninfected children. *Pediatr Infect Dis J*, 25(1): 65–69. doi: 10.1097/01.inf.0000183751.75880.f8.

van Toorn R, Rabie H, Dramowski A et al. (2012) Neurological manifestations of TB-IRIS: A report of 4 children. *Eur J Paediatr Neurol*, 16(6): 676–682. doi: 10.1016/j.ejpn.2012.04.005.

van Toorn R, Schaaf HS, Laubscher JA et al. (2014) Short intensified treatment in children with drug-susceptible tuberculous meningitis. *Pediatr Infect Dis J*, 33(3): 248–252. doi: 10.1097/INF.0000000000000065.

van Toorn R, Solomons R (2014) Update on the diagnosis and management of tuberculous meningitis in children. *Semin Pediatr Neurol*, 21(1): 12–18. doi: 10.1016/j.spen.2014.01.006.

Walker M, Kublin JG, Zunt JR (2006) Parasitic central nervous system infections in immunocompromised hosts: Malaria, microsporidiosis, leishmaniasis, and African trypanosomiasis. *Clin Infect Dis*, 42(1): 115–125. doi: 10.1086/498510.

Wasserman S, Meintjes G (2014) The diagnosis, management and prevention of HIV-associated tuberculosis. *S Afr Med J*, 104(12): 886–893. doi: 10.7196/SAMJ.9090.

Whitley RJ (2014) Herpes simplex virus infections. In: Singhi P, Griffin DE, Newton CR, editors, *Central Nervous System Infections in Childhood* (International Review of Child Neurology Series). London: Mac Keith Press, pp. 115–125.

Whitworth J, Morgan D, Quigley M et al. (2000) Effect of HIV-1 and increasing immunosuppression on malaria parasitaemia and clinical episodes in adults in rural Uganda: A cohort study. *Lancet*, 356(9235): 1051–1056. doi: 10.1016/S0140-6736(00)02727-6.

WHO (2000) Severe falciparum malaria. *Trans R Soc Trop Med & Hyg*, 94(Suppl 1): 1–90. doi: 10.1016/S0035-9203(00)90300-6.

WHO (2010) Antiretroviral therapy for HIV infection in infants and children: Towards universal access. Recommendations for a public health approach, 2010 revision. URL: http://apps.who.int/iris/bitstream/10665/164255/1/9789241599801_eng.pdf?ua=1 [accessed 5 August 2010].

WHO (2011) Rapid advice: Diagnosis, prevention and management of cryptococcal disease in HIV-infected adults, adolescents and children, December, 2011. URL: http://apps.who.int/iris/bitstream/10665/44786/1/9789241502979_eng.pdf [accessed: 26 January 2012].

WHO (2014) *Guidance for National Tuberculosis Programmes on the Management of Tuberculosis in Children. 2nd Edition*. ISBN: 978 92 4 154874 8. URL: http://apps.who.int/iris/bitstream/10665/112360/1/9789241548748_eng.pdf?ua=1 [accessed 15 January 2015].

WHO (2015) *Guidelines for the Treatment of Malaria. 3rd Edition*. http://apps.who.int/iris/bitstream/10665/162441/1/9789241549127_eng.pdf [accessed 07 December 2016].

WHO (2016) Malaria vaccine: WHO position paper – January 2016. *Wkly Epidemiol Rec* 2016, 91(4): 33–52. URL: https://fctc.who.int/publications/i/item/who-position-paper-on-malaria-vaccines [accessed 8 February 2017].

WHO (2019) *Guide to Introducing Meningococcal A: Conjugate Vaccine into the Routine Immunization Programme*. https://www.who.int/publications/i/item/9789241516860 [accessed 25 January 2021].

WHO (2020) *World Malaria Report 2020: 20 Years of Global Progress and Challenges*. https://www.who.int/teams/global--malaria--programme/reports/world--malaria--report--2020. [accessed 27 January 2021].

Wilmshurst JM, Burgess J, Hartley P et al. (2006) Specific neurologic complications of human immunodeficiency virus type 1 (HIV-1) infection in children. *J Child Neurol*, 21(9): 788–794. doi: 10.1177/08830738060210091901.

Wilmshurst JM, Eley BS, Brew BJ (2014) HIV infections of the CNS. In: Singhi P, Griffin DE, Newton CR, editors, *Central Nervous System Infections in Childhood* (International Review of Child Neurology Series). London: Mac Keith Press, pp. 147–159.

Wilmshurst JM, Hammond CK, Donald K et al. (2018) NeuroAIDS in children. *Handbook of Clinical Neurology* 152: 99–116. doi: 10.1016/B978-0-444-63849-6.00008-6.

Xu Z, Zhang C, Wang F-S (2020) COVID-19 in people with HIV. *The Lancet HIV*, 7(8): e524–e526. doi: 10.1016/S2352-3018(20)30163-6.

Yansouni CP, Bottieau E, Lutumba P et al. (2013) Rapid diagnostic tests for neurological infections in central Africa. *Lancet Infect Dis*, 13(6): 546–558. doi: 10.1016/S1473-3099(13)70004-5.

Yin L, Kou ZC, Rodriguez C et al. (2009) Antiretroviral therapy restores diversity in the T-cell receptor Vbeta repertoire of CD4 T-cell subpopulations among human immunodeficiency virus type 1-infected children and adolescents. *Clin Vaccine Immunol*, 16(9): 1293–1301. doi: 10.1128/CVI.00074-09.

Zaknun D, Zangerle R, Kapelari K et al. (1997) Concurrent ganciclovir and foscarnet treatment for cytomegalovirus encephalitis and retinitis in an infant with acquired immunodeficiency syndrome: Case report and review. *Pediatr Infect Dis J*, 16(8): 807–811. doi: 10.1097/00006454--199708000-00014.

Zhao BC, Jiang HY, Ma WY et al. (2016) Albendazole and corticosteroids for the treatment of solitary cysticercus granuloma: A network meta-analysis. *PLoS Negl Trop Dis*, 10(2): e0004418. doi: 10.1371/journal.pntd.0004418.

Cerebrovascular Disease

Charles K Hammond and Alvin Ndondo

INTRODUCTION

Human immunodeficiency virus (HIV) infection may be complicated by cerebrovascular diseases in both children and adults. These may manifest as focal neurological deficits, encephalopathy, or may be asymptomatic. Throughout this chapter, the term stroke is used to refer to a focal neurological deficit lasting more than 24 hours with imaging correlation, while cerebrovascular disease refers to the broader category with or without clinical correlation. Transient ischaemic attack (TIA) refers to focal deficit lasting less than 24 hours.

Childhood stroke is defined as a stroke occurring in children aged 29 days after birth to 18 years (Mirsky et al. 2017) and is traditionally classified as ischaemic or haemorrhagic. Ischaemic stroke is further subdivided into arterial ischaemic stroke (AIS) and cerebral sinovenous thrombosis (CSVT). Haemorrhagic stroke in children includes spontaneous intracerebral haemorrhage with or without intraventricular extension, intraventricular haemorrhage, or non-traumatic subarachnoid haemorrhage (SAH) (Mirsky et al. 2017).

The annual incidence of stroke in all children under 18 years of age is reported as 1.72 to 2.70 per 100 000 per year (Broderick et al. 1993; Fullerton et al. 2003; deVeber et al. 2017) with almost equal incidence of ischaemic stroke and haemorrhagic stroke (Fullerton et al. 2003). The risk of stroke in children varies among different ethnic groups and sex. Black children are at increased risk than White and Asian children (Broderick et al. 1993; Fullerton et al. 2003). There is also a higher incidence in males than females (Fullerton et al. 2003).

The prevalence of cerebrovascular disease in HIV-infected children may be underestimated because of limited neuroimaging, especially in low- and middle-income countries (LMICs), which is where the majority of these children reside (Kolapo and Vento 2011). These areas also have limited access to antiretroviral drugs (Kolapo and Vento 2011). In well-resourced countries, the prevalence of stroke in HIV-infected children in clinical series is reported to be between 1.3% and 2.6% (Park et al. 1990; Patsalides et al. 2002), although at autopsy a higher prevalence of cerebral ischaemia (4–36%) is reported (Rabinstein 2003; Benjamin et al. 2012).

This chapter discusses the risk factors, pathophysiology and pattern of vascular involvement, clinical presentation, and radiological presentation of strokes in children with HIV infection. It also discusses an approach to the HIV-infected child presenting with stroke in a resource-limited setting. The discussion in this chapter does not include venous, perinatal, neonatal, or traumatic arterial stroke.

RISK FACTORS AND PATHOGENESIS

The risk factors for the development of cerebrovascular disease in HIV-infected individuals are varied. In any particular child presenting with stroke, whether HIV-infected or uninfected, there are often multiple factors that together determine the risk of stroke or stroke recurrence (Roach et al. 2008; Benjamin et al. 2012; Hammond et al. 2016a). In the era before antiretroviral therapy (ART), cerebrovascular disease in HIV-infected individuals was largely attributed to opportunistic infections and malignancies (Engstrom, Lowenstein, and Bredesen 1989). Following the introduction of combination antiretroviral therapy (cART), there has been a decline in the incidence of opportunistic infections and neoplasms but no corresponding decline in the incidence of HIV-associated cerebrovascular disease (Rabinstein 2003). In the USA, between 1997 and 2006, stroke admissions declined by 7% in the general population but increased by 60% in HIV-infected individuals (Ovbiagele and Nath 2011).

Further studies have identified other causes and risk factors besides opportunistic infections and malignancy. Important aetiologies for stroke in HIV-infected children include the direct effect of HIV on cerebral vasculature (a condition termed HIV-associated cerebral vasculopathy), opportunistic infections, malignancies, cardioembolism, coagulopathies, and the effect of treatment (Evers et al. 2003; Rabinstein 2003; Benjamin et al. 2012; Arvind et al. 2013; Singer et al. 2013; Hammond et al. 2016a; Ismael et al. 2020). These risk factors are summarised in Table 8.1.

HIV-associated cerebral vasculopathy is defined as cerebral vasculopathy/arteriopathy affecting predominantly medium-sized cerebral vessels with radiological evidence of vessel stenosis, occlusion, or aneurysmal dilatation without any identifiable cause other than the HIV infection (Connor 2009; Pillay, Ramdial, and Naidoo 2015). It includes abnormalities of the intracranial or extracranial cerebral blood vessels that result directly or indirectly from HIV infection, excluding vasculitis associated with opportunistic infection or neoplastic involvement of the vessels (Benjamin et al. 2012; Pillay, Ramdial, and Naidoo 2015). The vasculopathy may be asymptomatic or cause stroke, encephalopathy, cognitive impairment, or non-specific neurological symptoms (Connor 2009; Pillay, Ramdial, and Naidoo 2015). The mechanism by which HIV induces arterial damage is largely unknown but is hypothesised to be either via direct HIV-1 infection of the vessel wall or via an indirect autoimmune process (Benjamin et al. 2012; Hammond et al. 2016a). In the direct mechanism, it is hypothesised that HIV directly infects the arterial smooth muscle of cerebral vessels, leading to damage to the endothelium and the vascular wall (Connor 2009; Benjamin et al. 2012). Histologic examinations have shown medial fibrosis and thinning, damage or loss of the muscularis and internal elastic lamina, and intimal hyperplasia of the vascular wall with a resultant aneurysmal dilatation or stenosis of the vessels (Gutierrez et al. 2012; Singer et al. 2013). Both fusiform and saccular aneurysms of the major vessels in the circle of Willis are described (see Chapter 4, Figures 4.6a–4.6e, 4.7a–4.7e, and 4.8a–4.8b) (Philippet et al. 1994; Shah et al. 1996; Dubrovsky et al. 1998; Mazzoni et al. 2000; Izbudak et al. 2013; Ismael et al. 2020). Furthermore, the direct role of HIV in vascular disease is supported by the identification of HIV viral antigen in the intima of affected parenchymal and leptomeningeal arteries using monoclonal antibodies to gp41 (Park et al. 1990).

In the other hypothesis, the virus is thought to indirectly damage cerebral blood vessels by triggering an autoimmune inflammatory response with resultant vasculitis or perivasculitis (Katsetos et al. 1999; Di Biagio et al. 2013). Supporting this hypothesis, inflammatory markers correlate with vascular intima-media thickness in perinatally HIV-1 infected children and adolescents who present with stroke (Katsetos et al. 1999; Di Biagio et al. 2013).

The risk of stroke and progressive cerebrovascular disease due to HIV-associated vasculopathy is high in patients with active infection, high HIV viral load, severe immunosuppression, or low CD4+ cell count (Patsalides et al. 2002; Mahadevan et al. 2008; Cutfield et al. 2009). In some of these reports, progression of cerebral vasculopathy is arrested or reversed with cART initiation (Mahadevan et al. 2008; Connor 2009; Cutfield et al. 2009). In a study in which carotid intima-media thickness was measured for HIV-infected children who were either ART-naïve or ART-exposed, results showed that ART-naïve HIV-infected children had increased carotid intima-media thickness compared to ART-exposed

Table 8.1 HIV-related risk factors for stroke (Rabinstein 2003; Benjamin et al. 2012; Singer et al. 2013; Hammond et al. 2016a).

HIV-associated vasculopathy
    Directly due to HIV infection of the cerebral vessels
    Indirectly due to vasculitis/perivasculitis

Opportunistic infections
    Tuberculous meningitis
    Varicella zoster virus vasculitis
    Herpes simplex virus types 1 and 2
    Meningovascular syphilis
    Cytomegalovirus infections
    Toxoplasmosis
    Cryptococcal meningitis
    Fungal infections (candida, aspergillus)

Neoplasia
    Primary central nervous system lymphomas
    Lymphomatoid granulomatosis
    Disseminated Kaposi sarcoma

Cardioembolism
    Bacterial endocarditis
    Mycotic aneurysm (secondary to bacterial endocarditis)
    Marantic endocarditis
    HIV-associated cardiac dysfunction (HIV myocarditis)

Coagulopathy (prothrombotic states)
    Protein S deficiency
    Protein C deficiency
    HIV-associated thrombocytopaenia
    Antiphospholipid antibodies
    Anticadiolipin antibodies
    Disseminated intravascular coagulation (in terminal patients)
    HIV-associated hyperviscosity

Treatment-related risk factors
    cART (especially protease inhibitors leading to accelerated atherosclerosis)
    Immune reconstitution inflammatory syndrome

HIV-infected children or HIV-uninfected children, suggesting that cART exposure may arrest or reverse HIV-associated vasculopathy (Idris et al. 2016).

Opportunistic vasculopathies were commonly reported in the pre-ART era. With most patients receiving cART early in the course of the disease, opportunistic infections have decreased significantly. However, opportunistic infections still remain an important cause of stroke in the severely immunocompromised child or in those with advanced disease due to limited access to cART. Common pathogens identified include varicella-zoster virus (VZV), cytomegalovirus (CMV), *Mycobacterium tuberculosis*, *Cryptococcus neoformans*, and *Candida albicans* (Engstrom, Lowenstein, and Bredesen 1989; Kieburtz et al. 1993; Patsalides et al. 2002; Rabinstein 2003; Ismael et al. 2020). Opportunistic pathogens cause vascular damage either by direct infection of the vascular wall or by a systemic immune-mediated mechanism (Pinto 1996; Tipping et al. 2007; Benjamin et al. 2012).

The common malignancies associated with stroke in HIV infection are primary central nervous system (CNS) lymphomas, lymphomatoid granulomatosis, and disseminated Kaposi sarcoma (Engstrom,

Lowenstein, and Bredesen 1989; Park et al. 1990; Kieburtz et al. 1993). Primary CNS lymphomas (see Chapter 4, Figures 4.13a and 4.13b) are mainly B-cell lymphomas associated with Epstein–Barr virus infection (Fallo et al. 2005; Little 2006). Lymphomatoid granulomatosis and disseminated Kaposi sarcoma have been associated with stroke in HIV-infected adults in pre-ART era reports (Engstrom, Lowenstein, and Bredesen 1989). Affected individuals often have severe immunosuppression mainly due to lack of access to cART. In these settings, there is either focal tumour infiltration of blood vessel walls with resultant vascular injury or invasion of the vascular lumen leading to focal thrombosis (Kieburtz et al. 1993).

Initiating cART in HIV-infected individuals should be approached with caution because it could lead to a rapid immune restoration over 1 to 2 months and subsequent robust immune response against pre-existing subclinical or partially treated opportunistic pathogens, which is a condition known as immune reconstitution inflammatory syndrome (IRIS). In neurological IRIS, the immune response leads to unmasking or paradoxical worsening of the underlying CNS opportunistic infection with associated cerebral vasculopathy leading to stroke (see Chapter 4, Figures 4.11a–4.11g and 4.12a–4.12d) (Bonkowsky et al. 2002; Lipman and Breen 2006; van Toorn et al. 2012). To prevent IRIS, it is important to actively search for opportunistic infections and treat them adequately before cART initiation (Lipman and Breen 2006).

Cardioembolism occurs due to various causes and may be a risk factor for cerebrovascular disease in an HIV-infected child. The risk of AIS from cardiac disorders is 31% in all children, with or without HIV infection (Mackay et al. 2011). There are no figures specific to HIV-infected children; however, in HIV-infected adults, cardioembolism accounts for 4% to 15% of ischaemic strokes (Benjamin et al. 2012). HIV-associated cardiac dysfunction is a condition in which the virus infects cardiac tissue and may lead to cardioembolic phenomena. This disorder might be associated with opportunistic infections and the pathogenesis is not well explained (Benjamin et al. 2012). Cardioembolism may also result from bacterial endocarditis or opportunistic infections of the cardiac tissue (Barbaro 2002; Hajjar et al. 2005; Benjamin et al. 2012; Ismael et al. 2020). Other cardiac conditions related to stroke in HIV-infected individuals are dilated cardiomyopathy, mural thrombi, and myxoid valvular degeneration (Berger et al. 1990; Rabinstein 2003; Ismael et al. 2020). Aortic root dilatation associated with left ventricular dilatation has been documented in HIV-infected children with high HIV viral load and low CD4+ cell count (Lai et al. 2001).

Coagulopathy in HIV infection may be due to various causes. The systemic HIV infection is thought to trigger consumptive coagulopathy and immune-mediated mechanisms (Saif and Greenberg 2001; Singer et al. 2013; Ismael et al. 2020). There are reports of protein S and protein C deficiencies (Patsalides et al. 2002; Goyal and Shah 2014) as well as immune and thrombotic thrombocytopaenia (Park et al. 1990; Rakhmanina et al. 2014) in HIV-infected children presenting with stroke without any other identifiable causes. HIV-infected individuals have a high prevalence of antiphospholipid and anticardiolipin antibodies (Brew and Miller 1996; Abuaf et al. 1997; Rabinstein 2003). In terminally ill patients, stroke can be precipitated by disseminated intravascular coagulation (Berger et al. 1990; Rabinstein 2003) or cerebral venous thrombosis as a consequence of dehydration (Berger et al. 1990).

A report from the International Pediatric Stroke Study (Mackay et al. 2011) indicates that prothrombotic states accounts for 13% of AIS in HIV-uninfected children. In this study, specific prothrombotic states identified include methyl tetrahydrofolate reductase mutation, elevated lipoprotein A, protein S and protein C deficiencies, prothrombin G20210A mutation, factor V Leiden mutation, antithrombin III deficiency, hyperhomocysteinaemia, and other genetic thrombophilias as well as acquired thrombophilias (Mackay et al. 2011).

THE ROLE OF COMBINATION ANTIRETROVIRAL THERAPY

The atherogenic effect of protease inhibitors as a potential risk for stroke is well described in adult studies (d'Arminio et al. 2004). A cART regimen containing protease inhibitors may increase the risk of stroke by elevating cholesterol and triglyceride levels (Rabinstein 2003; Calza et al. 2004). Dyslipidaemia occurs in up to 70% to 80% of HIV-infected individuals receiving cART (Calza, Manfredi, and Chiodo 2004), and is more pronounced after prolonged use of protease inhibitors, usually over 6 years (d'Arminio et al. 2004). Report from studies that assessed the effect of cART on childhood vasculature suggest that HIV-infected children exposed to cART may have increased arterial stiffness compared with uninfected and cART-naïve children (McComsey et al. 2007; Idris et al. 2016).

CONSIDERATIONS FOR NON-HIV-RELATED COMORBIDITIES

Besides HIV infection, sub-Saharan Africa (SSA) is home to sickle cell disease (SCD). It is estimated that 75% of the world's patients with SCD live in SSA (Kato et al. 2018; Esoh, Wonkam-Tingang, and Wonkam 2021). These patients may present with acute and life-threatening vaso-occlusive and hypoxic events including stroke. It is therefore important to consider the impact of SCD on the presentation and progression of cerebrovascular disease in HIV-infected individuals.

Both HIV and SCD lead to immune dysregulation, although the mechanisms are different. In SCD, the shortened red cell lifespan and decreased oxygen-carrying capacity predisposes the patient to tissue hypoxia and end organ dysfunction. Defective splenic function and immune response make the patient susceptible to infections, including pneumonia, meningitis, and severe malaria. Acute ischaemic stroke in patients with SCD is usually caused by occlusion of a large cerebral artery and can manifest as a TIA, sudden weakness, or impaired consciousness. Haemorrhagic stroke may also occur, presenting with severe headaches with hemiparesis or impaired consciousness (Kato et al. 2018).

Thus, in HIV-infected patients with coexisting SCD, it is expected that the severity and outcomes of cerebrovascular disease may differ from those without SCD. There have been no rigorous studies to test this hypothesis. However, findings from some observational studies of HIV-infected children and adults who also had SCD suggest that SCD does not adversely affect the progression of HIV in patients on cART (Bagasra et al. 1998; Kourtis et al. 2007; Ssenyondwa et al. 2020). Another study, evaluating the impact of sickle cell trait on the clinical and laboratory parameters of HIV infection, showed that children with sickle cell trait and coexisting HIV infection had lower mean HIV ribonucleic acid viral load (David et al. 2018). The mechanism by which SCD or trait mitigate the progression of HIV is not clearly understood and needs to be studied further.

Malaria is another important endemic disease in SSA, with potential impact on the presentation and progression of paediatric HIV infection. The most severe neurological complication is cerebral malaria, caused by *Plasmodium falciparum.* It affects more than 500 000 children annually, mainly in SSA. The highest mortality is seen in children under 5 years of age (Idro et al. 2010). Children with cerebral malaria present with coma and carry a high (15–20%) risk of mortality. About 11% of survivors sustain significant brain injury and have various neurological deficits, including cortical visual impairment, seizures, and motor, cognitive, and behavioural deficits (Newton 2005; Idro et al. 2010).

The mechanisms of brain injury in cerebral malaria are poorly understood but are thought to be due to parasite sequestration in the brain, the effects of cytokines and inflammatory metabolites, as well as endothelial cell damage and disruption of the blood–brain barrier (Idro et al. 2010).

The socioeconomic conditions in many parts of SSA also presents a challenge to the HIV-infected child. Many of these children live under difficult circumstances and are plagued by malnutrition, anaemia, and micronutrient deficiency, all of which may influence their neurodevelopment.

In HIV-infected adults, the traditional risk factors for stroke, such as hypertension, diabetes, dyslipidaemia, coronary artery disease, and atrial fibrillation, are still important. These risk factors become more pronounced with increasing age (Ismael et al. 2020). However, there are increasing numbers of children and adolescents who are recently being diagnosed with these lifestyle diseases. Thus, for the HIV-infected child living in SSA, the risk for cerebrovascular disease and subsequent neurocognitive challenges may be influenced by non-HIV comorbidities, including SCD and cerebral malaria, as well as malnutrition, anaemia, and micronutrient deficiencies (Newton 2005; Idro et al. 2010; David et al. 2018; Ssenyondwa et al. 2020). Lifestyle modifications have also led to increasing incidence of traditional risk factors for stroke in children (Ismael et al. 2020).

THE PATTERN OF CEREBROVASCULAR INVOLVEMENT

Both ischaemic and haemorrhagic strokes occur in children with HIV infection, but ischaemic strokes are more common (Park et al. 1990; Pinto 1996). Ischaemic infarcts occur in the cerebral cortex, internal capsule, or basal ganglia and commonly in the territories of the middle cerebral artery (MCA) or the anterior cerebral artery (ACA) (see Chapter 4, Figures 4.5, 4.6a, 4.6c, 4.7a–4.7b, and 4.8a–4.8b) (Patsalides et al. 2002; Izbudak et al. 2013; Hammond et al. 2016a).

Cases of transient cerebral arteriopathy have been reported in which non-progressive unilateral stenosis or occlusion of the distal internal carotid artery, proximal MCA, or ACA have resulted in lenticulostriate infarcts (Evers et al. 2003; Leeuwis, Wolfs, and Braun 2007). Transient cerebral arteriopathy can be indicative of an inflammatory response to HIV or VZV infection and lead to focal or multifocal infarcts. On magnetic resonance angiogram (MRA), the vascular abnormalities are non-progressive and remain unchanged over a period of time (Leeuwis, Wolfs, and Braun 2007). Besides the large vessels, microinfarcts in the small and medium vessels have also been noted at autopsy (Park et al. 1990).

Aneurysmal dilatations of the major vessels of the circle of Willis have been reported (Park et al. 1990). Aneurysmal arteriopathy may cause ischaemic stroke by focal thrombosis or may rupture leading to intracerebral or subarachnoid haemorrhage (Park et al. 1990; Philippet et al. 1994; Shah et al. 1996; Dubrovsky et al. 1998; Fulmer et al. 1998; Mazzoni et al. 2000; Nunes, Pinho, and Sfoggia 2001; Martinez-Longoria et al. 2004; Mahadevan et al. 2008; Gutierrez et al. 2012; Izbudak et al. 2013; Dhawan et al. 2016). Intracerebral haemorrhage may also be associated with CNS opportunistic vasculitis, thrombocytopaenia, or disseminated intravascular coagulation (Pinto 1996; Roquer et al. 1998; Rabinstein 2003; Cole et al. 2004; Rakhmanina et al. 2014).

Cases of progressive vasculopathy have been reported in some children with poor virologic suppression who presented with recurrent strokes or TIAs and were diagnosed as moyamoya syndrome (see Chapter 4, Figures 4.7a–4.7e). In these cases, serial imaging shows progressive occlusion of the distal internal carotid arteries and proximal MCAs or ACAs with development of collateral circulation (Hsiung and Sotero de Menezes 1999; Narayan, Samuels, and Barrow 2002; Hammond et al. 2016b).

CLINICAL MANIFESTATION

The presentations of cerebrovascular disease in HIV-infected children do not differ from uninfected children. Cerebrovascular disease may manifest overtly as strokes or TIAs, or may have subtle manifestations such as neurobehavioural problems, learning difficulties, or developmental regression which, in the HIV-infected child, can be misdiagnosed as HIV encephalopathy (Izbudak et al. 2013; Hammond et al. 2016a). This is even more challenging in LMICs, where access to neuroimaging is limited. TIAs may not be investigated due to limited resources or lack of recognition.

In overt stroke, common manifestations include hemiparesis, facial weakness, seizures, aphasia, or impaired consciousness (Park et al. 1990; Moriarty et al. 1994; Hammond et al. 2016a). In addition, neonates and young infants may present with non-specific clinical features such as vomiting or refusal of feeds, while older children may report headache or visual field defects. Transient ischemic attacks are common and may be recurrent. Additionally, some recurrent strokes or TIAs in HIV-infected children have been identified as moyamoya syndrome upon neuroimaging (Hsiung and Sotero de Menezes 1999; Narayan, Samuels, and Barrow 2002; Hammond et al. 2016b).

Patients may present with soft signs, which may initially be attributed to other conditions rather than stroke until they are sent for neuroimaging. These misleading presentations – so called stroke chameleons – may include acute mental status change, amnesia, hypertension, sensory symptoms, abnormal movement, psychiatric symptoms, vertigo, and syncope among others.

In haemorrhagic stroke, the most frequent presenting symptom in children is headache, especially in non-traumatic subarachnoid haemorrhage. Other symptoms include altered mental status, nausea and vomiting, neck pain, seizures, and focal neurological deficits such as hemiparesis, aphasia, or ataxia. In intraventricular haemorrhage, hydrocephalus may develop acutely or insidiously (Dhawan et al. 2016; Mirsky et al. 2017).

THE CONCEPT OF 'SILENT' STROKE

It is important to note that some cases of cerebrovascular diseases in children are asymptomatic and are only diagnosed either incidentally on neuroimaging or at autopsy (Berger et al. 1990; Kieburtz et al. 1993; Pinto 1996; Rabinstein 2003). In hindsight, many of these 'silent' strokes had subtle presentations that often escape medical attention for various reasons. In a case series of moyamoya syndrome in HIV-1 infected children, some children had misleading phenotypes such as cognitive delay or regression which were initially attributed to HIV encephalopathy until neuroimaging was performed showing evidence of preceding vascular events (Hammond et al. 2016b). However, there are instances when a stroke is truly silent and may only be recognised later on neuroimaging (Patsalides et al. 2002).

INVESTIGATIONS

In resource-limited settings, investigations after clinically diagnosed stroke or TIA in an HIV-infected child should be carefully selected to confirm the stroke, identify other risk factors besides HIV infection, recognise the pattern of cerebrovascular disease, and monitor disease progression. Stroke mimics are common in people with HIV infection and so brain imaging in an HIV-infected child presenting with sudden-onset focal signs is essential to aid diagnosis, rule out mimics, and to distinguish between haemorrhagic and ischaemic stroke (Benjamin et al. 2012). If available, magnetic resonance imaging (MRI) of the brain with angiography (MRA) of the cerebral and neck vessels should be done. However, in most LMICs this is not readily available. When it is available it often requires anaesthesia, so may delay diagnosis and treatment in the unstable child. Thus, obtaining a computerised tomography (CT) scan of the brain is a reasonable approach. However, a non-contrasted head CT scan has limited sensitivity for the detection of acute childhood AIS and stroke mimics, failing to identify the diagnosis in more than 40%

of children (Mirsky et al. 2017). Thus, MRI/MRA is superior to CT scanning in revealing intracranial details and, if available, should be undertaken as early as possible.

In well-resourced centres, the 'rapid brain' or hyperacute MRI protocol for stroke is not different in HIV-infected and uninfected children. It includes axial diffusion-weighted imaging, apparent diffusion coefficient maps, fluid attenuation inversion recovery, and either susceptibility-weighted imaging or gradient echo sequences to confirm the diagnosis of stroke and to assess for haemorrhage. If a stroke is confirmed on the rapid brain MRI study, a full protocol including T1- and T2-weighted MRI with time-of-flight MRA of the head and neck is performed. In CSVT, a head CT scan may demonstrate the venous thrombus as a hyperdensity within the intracranial dural sinuses, and contrast-enhanced CT may reveal a filling defect. However, if available, magnetic resonance venography with or without gadolinium should be undertaken for suspected CSVT (Rivkin et al. 2016; Mirsky et al. 2017). In haemorrhagic stroke, a head CT scan is often the first neuroimaging modality performed because of its sensitivity for detecting haemorrhage, its short scan time, and its availability in the emergency setting. Urgent neuroimaging is important for children with altered mental status, coma, or in whom the airway is not stable. However, in a stable and cooperative child, brain MRI with MRA and magnetic resonance venography can diagnose haemorrhage (Mirsky et al. 2017).

Besides neuroimaging, standard basic investigations for all children with strokes should include (Benjamin et al. 2012; Hammond et al. 2016a):

1. Basic blood tests: full blood count, glucose, urea and electrolytes, liver function tests, and erythrocyte sedimentation rate.
2. Chest radiograph to look specifically for infection (i.e. tuberculosis) and tumours. It may also identify cardiac diseases and blood vessel abnormalities.
3. Infection screen inclusive of urine dipstick with microscopy and culture, blood cultures, nasopharyngeal aspirates for cultures and viral studies, Mantoux skin test, sputum (or gastric washing) for acid-fast bacilli, nucleic acid amplification testing, and tuberculosis (TB) cultures.
4. Lumbar puncture: if not contraindicated, lumbar puncture should be done for cerebrospinal fluid (CSF) cell count, protein and glucose concentrations, Gram stain, and bacterial cultures. In TB endemic regions, acid-fast bacilli stain, nucleic acid amplification testing, and TB cultures are standard.
5. Cardiovascular assessment: 4-limb blood pressure monitoring provides a quick screen for defects such as coarctation. Electrocardiography may help detect conduction defects while an echocardiogram is useful in identifying valvular lesions.
6. Coagulation screen inclusive of platelet count and basic clotting screen. The clotting screen should include partial thromboplastin time, prothrombin time, international normalised ratio, fibrinogen level, thrombin time, and bleeding time.

Additional testing specific to children with HIV infection should include (Benjamin et al. 2012; Hammond et al. 2016a):

1. Blood testing, including CD4+ cell count, HIV viral load, cholesterol levels (especially if patient is taking antiretroviral regime containing protease inhibitors), polymerase chain reaction with antigen tests for herpes simplex virus types 1 and 2, VZV, CMV, mycoplasma, syphilis, toxoplasma, and *Cryptococcus*.
2. CSF testing, including polymerase chain reaction testing for herpes simplex virus types 1 and 2, VZV, CMV, human herpes virus types 6 and 7, John Cunningham virus, enteroviruses, and adenovirus. Also, CSF should be tested for *Cryptococcus*, toxoplasma, treponema, borrelia, and aspergillus.

The basic requirements for all children presenting with stroke in a resource-limited setting and the additional basic requirements in the HIV-infected child are shown in a stepwise approach in Figure 8.1.

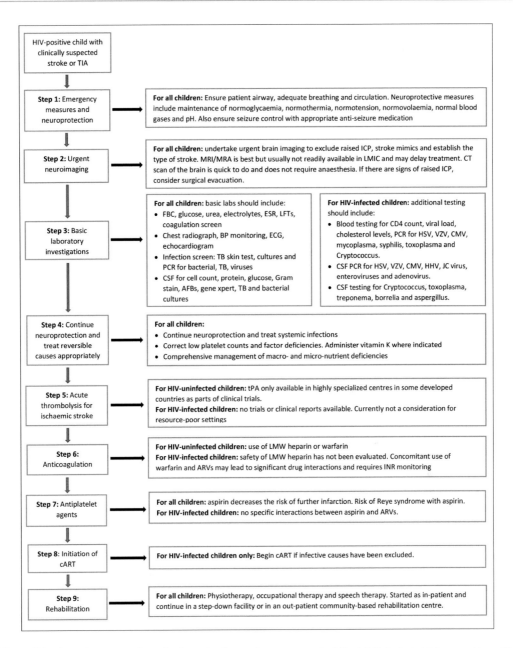

Figure 8.1 Stepwise approach to the investigation and management of the HIV-infected child presenting with stroke or TIA in a resource-limited setting (Benjamin et al. 2012; Hammond et al. 2016a).

Abbreviations: AFB, acid-fast bacilli; ARV, antiretroviral drugs; BP, blood pressure; cART, combination antiretroviral therapy; CMV, cytomegalovirus; CSF, cerebrospinal fluid; CT, computerised tomography; ECG, electrocardiogram; ESR, erythrocyte sedimentation rate; FBC, full blood count; HHV, human herpes virus; HSV, herpes simplex virus; ICP, intracranial pressure; INR, international normalised ratio; JC, John Cunningham; LFTs, liver function tests; LMW, low molecular weight; MRA, magnetic resonance angiography; MRI, magnetic resonance imaging; PCR, polymerase chain reaction; PT, prothrombin time; PTT, partial thromboplastin time; TIA, transient ischaemic attack; TB, tuberculosis; tPA, tissue plasminogen activator; VZV, varicella-zoster virus.

In some instances, specific further investigations beyond those listed above may also be required. However, in most LMICs these investigations would not be feasible due to non-availability, inaccessibility, and/or lack of capacity. Where available these should be carefully selected and guided by the outcomes of the initial clinical assessment and basic investigations (Hammond et al. 2016a). The specific further investigations include:

1. Coagulation screening for suspected thromboembolic events. This should include proteins S and C levels (done at least 3 months after the acute event, as levels around the time of the stroke may not reflect the patient's true levels due to consumptive coagulopathy), antithrombin III, factor V Leiden mutation, antiphospholipid antibodies, and anticardiolipin antibodies (Tipping et al. 2007; Cutfield et al. 2009; Hammond et al. 2016a).
2. Further cardiovascular workup including bubble gram echocardiogram to exclude pulmonary arteriovenous malformations, MRA of the neck to outline the carotid and the vertebral arteries, and abdominal Doppler ultrasound to identify renal vessel abnormalities (Cutfield et al. 2009; Hammond et al. 2016a).
3. Metabolic screening including blood and CSF lactate to screen for evidence of mitochondrial pathology such as mitochondrial encephalopathy with lactic acidosis and stroke-like events. Also, urinary organic and amino acids panel may be sent to exclude homocystinuria (Hammond et al. 2016a).
4. Nuclear medicine studies including single-photon emission CT and positron emission topography scans may be done to define cerebral perfusion and metabolism in patients being considered for revascularisation surgery (d'Arminio et al. 2004; Roach et al. 2008; Hammond et al. 2016b).
5. Brain biopsy is highly invasive and rarely done. However, when other screens have failed to elucidate an aetiology, it may be done to identify emboli, features of vasculitis, or additional pathology such as concomitant mycobacterial infection, fungal infection, lymphoma, or viral inclusions (Cutfield et al. 2009; Ferenczy et al. 2012; Hardie et al. 2013).

TREATMENT

All children with stroke should ideally be managed in a stroke unit equipped with facilities and skilled personnel able to undertake a comprehensive assessment of the patient's medical problems, disabilities, and psychosocial concerns. The multidisciplinary stroke team should include physicians, nursing staff, therapists, social workers, and psychologists and should have established pathways and management guidelines for the acute and post-acute management of stroke in children (Rivkin et al. 2016). In resource-limited settings such as SSA and Southeast Asia, where most HIV-infected children reside, lack of finances, shortages in skilled personnel, and a limited number of paediatric beds preclude such an establishment even at tertiary level hospitals. In some countries, adult stroke units exist that could serve as models for the reorganisation of existing resources to provide more efficient stroke care without necessarily incurring additional cost (Bryer et al. 2011).

Acute Management

The acute treatment approach to any child diagnosed with acute ischaemic stroke includes initial supportive treatment, such as neuroprotection, and anticoagulation. Surgical evacuation is done for intracranial haematomas to relieve intracranial pressure. A few highly specialised centres in well-resourced countries – mainly in North America and Europe – have introduced acute thrombolysis in carefully selected children presenting with acute AIS, but these do not include HIV-infected children and will not be discussed in this chapter.

The aim of neuroprotection is, first, to deliver adequate oxygen and glucose to the brain by optimising oxygen, blood glucose, blood pressure, and cerebral perfusion, and, second, to reduce neuronal metabolic demands by controlling fever and seizures (Rivkin et al. 2016). These measures do not differ between HIV-infected and uninfected children. Initial neuroprotective measures after acute stroke should include clearing the airway and proper positioning (e.g. keeping the head of the bed flat) to ensure adequate cerebral perfusion. Secure the airway in ICU for the comatose patient and treat any suspected seizure activity with appropriate anti-convulsants. Then, check arterial blood gases, pH, and administer supplemental oxygen if required. It is important to correct hypoglycaemia with glucose-containing fluids and maintain normoglycaemia. Significant hypertension should be treated to safely lower the systolic blood pressure by about 25% over 24 hours. Target systolic blood pressure should be between the 50th and 90th percentile for age. It is also important to maintain normovolemia with isotonic fluid at maintenance rate, giving boluses if necessary. Anaemia, if present, should be corrected with appropriate haemotransfusions. Fever should be adequately treated with acetaminophen (Hammond et al. 2016a; Rivkin et al. 2016).

In haemorrhagic stroke, acute management may include surgical evacuation of intracranial haematoma to reduce intracranial pressure. Thus, if there are persistent signs of raised intracranial pressure supported by imaging findings, urgent neurosurgical consultation should be sought. Ventricular drainage and, if indicated, ventriculo-peritoneal shunting for progressive hydrocephalus may be necessary (Roach et al. 2008).

Anticoagulation in the HIV-uninfected child with ischaemic stroke involves the use of low molecular weight heparins or warfarin. In the HIV-infected child presenting with ischaemic stroke, the safety and efficacy of low molecular weight heparins has not been evaluated (Roach et al. 2008). Warfarin is metabolised by the CYP450 enzyme system and, thus, concomitant use with cART requires strict international normalised ratio monitoring due to potential drug interactions, especially with protease inhibitors and non-nucleoside reverse transcriptase inhibitors (Liedtke, Vanguri, and Rathburn 2012).

In patients with SCD, rapid exchange transfusion is the treatment of choice (Kato et al. 2018). In LMIC, this may not be readily available. Blood transfusions, rehydration, and treatment of intercurrent infections are standard. In addition, chronic transfusions decrease stroke recurrence. Also, transcranial Doppler screening to detect increased vascular velocity helps to identify children at high risk of stroke, who should then be offered chronic transfusions. Hydroxyurea therapy is effective in reducing the transcranial Doppler vascular velocity and has the potential to prevent stroke in SCD and HIV-infected patients (Kato et al. 2018).

Long-term Management

The long-term management of ischaemic stroke includes medical and non-medical treatments. Medical treatment includes the use of anti-platelet agents for secondary prevention. Aspirin is the most common and widely used anti-platelet agent and may decrease the risk of further infarctions. It has no specific interactions with antiretroviral drugs and is safe to use in HIV-infected children; however, Reyes syndrome remains a concern (Singer et al. 2013). Thus, it is appropriate to immunise against influenza and varicella before starting aspirin. Other anti-platelet agents such as clopidogrel have not been trialled in HIV-infected children.

In HIV-infected children who present with HIV-associated cerebral vasculopathy leading to stroke, initiation of cART results in decreased HIV viral load and may improve the arteriopathy, with or without corticosteroids (Bhagavati and Choi 2008; Cutfield et al. 2009). Prior to cART initiation, it is important to identify and treat opportunistic infections adequately to prevent IRIS from occurring (Lipman and Breen 2006).

Surgical revascularisation procedures could be an option for children with moyamoya syndrome and those who continue to have cerebrovascular dysfunction despite optimal medical management (Roach et al. 2008). Revascularisation procedures utilise the extracranial circulation to perfuse the brain through the formation of anastomosis. These revascularisation procedures may be direct or indirect. In direct revascularisation, anastomotic connections are created between a donor vessel (usually the superficial temporal branch of the external carotid) and a recipient intracranial vessel. This is technically difficult to perform in young children due to the child's own small scalp donor vessels or the intracranial recipient vessels. Thus, the indirect revascularisation procedures, such as the drilling of burr holes with inversion of the dura in order to enhance new dural revascularisation of the brain without vessel synangiosis and craniotomy, are a preferred option in young children (Roach et al. 2008). However, the effectiveness of these procedures in HIV-infected children is not reported.

In HIV-infected adults presenting with stroke, newer focused vascular surgeries are reported with successful outcomes. The pipeline embolisation technique utilises a wire mesh cylindrical implanted device, which is placed within a cerebral artery and allows flow diversion when the location of the cerebral aneurysm precludes parent vessel sacrifice or surgical bypass (Delgado Almandoz et al. 2013).

Stroke Rehabilitation

Stroke rehabilitation is a goal-oriented process that attempts to obtain maximum function in patients who have had strokes and have physical, cognitive, and language disability. It is best performed by a multidisciplinary team of experienced therapists, who should bear in mind the peculiar issues facing the HIV-infected child with stroke. For any child who has a stroke, the definitive aim of rehabilitation should be to assist them to resume their premorbid function within the family, school, and community. Where there is significant permanent disability, the goal should be to reduce the burden of care for the family and to help the child become as independent as possible. For children, the parents or caregivers should be trained by the rehabilitation team. Institutionalisation may be required for children with poor outcomes, and decisions about home care versus institutionalisation must involve parents or caregivers and should take into account financial and social circumstances (Bryer et al. 2011).

In LMICs where in-patient beds for stroke rehabilitation are scarce, community-based rehabilitation or step-down facilities may be employed. This is especially true for stable patients who have a definite diagnosis, treatment plan, and prescribed medication and who no longer require an acute intervention and can be cared for mostly by nurses and allied health professionals (Bryer et al. 2011).

OUTCOME AND RECURRENCE RISK

In many patients with focal cerebral arteriopathy, strokes are non-progressive and do not recur (Leeuwis, Wolfs, and Braun 2007). However, there are reports of recurrent strokes or TIAs in HIV-infected patients with poor virologic suppression or a low CD4+ cell count. In these cases recurrence may be related to opportunistic vasculitis (Baily and Mandal 1995; Inglot et al. 2013), prothrombotic state (Gorczyca et al. 2005), progressive vasculopathy (Nogueras et al. 2002; Bhagavati and Choi 2008), or moyamoya syndrome (Hsiung and Sotero de Menezes 1999; Hammond et al. 2016b). Recurrence may also result from immune reconstitution (IRIS) following cART initiation (Lipman and Breen 2006). The outcome for most patients reported in the literature has been favourable following appropriate treatment of opportunistic infections, proper timing of cART initiation, and aspirin prophylaxis (Connor 2009; Cutfield et al. 2009).

SUMMARY AND FUTURE PERSPECTIVE

HIV infection in children is associated with increased risk of cerebrovascular disease. Vascular damage may result directly from HIV-associated vasculopathy or indirectly from opportunistic vasculopathy. The evidence suggests that there is a higher incidence of vasculopathy in children with poor virologic suppression. Apart from vasculopathy, cardioembolism and prothrombotic states from various causes also predispose the HIV-infected child to stroke. The treatment of HIV-infected children with cART exposes them to metabolic changes that also increase the cerebrovascular risk. Immune reconstitution following treatment initiation may also lead to vascular damage. As more HIV-infected children are receiving cART for long periods and surviving into adulthood, attention should be given to the management of these complications of treatment. Thus, in the management of the HIV-infected child, vascular risk factors must be identified and managed alongside the management of the HIV infection and immunosuppression.

REFERENCES

Abuaf N, Laperche S, Rajoely B AM et al. (1997) Autoantibodies to phospholipids and to the coagulation proteins in AIDS. *Thrombosis and Haemostasis*, 77(5): 856–861.

Arvind G, Evangelyne S, Limanukshi A, Devi SB, Singh WJ (2013) Human immunodeficiency virus-associated stroke: An aetiopathogenesis study. *The Journal of the Association of Physicians of India*, 61(11): 793–797.

Bagasra O, Steiner RM, Ballas SK et al. (1998) Viral burden and disease progression in HIV-1-infected patients with sickle cell anemia. *American Journal of Hematology*, 59(3): 199–207. https://doi.org/10.1002/(sici)1096-8652(199811)59:3<199::aid-ajh4>3.0.co;2-l.

Baily GG, Mandal BK (1995) Recurrent transient neurological deficits in advanced HIV infection. *AIDS (London, England)*, 9(7): 709–712.

Barbaro G (2002) Cardiovascular manifestations of HIV infection. *Circulation*, 106(11)L 1420–1425.

Benjamin LA, Bryer A, Emsley HCA, Khoo S, Solomon T, Connor MD (2012) HIV infection and stroke: Current perspectives and future directions. *The Lancet. Neurology*, 11(10): 878–890. https://doi.org/10.1016/S1474-4422(12)70205-3.

Berger JR, Harris JO, Gregorios J, Norenberg M (1990) Cerebrovascular disease in AIDS: A case-control study. *AIDS (London, England)*, 4(3): 239–244.

Bhagavati S, Choi J (2008) Rapidly progressive cerebrovascular stenosis and recurrent strokes followed by improvement in HIV vasculopathy. *Cerebrovascular Diseases (Basel, Switzerland)*, 26(4): 449–452. https://doi.org/10.1159/000157632.

Bonkowsky JL, Christenson JC, Nixon GW, Pavia AT (2002) Cerebral aneurysms in a child with acquired immune deficiency syndrome during rapid immune reconstitution. *Journal of Child Neurology*, 17(6): 457–460.

Brew BJ, Miller J (1996) Human immunodeficiency virus type 1-related transient neurological deficits. *The American Journal of Medicine*, 101(3) 257–261. https://doi.org/10.1016/S0002-9343(96)00123-4.

Broderick J, Talbot GT, Prenger E, Leach A, Brott T (1993) Stroke in children within a major metropolitan area: The surprising importance of intracerebral hemorrhage. *Journal of Child Neurology*, 8(3): 250–255. https://doi.org/10.1177/088307389300800308.

Bryer A, Connor MD, Haug P et al. (2011) The South African guideline for the management of ischemic stroke and transient ischemic attack: Recommendations for a resource-constrained health care setting. *International Journal of Stroke: Official Journal of the International Stroke Society*, 6(4): 349–354. https://doi.org/10.1111/j.1747-4949.2011.00629.x.

Calza L, Manfredi R, Chiodo F (2004) Dyslipidaemia associated with antiretroviral therapy in HIV-infected patients. *The Journal of Antimicrobial Chemotherapy*, 53(1): 10–14. https://doi.org/10.1093/jac/dkh013.

Cole JW, Pinto AN, Hebel JR et al. (2004) Acquired immunodeficiency syndrome and the risk of stroke. *Stroke; a Journal of Cerebral Circulation*, 35(1): 51–56. https://doi.org/10.1161/01.STR.0000105393.57853.11.

Connor MD (2009) Treatment of HIV-associated cerebral vasculopathy. *Journal of Neurology, Neurosurgery, and Psychiatry*, 80(8): 831. https://doi.org/10.1136/jnnp.2008.169490.

Cutfield NJ, Steele H, Wilhelm T, Weatherall MW (2009) Successful treatment of HIV-associated cerebral vasculopathy with HAART. *Journal of Neurology, Neurosurgery, and Psychiatry*, 80(8): 936–937. https://doi.org/10.1136/jnnp.2008.165852.

d'Arminio A, Sabin CA, Phillips AN et al. (2004) Cardio- and cerebrovascular events in HIV-infected persons. *AIDS (London, England)*, 18(13): 1811–1817.

David AN, Jinadu MY, Wapmuk AE et al. (2018) Prevalence and impact of sickle cell trait on the clinical and laboratory parameters of HIV-infected children in Lagos, Nigeria. *The Pan African Medical Journal*, 31: 113. https://doi.10.11604/pamj.2018.31.113.15097.

Delgado Almandoz JE, Crandall BM, Fease JL et al. (2013) Successful endovascular treatment of three fusiform cerebral aneurysms with the Pipeline Embolization Device in a patient with dilating HIV vasculopathy. *BMJ Case Reports*, 2013. https://doi.org/10.1136/bcr-2012-010634.

deVeber GA, Kirton A, Booth FA et al. (2017) Epidemiology and outcomes of arterial ischemic stroke in children: The Canadian Pediatric Ischemic Stroke Registry. *Pediatric Neurology*. https://doi.org/10.1016/j.pediatrneurol.2017.01.016.

Dhawan SR, Gupta A, Gupta V, Singhi PD (2016) Multiple intracranial aneurysms in HIV infection. *Indian Journal of Pediatrics*, 83(8): 852–854. https://doi.org/10.1007/s12098-016-2073-7.

Di Biagio A, Rosso R, Maggi P et al. (2013) Inflammation markers correlate with common carotid intima-media thickness in patients perinatally infected with human immunodeficiency virus 1. *Journal of Ultrasound in Medicine: Official Journal of the American Institute of Ultrasound in Medicine*, 32(5): 763–768. https://doi.org/10.7863/ultra.32.5.763.

Dubrovsky T, Curless R, Scott G et al. (1998) Cerebral aneurysmal arteriopathy in childhood AIDS. *Neurology*, 51(2): 560–565.

Engstrom JW, Lowenstein DH, Bredesen DE (1989) Cerebral infarctions and transient neurologic deficits associated with acquired immunodeficiency syndrome. *The American Journal of Medicine*, 86(5): 528–532.

Esoh K, Wonkam-Tingang E, Wonkam A (2021) Sickle cell disease in sub-Saharan Africa: Transferable strategies for prevention and care. *The Lancet. Haematology*, 8(10): e744–e755. https://doi.org/10.1016/S2352-3026(21)00191-5.

Evers S, Nabavi D, Rahmann A, Heese C, Reichelt D, Husstedt I-W (2003) Ischaemic cerebrovascular events in HIV infection: A cohort study. *Cerebrovascular Diseases (Basel, Switzerland)*, 15(3): 199–205. https://doi.org/68828.

Fallo A, De Matteo E, Preciado MV et al. (2005) Epstein-Barr virus associated with primary CNS lymphoma and disseminated BCG infection in a child with AIDS. *International Journal of Infectious Diseases: IJID: Official Publication of the International Society for Infectious Diseases*, 9(2): 96–103. https://doi.org/10.1016/j.ijid.2004.05.008.

Ferenczy MW, Marshall LJ, Nelson CDS et al. (2012) Molecular biology, epidemiology, and pathogenesis of progressive multifocal leukoencephalopathy, the JC virus-induced demyelinating disease of the human brain. *Clinical Microbiology Reviews*, 25(3): 471–506. https://doi.org/10.1128/CMR.05031-11.

Fullerton HJ, Wu YW, Zhao S, Johnston SC (2003) Risk of stroke in children: Ethnic and gender disparities. *Neurology*, 61(2): 189–194.

Fulmer BB, Dillard SC, Musulman EM, Palmer CA, Oakes J (1998) Two cases of cerebral aneurysms in HIV+ children. *Pediatric Neurosurgery*, 28(1): 31–34.

Gorczyca I, Stanek M, Podlasin B, Furmanek M, Pniewski J (2005) Recurrent cerebral infarcts as the first manifestation of infection with the HIV virus. *Folia Neuropathologica*, 43(1): 45–49.

Goyal A, Shah I (2014) HIV-associated thromboembolic phenomenon due to protein C deficiency. *Journal of the International Association of Providers of AIDS Care*, 13(4): 316–317. https://doi.org/10.1177/2325957413508318.

Gutierrez J, Glenn M, Isaacson RS, Marr AD, Mash D, Petito C (2012) Thinning of the arterial media layer as a possible preclinical stage in HIV vasculopathy: A pilot study. *Stroke; a Journal of Cerebral Circulation*, 43(4): 1156–1158. https://doi.org/10.1161/STROKEAHA.111.643387.

Hajjar LA, Calderaro D, Yu PC et al. (2005) Cardiovascular manifestations in patients infected with the human immunodeficiency virus. *Arquivos Brasileiros de Cardiologia*, 85(5): 363–377. https://doi.org/10.1590/S0066-782X2005001800013.

Hammond CK, Eley B, Wieselthaler N, Ndondo A, Wilmshurst JM (2016a) Cerebrovascular disease in children with HIV-1 infection. *Developmental Medicine and Child Neurology*, 58(5): 452–460. https://doi.org/10.1111/dmcn.13080.

Hammond CK, Shapson-Coe A, Govender R et al. (2016b) Moyamoya syndrome in South African children with HIV-1 infection. *Journal of Child Neurology*, 31(8): 1010–1017. https://doi.org/10.1177/0883073816635747.

Hardie DR, Albertyn C, Heckmann JM, Smuts HEM (2013) Molecular characterisation of virus in the brains of patients with measles inclusion body encephalitis (MIBE). *Virology Journal*, 10: 283. https://doi.org/10.1186/1743-422X-10-283.

Hsiung GY, Sotero de Menezes M (1999) Moyamoya syndrome in a patient with congenital human immunodeficiency virus infection. *Journal of Child Neurology*, 14(4): 268–270.

Idri NS, Grobbee DE, Burgner D, Cheung MMH, Kurniati N, Uiterwaal CSPM (2016) Effects of paediatric HIV infection on childhood vasculature. *European Heart Journal*, 37(48): 3610–3616. https://doi.org/10.1093/eurheartj/ehv702.

Idro R, Marsh K, John CC, Newton CR (2010) Cerebral malaria: Mechanisms of brain injury and strategies for improved neuro-cognitive outcome. *Pediatric Research*, 68(4): 267–274. https://doi.org/10.1203/PDR.0b013e3181eee738.

Inglot M, Szymanek A, Szymczak AP et al. (2013) Three episodes of brain stroke as a manifestation of neurosyphilis in an HIV-infected man. *Acta Dermato-Venereologica*, 93(2), 234–235. https://doi.org/10.2340/00015555-1482.

Ismael S, Moshahid Khan M, Kumar P et al. (2020) HIV-associated risk factors for ischemic stroke and future perspectives. *International Journal of Molecular Sciences*, 21(15): 5306. https://doi.org/10.3390/ijms21155306.

Izbudak I, Chalian M, Hutton N et al. (2013) Perinatally HIV-infected youth presenting with acute stroke: Progression/evolution of ischemic disease on neuroimaging. *Journal of Neuroradiology. Journal De Neuroradiologie*, 40(3)|: 172–180. https://doi.org/10.1016/j.neurad.2012.08.001.

Kato GJ, Piel FB, Reid CD et al. (2018) Sickle cell disease. *Nature Reviews. Disease Primers*, 4: 18010. https://doi.org/10.1038/nrdp.2018.10.

Katsetos CD, Fincke JE, Legido A et al. (1999) Angiocentric CD3(+) T-cell infiltrates in human immunodeficiency virus type 1-associated central nervous system disease in children. *Clinical and Diagnostic Laboratory Immunology*, 6(1): 105–114.

Kieburtz KD, Eskin TA, Ketonen L, Tuite MJ (1993) Opportunistic cerebral vasculopathy and stroke in patients with the acquired immunodeficiency syndrome. *Archives of Neurology*, 50(4): 430–432.

Kolapo KO, Vento S (2011) Stroke: A realistic approach to a growing problem in sub-Saharan Africa is urgently needed. *Tropical Medicine & International Health: TM & IH*, 16(6), 707–710. https://doi.org/10.1111/j.1365-3156.2011.02759.x.

Kourtis AP, Bansil P, Johnson C, Meikle SF, Posner SF, Jamieson DJ (2007) Children with sickle cell disease and human immunodeficiency virus-1 infection: Use of inpatient care services in the United States. *The Pediatric Infectious Disease Journal*, 26(5): 406–410. https://doi.org/10.1097/01.inf.0000259953.79654.d0.

Lai WW, Colan SD, Easley KA et al. (2001) Dilation of the aortic root in children infected with human immunodeficiency virus type 1: The Prospective P2C2 HIV Multicenter Study. *American Heart Journal*, 141(4): 661–670. https://doi.org/10.1067/mhj.2001.113757.

Leeuwis JW, Wolfs TFW, Braun KPJ (2007) A child with HIV-associated transient cerebral arteriopathy. *AIDS (London, England)*, 21(10): 1383–1384. https://doi.org/10.1097/QAD.0b013e3281053a30.

Liedtke MD, Vanguri A, Rathbun RC (2012) A probable interaction between warfarin and the antiretroviral TRIO study regimen. *The Annals of Pharmacotherapy*, 46(11): e34. https://doi.org/10.1345/aph.1R290.

Lipman M, Breen R (2006) Immune reconstitution inflammatory syndrome in HIV. *Current Opinion in Infectious Diseases*, 19(1): 20–25.

Little R (2006) Neoplastic disease in pediatric HIV infection. In: Zeichner SL, Read JS, editors, *Handbook of Pediatric HIV Care*. Cambridge: Cambridge University Press, pp. 637–649.

Mackay MT, Wiznitzer M, Benedict SL et al. (2011) Arterial ischemic stroke risk factors: The International Pediatric Stroke Study. *Annals of Neurology*, 69(1): 130–140. https://doi.org/10.1002/ana.22224.

Mahadevan A, Tagore R, Siddappa NB et al. (2008) Giant serpentine aneurysm of vertebrobasilar artery mimicking dolichoectasia – An unusual complication of pediatric AIDS. Report of a case with review of the literature. *Clinical Neuropathology*, 27(1): 37–52.

Martínez-Longoria CA, Morales-Aguirre JJ, Villalobos-Acosta CP, Gómez-Barreto D, Cashat-Cruz M (2004) Occurrence of intracerebral aneurysm in an HIV-infected child: A case report. *Pediatric Neurology*, 31(2): 130–132. https://doi.org/10.1016/j.pediatrneurol.2004.02.008.

Mazzoni P, Chiriboga CA, Millar WS, Rogers A (2000) Intracerebral aneurysms in human immunodeficiency virus infection: Case report and literature review. *Pediatric Neurology*, 23(3): 252–255.

McComsey GA, O'Riordan M, Hazen SL et al. (2007) Increased carotid intima media thickness and cardiac biomarkers in HIV-infected children. *AIDS (London, England)*, 21(8), 921–927. https://doi.org/10.1097/QAD.0b013e328133f29c.

Mirsky DM, Beslow LA, Amlie-Lefond C et al. (2017) Pathways for Neuroimaging of Childhood Stroke. *Pediatric Neurology*, 69: 11–23. https://doi.org/10.1016/j.pediatrneurol.2016.12.004.

Moriarty DM, Haller JO, Loh JP, Fikrig S (1994) Cerebral infarction in pediatric acquired immunodeficiency syndrome. *Pediatric Radiology*, 24(8): 611–612.

Narayan P, Samuels OB, Barrow DL (2002) Stroke and pediatric human immunodeficiency virus infection. Case report and review of the literature. *Pediatric Neurosurgery*, 37(3): 158–163.

Newton CRJC (2005) Interaction between Plasmodium falciparum and human immunodeficiency virus type 1 on the central nervous system of African children. *Journal of Neurovirology*, 11(Suppl 3): 45–51. https://doi.org/10.1080/13550280500511881.

Nogueras C, Sala M, Sasal M et al. (2002) Recurrent stroke as a manifestation of primary angiitis of the central nervous system in a patient infected with human immunodeficiency virus. *Archives of Neurology*, 59(3): 468–473.

Nunes ML, Pinho AP, Sfoggia A (2001) Cerebral aneurysmal dilatation in an infant with perinatally acquired HIV infection and HSV encephalitis. *Arquivos De Neuro-Psiquiatria*, 59(1): 116–118.

Ovbiagele B, Nath A (2011) Increasing incidence of ischemic stroke in patients with HIV infection. *Neurology*, 76(5): 444–450. https://doi.org/10.1212/WNL.0b013e31820a0cfc.

Park YD, Belman AL, Kim TS et al. (1990) Stroke in pediatric acquired immunodeficiency syndrome. *Annals of Neurology*, 28(3): 303–311. https://doi.org/10.1002/ana.410280302.

Patsalides AD, Wood LV, Atac GK, Sandifer E, Butman JA, Patronas NJ (2002) Cerebrovascular disease in HIV-infected pediatric patients: Neuroimaging findings. *AJR. American Journal of Roentgenology*, 179(4): 999–1003. https://doi.org/10.2214/ajr.179.4.1790999.

Philippet P, Blanche S, Sebag G, Rodesch G, Griscelli C, Tardieu M (1994) Stroke and cerebral infarcts in children infected with human immunodeficiency virus. *Archives of Pediatrics & Adolescent Medicine*, 148(9): 965–970.

Pillay B, Ramdial PK, Naidoo DP (2015) HIV-associated large-vessel vasculopathy: A review of the current and emerging clinicopathological spectrum in vascular surgical practice. *Cardiovascular Journal of Africa*, 26(2): 70–81. https://doi.org/10.5830/CVJA-2015-017.

Pinto AN (1996) AIDS and cerebrovascular disease. *Stroke; a Journal of Cerebral Circulation*, 27(3): 538–543.

Rabinstein AA (2003) Stroke in HIV-infected patients: A clinical perspective. *Cerebrovascular Diseases (Basel, Switzerland)*, 15(1–2): 37–44. https://doi.org/67120.

Rakhmanina N, Wong EC, Davis JC, Ray PE (2014) Hemorrhagic stroke in an adolescent female with HIV-associated thrombotic thrombocytopenic purpura. *Journal of AIDS & Clinical Research*, 5(6). https://doi.org/10.4172/2155-6113.1000311.

Rivkin MJ, Bernard TJ, Dowling MM, Amlie-Lefond C (2016) Guidelines for urgent management of stroke in children. *Pediatric Neurology*, 56: 8–17. https://doi.org/10.1016/j.pediatrneurol.2016.01.016.

Roach ES, Golomb MR, Adams R et al. (2008) Management of stroke in infants and children: A scientific statement from a Special Writing Group of the American Heart Association Stroke Council and the Council on Cardiovascular Disease in the Young. *Stroke; a Journal of Cerebral Circulation*, 39(9): 2644–2691. https://doi.org/10.1161/STROKEAHA.108.189696.

Roquer J, Palomeras E, Knobel H, Pou A (1998) Intracerebral haemorrhage in AIDS. *Cerebrovascular Diseases (Basel, Switzerland)*, 8(4): 222–227.

Saif MW, Greenberg B (2001) HIV and thrombosis: A review. *AIDS Patient Care and STDs*, 15(1): 15–24. https://doi.org/10.1089/108729101460065.

Shah SS, Zimmerman RA, Rorke LB, Vezina LG (1996) Cerebrovascular complications of HIV in children. *AJNR. American Journal of Neuroradiology*, 17(10): 1913–1917.

Singer EJ, Valdes-Sueiras M, Commins DL, Yong W, Carlson M (2013) HIV stroke risk: Evidence and implications. *Therapeutic Advances in Chronic Disease*, 4(2): 61–70. https://doi.org/10.1177/2040622312471840.

Ssenyondwa J, George PE, Bazo-Alvarez JC et al. (2020) Impact of sickle cell disease on presentation and progression of paediatric HIV: A retrospective cohort study. *Tropical Medicine & International Health*, 25(7): 897–904. https://doi.org/10.1111/tmi.13408.

Tipping B, de Villiers L, Wainwright H, Candy S, Bryer A (2007) Stroke in patients with human immunodeficiency virus infection. *Journal of Neurology, Neurosurgery, and Psychiatry*, 78(12): 1320–1324. https://doi.org/10.1136/jnnp.2007.116103.

van Toorn R, Rabie H, Dramowski A, Schoeman JF (2012) Neurological manifestations of TB-IRIS: A report of 4 children. *European Journal of Paediatric Neurology: EJPN: Official Journal of the European Paediatric Neurology Society*, 16(6): 676–682. https://doi.org/10.1016/j.ejpn.2012.04.005.

Tumours of the Central Nervous System in Children with HIV

Rajeshree Govender, Alan Davidson, and Beverley G Neethling

INTRODUCTION

The human immunodeficiency virus type 1 (HIV-1) epidemic has complicated the diagnosis and management of children with comorbid malignancies. The incidence rate of malignancies in the HIV-1-infected population is higher than in the HIV-negative population (Granovsky et al. 1998; Mueller 1999b; Biggar et al. 2000). The incidence of cancer in HIV-negative children is reported at 0.13 to 0.15 per 1000 children between birth and 15 years of age (Stack et al. 2007). HIV-1-positive children are at higher risk for both AIDs-defining malignancies and non-HIV-defining cancers. Tumours represent about 2% of the AIDS-defining events in children, as listed by the Centres for Disease Control and Prevention (CDC). The most common malignancies in HIV-1-positive children are Kaposi sarcoma and non-Hodgkin lymphoma (NHL). A South African study showed that HIV-infected children were at a high risk of developing cancer, with an overall incidence rate of 82 per 100 000 person-years. The majority of cancers were AIDS-defining, with an incidence rate of 34 per 100 000 person-years for Kaposi sarcoma and 31 per 100 000 person-years for NHL. The incidence rate of non-AIDs-defining malignancies was 17 per 100 000 person-years (Bohlius et al. 2016). Data from various settings have shown that the incidence rate of cancer has declined with the introduction of highly active antiretroviral therapy (HAART) (Kest et al. 2005; Simard et al. 2012; Bohlius et al. 2016). An Italian pediatric population of 1190 perinatally HIV-infected children had increased survival and decreased CDC class B and C clinical events documented during the HAART era (Chiappini et al. 2007). In the same population, significantly decreased cancer rates were observed from pre- to late-HAART periods, from 4.49 to 0.76 per 1000 person-years (Chiappini et al. 2006). Results from the study of Kest et al. (2005) that followed up on 2969 children in the Pediatric AIDS Clinical Trials Group (PACTG) from 1993 to 2003 revealed a lower incidence rate of cancer in HIV-infected children who received HAART for a prolonged period (more than 2 years) than in those treated for a shorter duration. In a Spanish study (Álvaro-Meca et al. 2011) the rates of AIDs-defining malignancies dropped in the post-HAART era, as opposed to the rates of non-AIDS-defining malignancies, which rose considerably.

There are multiple new genetic biomarkers included in the 2021 World Health Organization (WHO) classification of brain tumours in children; however, none are specific to HIV-positive children (Louis et al. 2021).

PATHOGENESIS OF MALIGNANCIES IN HIV-1 INFECTION

The higher incidence rate of cancer in HIV-1-infected children is associated with immune system impairment due to the progressive depletion of CD4+ lymphocytes and loss of immune functions, chronic immune activation, and coinfection with oncogenic viruses (Flint et al. 2009; Stefan et al. 2014; Goncalves et al. 2016). Features of chronic immune activation include increased levels of pro-inflammatory cytokines and chemokines, polyclonal B-cell activation, increased cell turnover, and accelerated immune senescence (Douek, Roederer, and Koup 2009; Desai and Landay 2010; Breen et al. 2011). All these factors are known to increase the risk of malignancies, and the association between viruses and tumours of the central nervous system (CNS) has been well described (Alibek et al. 2013). The association between Epstein–Barr virus (EBV) and malignancies like lymphomas (Alibek et al. 2013), acute lymphoblastic leukaemia (Tedeschi et al. 2006), and leiomyosarcomas, is well known. Polyomavirus simian virus 40 and John Cunningham virus (JCV) are implicated in the pathogenesis of CNS malignancies (Alibek et al. 2013). The JCV infects glial cells such as astrocytes and oligodendrocytes. When patients are immunosuppressed (such as in HIV infection), JCV can become reactivated leading to increased viral replication and cytolytic destruction of oligodendroglia, resulting in the well described entity of progressive multifocal leukoencephalopathy (Dubois et al. 1997). The oncogenic potential of JCV, especially in humans, is controversial. JCV-induced tumours in animal models include medulloblastomas, gliomas, and neuroblastomas (Maginnis and Atwood 2009). In humans, there are conflicting reports of JCV associated with oligoastrocytomas (Rencic et al. 1996), glioblastomas, oligodendrogliomas, and medulloblastomas (Pina-Oviedo et al. 2006). In a series of patients with a variety of CNS tumours, JCV DNA was found in 28% of the ependymomas and in 20% of the choroid plexus papillomas (Okamoto et al. 2005). Cytomegalovirus DNA has also been implicated in the genesis of medulloblastomas (Baryawno et al. 2011) and glioblastoma multiforme (Lucas et al. 2010).

Children with HIV-1 infection have a higher risk of coinfection with other viruses, so they are likely at a greater risk for development of these tumours. Children exposed to HIV-1 and didanosine in utero (as part of the prevention of mother-to-child transmission of HIV-1) are also at a higher risk of developing cancers (Hleyhel et al. 2016). Transplacental exposure to 3′-azido-2′, 3′-dideoxythymidine in mice has also been shown to have carcinogenic effects (Olivero et al. 1997). A number of genotoxic markers have been identified in humans and animals that are implicated in causing nuclear and mitochondrial damage secondary to perinatal nucleoside reverse transcriptase inhibitor (NRTI) exposure (Olivero et al. 1997). However, results of the PACTG 219 study showed no increase in the rates of malignancy in 2077 children exposed to NRTIs in utero (Olivero et al. 1997). Long-term follow-up studies are needed to conclusively prove or disprove the link between NRTI exposure and malignancy risk.

BRAIN: HIV-1-ASSOCIATED MALIGNANCIES

Primary CNS Lymphomas: Presentation, Imaging, Treatment

Primary CNS lymphomas (PCNSL) may be the presenting feature of AIDS in up to 0.6% of all patients. There has been a decline in the incidence of HIV-associated CNS lymphoma since the rollout of HAART. Interestingly, PCNSL was unusual in South Africa before the introduction of HAART. A national study showed that only 2 out of 220 (or just under 1%) of patients with AIDS-defining malignancy had PCNSL (Davidson et al. 2014).

PCNSL in HIV-1-positive populations are usually diffuse, large-cell, NHL of B-cell origin that occur in the brain (rarely in the spinal cord). Most patients have evidence of EBV coinfection in either the lesion or the cerebrospinal fluid (CSF). The pathogenesis is related to an impaired T-cell response to the EBV-infected B cells. These tumours are usually associated with severe immunosuppression and a CD4+ lymphocyte count of less than 100 cells/µL (Gasser et al. 2007). However, PCNSL can rarely manifest in HIV-1-infected children with a preserved immune status (Mueller 1999a).

The presence of PCNSL is indicative of a WHO stage 4, or CDC category C, condition. Clinical presentation is variable, and includes focal neurological signs (facial nerve palsy, diplopia, dysarthria, ataxia, bulbar palsy, quadriparesis), encephalopathy, and seizures. More insidious PCNSL presents with headaches, vomiting, and lethargy. Children with PCNSL may also present solely with diabetes insipidus and progressive panhypopituitarism due to pituitary and hypothalamic involvement (Baleydier et al. 2001). Fundoscopy is important, as some patients may have concomitant ocular involvement.

On computed tomography (CT) scans, a hypodense or hyperdense lesion that enhances in a ring-like pattern is often seen. Surrounding oedema and mass effect may also be observed. Magnetic resonance imaging (MRI) may assist in identifying additional lesions not seen on the CT scan. MRI (Figure 9.1) of CNS lymphoma typically shows a lesion that is hypointense to grey matter on T1- and T2-weighted imaging (Chapter 5, Figure 5.13). If the tumour is undergoing active necrosis, it may

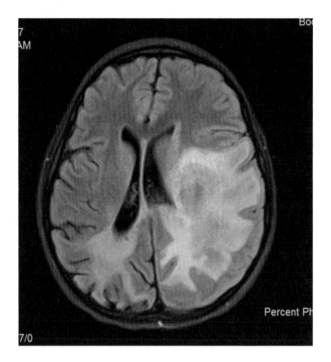

Figure 9.1   Axial fluid attenuated inversion recovery sequence of a magnetic resonance imaging scan of a 5-year-old HIV-positive female who presented with a left hemiplegia demonstrating an ovoid lesion in the left cerebral hemisphere with extensive surrounding vasogenic oedema that extends to the right hemisphere. The histological diagnosis was that of a central nervous system lymphoma.

appear hyperintense on T2-weighted scans. Post-contrast scans typically show intense homogeneous enhancement in high-grade tumours, while low-grade tumours have absent-to-moderate enhancement. Peripheral ring enhancement may be seen in immunocompromised patients. Less commonly, the tumour may present with prominent leptomeningeal involvement and no evidence of an intracranial mass. The most frequent tumour locations in children are in the parietal and frontal lobes, the cerebellum, the pituitary stalk, and the hypothalamus (Alba et al. 2006). The differential diagnosis for these lesions includes toxoplasmosis, cryptococcomas, tuberculomas, meningiomas, metastases from a systemic lymphoma, or glioblastoma multiforme. Magnetic resonance spectroscopy (MRS) in PCNSL typically shows decreased N–acetyl-aspartate and creatine, as well as a choline peak. A thallium-201 single-photon emission CT (SPECT) scan may be useful in distinguishing between lymphoma and toxoplasmosis (which is the main differential diagnosis for the lesion on neuroimaging). Increased thallium uptake by the lesion is suggestive of a PCNSL. An 18-fluorodeoxyglucose positron emission tomography (PET) scan can be used as an alternative to the SPECT scan to assist in differentiating CNS lymphomas from toxoplasmosis. A 2017 systematic review and meta-analysis to assess the roles of SPECT, PET, and MRS in distinguishing PCNSL from other focal brain lesions in HIV-infected patients found that SPECT has good diagnostic accuracy for discriminating PCNSL from other focal brain lesions in the study population. SPECT was, however, less sensitive and specific than pathology/serology for diagnosis. PET was found to be superior but was more expensive, while MRS had modest sensitivity and specificity (Yang et al. 2017).

CSF analysis in patients with CNS lymphoma and associated leptomeningeal disease shows pleocytosis and elevated protein levels. Flow cytometry studies, B-cell re-arrangements (to assess monoclonality) and MYC analysis (for translocations) should also be undertaken on the CSF to assist in sub-typing CNS lymphomas. Studies utilising the amplification of EBV DNA in CSF using the polymerase chain reaction will support the diagnosis of a CNS lymphoma. Quantitative polymerase chain reaction with a cut-off of 10 000 EBV DNA copies/mL increases the specificity and predictive value of the test (Corcoran et al. 2008).

Definitive diagnosis is made by stereotactic brain biopsy. Because this is an invasive procedure, it is usually done after pre-emptive treatment for toxoplasmosis with no response in adults. This approach of treating empirically for toxoplasmosis is less well defined in children. Histological diagnosis shows either a small, non-cleaved type or a large, immunoblastic type.

There are no consensus guidelines for the treatment of CNS lymphomas, so HAART remains the mainstay of treatment. Improved survival rates have been demonstrated with the concomitant use of chemotherapy and brain irradiation. Because of the frequent association with EBV infection, antivirals and other immunomodulatory therapies have been attempted. Treatment with ganciclovir has been associated with improved survival rates (Bossolasco et al. 2006). Other immunomodulating agents that have been used include interleukin-2, intra-thecal methotrexate, and procarbazine (Aboulafia et al. 2006). The CNS is a sanctuary site for lymphoma, and these lymphomas can be difficult to eradicate. CNS prophylaxis is recommended for all patients with HIV-associated lymphoma, even those without current clinical CNS involvement.

Non-lymphomatous Brain Tumours

Since brain tumours (of non-lymphoid origin) are the second most common cancer in non-HIV-infected children, they often occur in HIV-1-positive children. The occurrence of glial neoplasms in the course of the HIV-1 infection could be coincidental. However, the possibility might exist that HIV-1 is directly involved in glial oncogenesis by promoting tumour formation by a yet unknown mechanism

(Tacconi et al. 1996). A French study found that the risk of non-AIDS-defining malignancies is about 5.4 times higher in HIV-1-infected patients than in the general population (Hajjar et al. 1992). The risk of death in the same study was found to 4 times higher in HIV-1-infected patients when compared to the general population. In all HIV-1-infected patients, the incidence of glial CNS tumours is about 0.05% (Hajjar et al. 1992). An American survey found that the overall incidence of primary brain tumours was higher in patients with AIDS than in the general population (Goedert et al. 1998). A broad spectrum of tumours has been described in the adult population with HIV infection, and these include astrocytomas, ependymomas, and embryonal tumours (Büttner and Weis 1999). Mandel et al. (1994) reported on a 13-year-old HIV-1-infected female with an ependymoblastoma. The patient experienced a positive outcome after surgical removal and craniospinal irradiation. Davidson et al. (2014) reported seven children (10%) with non-AIDs-defining CNS tumours in their series of South African children with HIV-1 infection.

SPINAL CORD TUMOURS

Spinal cord tumours in HIV-1 infection are very rare. Weill et al. described two HIV-1-infected patients with glial tumours of the spinal cord (Weill et al. 1987). Both were adult patients, and one patient had an intra-medullary astrocytoma at T12 (WHO Grade 3) while the other patient had a glioblastoma of the medullary conus.

EBV-associated smooth muscle tumours are not uncommon in children with HIV-1 infection (Mueller 1999b). The presence of EBV in both leiomyoma and leiomyosarcoma suggests that EBV infection precedes malignant transformation. The prevalence of leiomyosarcoma among HIV-infected children who had a tumour was only 3% (Biggar et al. 2000). EBV-associated smooth muscle tumour usually presents late in the course of children with AIDS, which is associated with a role of chronic immune suppression in tumour pathogenesis. Leiomyosarcomas of CNS origin are extremely rare. Wilaisakditipakorn et al. (2015) describe an 11-year-old male with slowly progressive HIV-1 disease who presented with quadriplegia and ventilator dependence secondary to an EBV-associated leiomyosar-coma of the cervical spinal cord. Another patient with this condition was an 11-year-old HIV-1-positive female (personal communication) with a CD4+ count of 15% who presented with paraparesis and kyphoscoliosis. The patient also experienced incontinence and had a vesicovaginal fistula. The MRI scan of her spine (Figure 9.2) showed heterogeneous enhanced intradural-extramedullary masses with extension into the T2–T5, L1–L2, and L4–S1 neural foraminae. Biopsy of one of the lesions showed a smooth muscle tumour (spindle cells) with EBV markers positive by immunochemical staining and in situ hybridisation (Wilaisakditipakorn et al. 2015). Treatment of choice for these patients is surgical removal (Chiappini et al. 2014).

TREATMENT OF MALIGNANCIES IN HIV INFECTION

The treatment of malignancies in children with HIV-1 infection is complex, and there is a lack of suffi-cient knowledge of the interactions between HAART and chemotherapy (Bower et al. 2004). Treatment is complicated by multiple comorbidities, including tuberculosis, cytomegalovirus infection, and chronic lung disease, as there are potential drug–drug interactions. In the South African series, 10% of the HIV-1-infected children treated for a comorbid malignancy died from toxicity (Davidson et al. 2014). This highlights the inherent risks of treating immunocompromised children with chemotherapy. If these

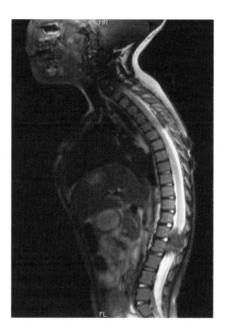

Figure 9.2   Sagittal T2-weighted magnetic resonance imaging scan that demonstrates a well circumscribed ovoid intradural-extra-medullary lesion at L1–L2 inter-vertebral level impinging on the cauda equine nerve roots.

children are HAART-naïve, they should be initiated on treatment, and the outcome can still be positive with optimal care.

Precision medicine is an emerging approach in oncology. Advances in molecular diagnostics (especially next generation sequencing) can characterise a tumour's genetic variability and direct therapy. Target therapies include signal transduction inhibitors, gene expression modulators, apoptosis inducers, angiogenesis inhibitors, and monoclonal antibodies (Pollack, Agnihotri, and Broniscer 2019). Pediatric tumours have a different genetic make-up, with different actionable targets (Seibel et al. 2017). Identification of specific mutations in pediatric high-grade gliomas (*PARP1* over-expression, *TP53* mutations, and *TOP2A* amplification) provides potential new therapeutic targets (Entz-Werlé et al. 2021). Drugs that inhibit the sonic hedgehog signalling pathways (Vismodegib) in medulloblastomas have long been recognised as a potential targeted therapy (Juraschka and Taylor 2019). Other advances in the treatment of CNS malignancies include intensity-modulated radiation therapy, volumetric modulated arc therapy, proton beam radiation therapy, and stereotactic radiosurgery (DeNunzio and Yock 2020). Many of these modalities are not accessible in low- and middle-income countries. With the advent of HAART, however, there are no differences in the treatment regimens for CNS tumours in HIV-positive versus HIV-negative children.

CONCLUSION

Early testing, diagnosis, and treatment of HIV-1-infected children is a useful strategy to prevent malignancies in this population. Children on HAART have a lower risk of developing cancer than children who were not on treatment. Children with more severe immunosuppression are also at higher risk for malignancies. This highlights the importance of developing guidelines for regular monitoring of HIV-1-infected children for the warning signs of malignancies. Infectious agents, as described above, are a significant and likely preventable cause of cancer. Therefore, identification of additional cancers with an infectious aetiology has important implications for public health (Bohlius et al. 2016).

REFERENCES

Abla O, Sandlund JT, Sung L et al. (2006) A case series of pediatric primary central nervous system lymphoma: Favorable outcome without cranial irradiation. *Ped Blood Cancer*, 47(7): 880–885. Available at: http://dx.doi.org/10.1002/pbc.20736.

Aboulafia DM, Ratner L, Miles SA, Harrington WJ (2006) Antiviral and immunomodulatory treatment for AIDS-related primary central nervous system lymphoma: AIDS Malignancies Consortium Pilot Study 019. *Clin Lymphoma Myeloma*, 6(5): 399–402. Available at: http://dx.doi.org/10.3816/clm.2006.n.017.

Alibek K, Mussabekova A, Kakpenova A et al. (2013) Childhood cancers: What is a possible role of infectious agents? *Infect Agents Cancer*, 8(1): 48. Available at: http://dx.doi.org/10.1186/1750-9378-8-48.

Álvaro-Meca A, Micheloud D, Jensen J, Díaz A, García-Alvarez M, Resino S (2011) Epidemiologic trends of cancer diagnoses among HIV-infected children in Spain from 1997 to 2008. *J Pediatric Infect Dis Soc*, 30(9): 764–768. Available at: http://dx.doi.org/10.1097/inf.0b013e31821ba148.

Baleydier F, Galambrun C, Manel AM, Guibaud L, Nicolino M, Bertrand Y (2001) Primary lymphoma of the pituitary stalk in an immunocompetent 9-year-old child. *Med Pediatr Oncol*, 36(3): 392–395. Available at: http://dx.doi.org/10.1002/mpo.1094.

Baryawno N, Rahbar A, Wolmer-Solberg N et al. (2011) Detection of human cytomegalovirus in medulloblastomas reveals a potential therapeutic target. *J Clin Invest*, 121(10): 4043–4055. Available at: http://dx.doi.org/10.1172/jci57147.

Biggar RJ, Frisch M, Goedert JJ, AIDS–Cancer Match Registry Study Group (2000) Risk of cancer in children with AIDS. *Jama*, 284(2): 205–209. Available at: http://dx.doi.org/10.1001/jama.284.2.205.

Bohlius J, Maxwell N, Spoerri A et al. (for IeDEA-Southern Africa) (2016) Incidence of AIDS-defining and other cancers in HIV-positive children in South Africa. *Pediatr Infect Dis J*, 35(6): e164–e170. Available at: http://dx.doi.org/10.1097/inf.0000000000001117.

Bossolasco S, Falk KI, Ponzoni M et al. (2006) Ganciclovir is associated with low or undetectable Epstein-Barr virus DNA load in cerebrospinal fluid of patients with HIV-related primary central nervous system lymphoma. *Clin Infect Dis*, 42(4): e21–e25. Available at: http://dx.doi.org/10.1086/499956.

Bower M, McCall-Peat N, Ryan N et al. (2004) Protease inhibitors potentiate chemotherapy-induced neutropenia. *Blood*, 104(9): 2943–2946. Available at: http://dx.doi.org/10.1182/blood-2004-05-1747.

Breen EC, Hussain S, Magpantay L et al. (2011) B-cell stimulatory cytokines and markers of immune activation are elevated several years prior to the diagnosis of systemic AIDS-associated non-Hodgkin B-cell lymphoma. *Cancer Epidemiology Biomarkers & Prevention*, 20(7): 1303–1314. Available at: http://dx.doi.org/10.1158/1055-9965.epi-11-0037.

Büttner A, Weis S (1999) Non-lymphomatous brain tumors in HIV-1 infection: A review. *J Neurooncol*, 41(1): 81–88. Available at: http://dx.doi.org/10.1023/a:1006137219766.

Chiappini E, Galli L, Tovo PA et al. (2006) Cancer rates after year 2000 significantly decrease in children with perinatal HIV infection: A study by the Italian register for HIV infection in children. *J Clin Oncol*, 25(1): 97–101. Available at: http://dx.doi.org/10.1200/jco.2006.06.6506.

Chiappini E, Galli L, Tovo PA et al. (2007) Changing patterns of clinical events in perinatally HIV-1-infected children during the era of HAART. *AIDS*, 21(12): 1607–1615. Available at: http://dx.doi.org/10.1097/qad.0b013e32823ecf5b.

Chiappini E, Berti E, Gianesin K et al. (2014) Pediatric human immunodeficiency virus infection and cancer in the highly active antiretroviral treatment (HAART) era. *Cancer Lett*, 347(1): 38–45. Available at: http://dx.doi.org/10.1016/j.canlet.2014.02.002.

Corcoran C, Rebe K, van der Plas H, Myer L, Hardie DR (2008) The predictive value of cerebrospinal fluid Epstein-Barr viral load as a marker of primary central nervous system lymphoma in HIV-infected persons. *J Clin Virol*, 42(4): 433–436. Available at: http://dx.doi.org/10.1016/j.jcv.2008.03.017.

Davidson A, Wainwright RD, Stones DK J et al. (2014) Malignancies in South African children with HIV. *J Pediatr Hematol Oncol*, 36(2): 111–117. Available at: http://dx.doi.org/10.1097/mph.0b013e31829cdd49.

DeNunzio NJ, Yock TI (2020) Modern radiotherapy for pediatric brain tumors. *Cancers* (Basel). 12(6): 1533, June 11. doi: 10.3390/cancers12061533; PMID: 32545204; PMCID: PMC7352417.

Desai S, Landay A (2010) Early immune senescence in HIV disease. *Current HIV/AIDS Reports*, 7(1): 4–10. Available at: http://dx.doi.org/10.1007/s11904-009-0038-4.

Douek DC, Roederer M, Koup RA (2009) Emerging concepts in the immunopathogenesis of AIDS. *Annual Review of Medicine*, 60(1): 471–484. Available at: http://dx.doi.org/10.1146/annurev.med.60.041807.123549.

Dubois V, Dutronc H, Lafon ME et al. (1997) Latency and reactivation of JC virus in peripheral blood of human immunodeficiency virus type 1-infected patients. *J Clin Microbiol*, 35(9): 2288–2292.

Entz-Werlé N, Poidevin L, Nazarov PV et al. (2021) A DNA repair and cell cycle gene expression signature in pediatric high-grade gliomas: Prognostic and therapeutic value. *Cancers*, 13 (9): 2252. https://doi.org/10.3390/cancers13092252.

Flint SJ, Enquist LW, Racaniello VR, Skalka AM (2009) Infection of a susceptible host. In: Flint SJ, Enquist LW, Racaniello VR, Skalka AM, editors, *Principles of Virology. Volume II: Pathogenesis and Control. 3rd edn*. Washington: ASM Press, pp. 3–27.

Gasser O, Bihl FK, Wolbers M et al. (2007) HIV patients developing primary CNS lymphoma lack EBV-specific CD4+ T cell function irrespective of absolute CD4+ T cell counts. *PLoS Med*, 4(3): e96. Available at: http://dx.doi.org/10.1371/journal.pmed.0040096.

Goedert JJ, Coté TR, Virgo P et al. (1998) Spectrum of AIDS-associated malignant disorders. *Lancet*, 351(9119): 1833–1839. Available at: http://dx.doi.org/10.1016/s0140-6736(97)09028-4.

Goncalves PH, Montezuma-Rusca JM, Yarchoan R, Uldrick TS (2016) Cancer prevention in HIV-infected populations. *Semin Oncol*, 43(1): 173–188. Available at: http://dx.doi.org/10.1053/j.seminoncol.2015.09.011.

Granovsky MO, Mueller BU, Nicholson HS, Rosenberg PS, Rabkin CS (1998) Cancer in human immunodeficiency virus-infected children: A case series from the Children's Cancer Group and the National Cancer Institute. *J Clin Oncol*, 16(5): 1729–1735. Available at: https://doi.org/10.1200/jco.1998.16.5.1729.

Hajjar M, Lacoste D, Brossard G, Dupon M, Salmi LR, Dabis F (1992) Non-acquired immune deficiency syndrome-defining malignancies in a hospital-based cohort of human immunodeficiency virus-infected patients: Bordeaux, France, 1985-1991. *J Natl Cancer Inst*, 84(20): 1593–1595. Available at: http://dx.doi.org/10.1093/jnci/84.20.1593.

Hleyhel M, Goujon S, Delteil C et al. (2016) Risk of cancer in children exposed to didanosine in utero. *AIDS*, 30(8): 1245–1256. Available at: http://dx.doi.org/10.1097/qad.0000000000001051.

Juraschka K, Taylor MD (2019) Medulloblastoma in the age of molecular subgroups: A review. *J Neurosurg Pediatr*, 24(4): 353–363. doi: 10.3171/2019.5; PEDS18381. PMID: 31574483.

Kest H, Brogly S, McSherry G, Dashefsky B, Oleske J, Seage GR (2005) Malignancy in perinatally human immunodeficiency virus-infected children in the United States. *Pediatr Infect Dis J*, 24(3): 237–242. Available at: http://dx.doi.org/10.1097/01.inf.0000154324.59426.8d.

Louis DN, Perry A, Wesseling P et al. (2021) The 2021 WHO classification of tumors of the central nervous system: A summary. *Neuro Oncol*, 23(8): 1231–1251. doi: 10.1093/neuonc/noab106; PMID: 34185076; PMCID: PMC8328013.

Lucas KG, Bao L, Bruggeman R, Dunham K, Specht C (2010) The detection of CMV pp65 and IE1 in glioblastoma multiforme. *J Neurooncol*, 103(2): 231–238. Available at: http://dx.doi.org/10.1007/s11060-010-0383-6.

Maginnis MS, Atwood WJ (2009) JC virus: An oncogenic virus in animals and humans? *Semin Cancer Biol*, 19(4): 261–269. doi: 10.1016/j.semcancer.2009.02.013; Epub 2009 Feb 24; PMID: 19505654; PMCID: PMC2694964.

Mandel M, Toren A, Hadani M, Engelberg I, Martinowitz U, Rechavi G (1994) Ependymoblastoma in an HIV-positive hemophilic girl. *Med Pediatr Oncol*, 23(5): 441–443. Available at: http://dx.doi.org/10.1002/mpo.2950230509.

Mueller BU (1999a) Cancers in children infected with the human immunodeficiency virus. *Oncologist*, 4(4): 309–317.

Mueller BU (1999b) HIV-associated malignancies in children. *AIDS Patient Care STDS*, 13(9): 527–533. Available at: http://dx.doi.org/10.1089/apc.1999.13.527.

Okamoto H, Mineta T, Ueda S et al. (2005) Detection of JC virus DNA sequences in brain tumors in pediatric patients. *J Neurosurg Pediatr*, 102(3): 294–298. Available at: http://dx.doi.org/10.3171/ped.2005.102.3.0294.

Olivero OA, Yuspa SH, Poirier MC et al. (1997) Transplacental effects of 3′-azido-2′, 3′-dideoxythymidine (AZT): Tumorigenicity in mice and genotoxicity in mice and monkeys. *J. Natl. Cancer Inst*, 89(21): 1602–1608. Available at: https://doi.org/10.1093/jnci/89.21.1602.

Pina-Oviedo S, de Leon-Bojorge B, Cuesta-Mejias T et al. (2006) Glioblastoma multiforme with small cell neuronal-like component: Association with human neurotropic JC virus. *Acta Neuropathol*, 111(4): 388–396.

Pollack IF, Agnihotri S, Broniscer A (2019) Childhood brain tumors: Current management, biological insights, and future directions. *Journal of Neurosurgery: Pediatrics*, 23(3): 261–273. https://doi.org/10.3171/2018.10.PEDS18377.

Rencic A, Gordon J, Otte J et al. (1996) Detection of JC virus DNA sequence and expression of the viral oncoprotein, tumor antigen, in brain of immunocompetent patient with oligoastrocytoma. *Proc Natl Acad Sci USA*, 93(14): 7352–7357.

Seibel NL, Janeway K, Allen CE et al. (2017) Pediatric oncology enters an era of precision medicine. *Curr Probl Cancer*, 41(3): 194–200. https://doi.org/10.1016/j.currproblcancer.2017.01.002.

Simard EP, Shiels MS, Bhatia K, Engels EA (2012) Long-term cancer risk among people diagnosed with AIDS during childhood. *Cancer Epidemiol Biomarkers Prev*, 21(1): 148–154. Available at: http://dx.doi.org/10.1158/1055-9965.epi-11-0823.

Stack M, Walsh P, Comber H, Ryan C, O'Lorcain P (2007) Childhood cancer in Ireland: A population-based study. *Arch Dis Childhood*, 92(10): 890–897. Available at: http://dx.doi.org/10.1136/adc.2005.087544.

Stefan DC (2014) Malignancies in children with HIV infection. In: Yarchoan R, editor. *Cancers in People with HIV and AIDS: Progress and Challenges.* New York: Springer, pp 349–357. Available from: http://dx.doi.org/10.1007/978-1-4939-0859-2_26.

Tacconi L, Stapleton S, Signorelli F, Thomas DG (1996) Acquired immune deficiency syndrome (AIDS) and cerebral astrocytoma. *Clin Neurol Neurosurg*, 98(2): 149–151. Available at: http://dx.doi.org/10.1016/0303-8467(96)00002-9.

Tedeschi R, Bloigu A, Ögmundsdottir HM et al. (2006) Activation of maternal Epstein-Barr virus infection and risk of acute leukemia in the offspring. *Am J Epidemiol*, 165(2): 134–137. Available at: http://dx.doi.org/10.1093/aje/kwj332.

Weill O, Finaud M, Bille F, Gastaut JL, Malca S, Vincentelli F (1987) Gliome malin médullaire. Une nouvelle complication de l'infection par le virus HIV? *La Presse médicale*, 16(39): 1997.

Wilaisakditipakorn T, Vilaisaktipakorn P, Bunupuradah T, Puthanakit T (2015) A slow progressor HIV-infected boy developing quadriplegia with evidence of Epstein-Barr virus associated smooth muscle tumour of the cervical spinal cord. *BMJ Case Reports*, 2015: bcr2015210133. Available at: http://dx.doi.org/10.1136/bcr-2015-210133.

Yang M, Sun J, Bai HX et al. (2017) Diagnostic accuracy of SPECT, PET, and MRS for primary central nervous system lymphoma in HIV patients: A systematic review and meta-analysis. *Medicine (Baltimore)*, 96(19): e6676. doi: 10.1097/MD.0000000000006676; PMID: 28489744; PMCID: PMC5428578.

HIV-associated Immune Reconstitution Inflammatory Syndrome of the Central Nervous System

Rajeshree Govender and James Nuttall

INTRODUCTION

Prevention of mother-to-child transmission programmes and antiretroviral therapy (ART) have had a major impact on reducing the number of children acquiring human immunodeficiency virus (HIV) infection and the morbidity and mortality of children who are HIV infected respectively (B-Lajoie et al. 2016; UNICEF 2019). Despite the overall success of ART, immune reconstitution inflammatory syndrome (IRIS) has been recognised as a complication of immunological recovery, particularly among individuals with advanced immunosuppression at the time of starting ART. This condition is associated with hyper-responsiveness of the innate immune system as T-cell function recovers and the ability to cause inflammation is restored but dysregulated (Barber et al. 2012; Bahr et al. 2013). Both ART-related and non-HIV forms of IRIS have been described in this book. The majority of ART-related IRIS cases are associated with an underlying opportunistic infection, although IRIS in the absence of opportunistic infections has also been reported (Johnson and Nath 2014). The clinical features may involve various organ systems, but IRIS involving the central nervous system (CNS) is the most serious – and potentially life-threatening – manifestation of the syndrome. The pathophysiology of IRIS is incompletely understood and there are significant diagnostic and management challenges, particularly in resource-constrained settings (Navis et al. 2020). There is a paucity of paediatric literature on IRIS and in particular on CNS IRIS (Link-Gelles et al. 2014).

DEFINITION

Before the development of case definitions for IRIS, two clinical scenarios of HIV-associated IRIS in the weeks or months following ART initiation were recognised. Paradoxical IRIS is characterised by clinical recrudescence of a successfully treated infection or symptomatic relapse despite initial clinical improvement and continued microbiological treatment success. This is thought to be due to antigen-driven immune activation often with a robust immune response in the setting of few or no detectable organisms. The other scenario of unmasking IRIS occurs as the result of an occult subclinical opportunistic infection that is unmasked by immune recovery following ART initiation and becomes detectable. Unmasking IRIS requires differentiation from incident opportunistic infections (Boulware, Callens, and Pahwa 2008; Speicher et al. 2013).

A consensus case definition of IRIS has been developed to facilitate identification of the condition and enable further study. Criteria include: (1) evidence of a clinical response to ART indicated by a >1 $\log_{10}$ decrease in HIV-1 ribonucleic acid (RNA) (if possible); (2) clinical deterioration from an infectious or inflammatory condition temporally related to the initiation of ART; and (3) if symptoms cannot be explained by an alternate infection or neoplasm, treatment failure of the opportunistic infection, an adverse drug reaction, or complete noncompliance to ART or antimicrobial treatment. Of note, in unmasking IRIS a new active diagnosis is required. Additional clinical criteria have been proposed for the paradoxical and unmasking forms of IRIS in relation to specific opportunistic infections. For example, major and minor clinical criteria for the diagnosis of paradoxical tuberculosis (TB) IRIS have been proposed. Since there are no confirmatory tests for IRIS, it remains a diagnosis of exclusion (Boulware, Callens, and Pahwa 2008).

Consensus case definitions of CNS IRIS include worsening neurological status that may be accompanied by either new or deteriorating neuroradiological findings ocurring within 3 months of ART initiation (Torok et al. 2011). As aforementioned, exclusion of other causes of clinical or radiological deterioration must be made before diagnosing CNS IRIS (Torok et al. 2011). Paradoxical CNS IRIS has been described in progressive multifocal leukoencephalopathy (PML) and clinical case definitions for specific forms of CNS IRIS – such as TB and cryptococcal infection – have been developed (Haddow et al. 2010; Torok et al. 2011; Meintjes et al. 2018; Frattaroli et al. 2021).

Case definitions for autoimmune and non-infective forms of HIV-associated IRIS have not been developed and there are few reports in the literature.

EPIDEMIOLOGY

The incidence of CNS IRIS in children is not known as the current paediatric literature is limited to case reports predominantly among children older than 10 years of age (adolescents) (Nuttall et al. 2004; Ch'ng and Dieudonne 2007; Zampoli, Kilborn, and Eley 2007; Oberdorfer et al. 2009; van Toorn et al. 2012; Iro et al. 2013; Kalk et al. 2013; Schwenk et al. 2014; Hassan, Cotton, and Rabie 2015). Interestingly, no CNS IRIS cases were reported from single-centre or regional retrospective analyses of all IRIS events among children initiating ART in either resource-rich or resource-constrained settings, which reported overall IRIS rates of 5.9% and 19% to 38% respectively (Puthanakit et al. 2006; Smith et al. 2009; Wang et al. 2009; Orikiiriza et al. 2010; Gkentzi et al. 2014). These rates are likely to be a reflection of differences in the burden of opportunistic infections, IRIS case definitions, and diagnostic resources. A number of reports of unmasking forms of IRIS highlight the difficulty of excluding certain opportunistic infections (including TB) before ART initiation, particularly among immunosuppressed children in resource-constrained settings (Ch'ng and Dieudonne 2007; Zampoli, Kilborn, and Eley 2007; Boulware, Callens, and Pahwa 2008; Oberdorfer et al. 2009; van Toorn et al. 2012; Iro et al. 2013; Schwenk et al. 2014; Hassan, Cotton, and Rabie 2015; Weld and Dooley 2018). Unrecognised IRIS may be responsible for a proportion of the high mortality rate reported during the first 3 to 6 months following ART initiation in some paediatric ART cohorts (Bong et al. 2007; Puthanakit et al. 2007; Boulware, Callens, and Pahwa 2008).

In adult patients, the overall incidence of CNS IRIS is estimated to be approximately 1%. However, in patients with an opportunistic infection of the CNS identified before ART initiation, it is considerably higher, ranging from 15% to 40% (Bicanic et al. 2009; McCombe et al. 2009; Pepper et al. 2009; Riveiro-Barcie et al. 2013). An adult study in Cape Town found that CNS TB IRIS accounted for greater than 10% of all TB-associated IRIS cases among hospital inpatients (Pepper et al. 2009). Seventeen per cent of HIV-infected adults with cryptococcal meningitis developed symptoms of paradoxical IRIS within 29 days of ART initiation (Bicanic et al. 2009).

Whereas a variety of mycobacterial infections (including *Bacillus Calmette-Guerin*-related complications, pulmonary or extrapulmonary TB, and *Mycobacterium avium intracellulare*) was the most common non-CNS IRIS manifestation reported across all settings, TB involving the CNS, PML secondary to John Cunningham polyoma virus, and cryptococcal infections were responsible for the majority of CNS IRIS cases reported in children (Nuttall et al. 2004; Ch'ng and Dieudonn 2007; Puthanakit et al. 2007; Zampoli, Kilborn, and Eley 2007; Oberdorfer et al. 2009; Smith et al. 2009; Wang et al. 2009; Orikiiriza et al. 2010; van Toorn et al. 2012; Iro et al. 2013; Kalk et al. 2013; Gkentzi et al. 2014; Schwenk et al. 2014; Hassan, Cotton, and Rabie 2015). CNS IRIS has been reported in association with a wide array of viral, fungal, bacterial, and parasitic pathogens (Table 10.1) (Bahr et al. 2013). Organisms associated with CNS IRIS include *Mycobacterium tuberculosis*, *Mycobacterium avium complex*, *Cryptococcus neoformans*, Coccidiomycoses, Candida, *Sporothrix schenckii*, John Cunningham virus, herpes simplex virus, cytomegalovirus, varicella-zoster virus, Epstein–Barr virus, parvovirus B19, HIV, and toxoplasma (Boulware et al. 2010; Agarwal et al. 2012; Bahr et al. 2013).

The degree of immune suppression and the presence of an opportunistic infection at the time of ART initiation are the main risk factors for the development of IRIS, whether IRIS occurs in the CNS or

Table 10.1 Infections associated with immune reconstitution inflammatory syndrome (IRIS) of the central nervous system (CNS) and their common manifestations.

Pathogen	CNS IRIS manifestation
Viruses	
John Cunningham virus	Progressive multifocal leukoencephalopathy
Varicella-zoster virus	Encephalitis, transverse myelitis, vasculopathy
Cytomegalovirus	Encephalitis, vasculitis, ventriculitis
Herpes simplex virus	Encephalitis
Epstein–Barr virus	Cerebral lymphoid granulomatosis
Parvovirus B19	Encephalitis
Human immunodeficiency virus	Encephalitis/encephalopathy
Bacteria	
Mycobacterium tuberculosis	Meningitis, intracerebral tuberculoma, radiculopathy, epidural abscess
Mycobacterium avium complex	Mass lesion
Fungi	
Cryptococcus neoformans	Meningitis, intracerebral abscess, cerebellitis
Coccidioidomycosis	Meningitis
Candida	Meningitis
Sporothrix schenckii	Meningitis
Parasites	
Toxoplasma	Encephalitis

elsewhere in the body (Shelburne et al. 2005; Johnson and Nath 2011). Immune suppression is indicated by the nadir CD4+ lymphocyte count and, notably, in the case of CNS IRIS the opportunistic infection will involve the CNS (Shelburne et al. 2005; Johnson and Nath 2011). In one paediatric study, severe malnutrition was identified as a significant risk factor for the development of IRIS (Wang et al. 2009).

The timing of ART initiation in severely immunosuppressed adult patients with underlying opportunistic infections has been identified as a risk factor for paradoxical forms of IRIS (Lawn, Torok, and Wood 2011). Among adults with TB meningitis (TBM), immediate initiation of ART at the same time as starting TB treatment was found to confer no advantage in reducing mortality but was associated with a higher incidence of CNS IRIS and serious adverse drug reactions compared to starting ART 2 months after starting TBM treatment. This study (Torok et al. 2011) also described a very high overall mortality rate (67%) regardless of ART timing. Similar studies have not been conducted in HIV-infected children with TB involving the CNS and the optimal timing of ART initiation in HIV-infected children with CNS TB is not known.

Cryptococcal infection, particularly cryptococcal meningitis, is considerably less common in children than adults and there are very few reports describing CNS cryptococcal IRIS among children (Bicanic et al. 2009; Meiring et al. 2012; Hassan, Cotton, and Rabie 2015). Both unmasking and paradoxical forms of CNS IRIS have been described and the risk factors in children appear to be similar to those in adults. Adult data have shown a 15% higher mortality in patients starting ART in hospital 1 to 2 weeks after diagnosis of cryptococcal meningitis than in patients starting ART 5 to 6 weeks after diagnosis of cryptococcal meningitis but paediatric data are lacking (Boulware et al. 2014). Since there is no effective antimicrobial treatment for John Cunningham virus, the timing of ART in patients with PML is not a major consideration and ART is usually initiated as soon as possible after PML diagnosis. Both paradoxical and unmasking forms of PML IRIS have been described (Bahr et al. 2013; Frattaroli et al. 2021).

Therapeutic strategies using drugs known to reactivate viral reservoirs, including in the CNS, with the aim of stimulating cytotoxic immune responses to eradicate viral reservoirs, may inadvertently increase the risk of severe CNS IRIS-like reactions (Nath and Clements 2011).

PATHOPHYSIOLOGY

Following a relatively anergic state, initiation of effective ART results in a dramatic reduction in circulating HIV-1 usually accompanied by an increase in circulating CD4+ T-cells. Among adults, the early stage of immune reconstitution is characterised by release of memory T-cells (CD45RO) from lymph nodes into the circulation, and during the later stages there is a gradual rise in naïve T-cell (CD45RA) production from the thymus (Lipman and Breen 2006). Children generally have more pronounced thymic activity than adults, leading to an early and sustained output of naïve T-cells during immune reconstitution (Gibb et al. 2000).

The development of IRIS is associated with a dysregulated immune response in reaction to an antigen from an opportunistic infection or a self-antigen resulting in an exaggerated inflammatory response (Kestens, Seddiki, and Bohjanen 2008). This is associated with a relative lack of regulatory T-cell function (Seddiki et al. 2009). Infiltration of activated T-cells into the meninges, parenchyma, and blood vessels of the CNS, along with significantly elevated levels of both pro- and anti-inflammatory cytokines and chemokines in both blood and cerebrospinal fluid (CSF), have been reported in patients with CNS IRIS compared to those without (Price et al. 2009; Tadokera et al. 2011). Tumour necrosis factor alpha, interleukin 6, and interferon gamma levels may be elevated (Price et al. 2009).

Activation of inflammasomes – immune complexes comprising receptors and sensors that mediate innate immune responses and induce inflammation – have been identified as integral to the immunopathogenesis of TB IRIS (Tan et al. 2016; Marais et al. 2017). Furthermore, dysregulated inter-actions between innate and adaptive immune responses with impaired homeostatic mechanisms have been implicated in both TB IRIS and cryptococcal meningitis IRIS (Meya et al. 2016; Walker et al. 2020). In TB IRIS, invariant natural killer T cells, a subgroup of T-cells that bridge the gap between innate and adaptive immunity, exhibit cytoxicity by releasing pro-inflammatory cytokines and are hypothesised to play a key role (Walker et al. 2020).

In the context of CNS IRIS, inflammation leads to oedema which, in the limited physical space of the brain or spinal cord, may cause raised intracranial pressure, compression, and damage to vital structures.

In CNS IRIS occurring without evidence of an opportunistic infection, the immune response is thought to be directed against residual virus in the CNS, when HIV-Tat protein is released from HIV-infected cells despite control of viral replication, or against self-antigens. Pathologically, these patients demonstrate CD8+ lymphocyte infiltration into the brain parenchyma, axonal and myelin damage, reactive astrocytosis, and microglial activation (Lindzen et al. 2008; Johnson and Nath 2011; Gray et al. 2013).

The pathogenesis of IRIS – particulalrly CNS IRIS – is not fully understood and the interaction between genetic factors, the innate immune system, dysregulated T-cell responses, and antigen burden is complex.

CLINICAL PRESENTATION

The clinical features of CNS IRIS usually result from inflammatory oedema or expansion of mass lesions within an enclosed space. Raised intracranial pressure frequently occurs. Symptoms and signs reported in children include headache, seizures, meningeal irritation, decreased level of consciousness, focal neu-rological deficits, ataxia, dysarthria, and dysphasia (Nuttall et al. 2004; Ch'ng and Dieudonne 2007; Zampoli, Kilborn, and Eley 2007; Oberdorfer et al. 2009; van Toorn et al. 2012; Iro et al. 2013; Kalk et al. 2013; Schwenk et al. 2014; Hassan, Cotton, and Rabie 2015). Similar clinical features have been reported for both paradoxical and unmasking forms of CNS IRIS.

The clinical manifestations of CNS TB IRIS in children include TBM, myeloradiculopathy, TB abscesses, and TB granulomas. Radiological features of CNS TB IRIS that have been described include ring-enhancing lesions (due to tuberculomas or cold abscesses), obstructive hydrocephalus, vasogenic oedema, and raised intracranial pressure with mass effect (van Toorn et al. 2012) (Chapter 4, Figures 4.11 and 4.12).

The most common clinical manifestation of IRIS due to CNS cryptococcal infection is recurrence of symptoms and signs of meningitis. Raised intracranial pressure is also common. Other manifestations include intracranial cryptococcoma or abscess, spinal cord abscess, cranial nerve lesions, hemiparesis, and paraparesis. Extracranial manifestations including pulmonary infiltrates, skin infiltrates, or lymphade-nopathy due to cryptococcal infection may support a diagnosis of cryptococcal IRIS involving the CNS (Boulware et al. 2010).

The clinical presentation of PML IRIS varies depending on the site of the brain lesions and may include cognitive defects, hemiplegia, focal sensory deficits, ataxia, and seizures. Larger lesions may result in cerebral oedema and herniation (Nuttall et al. 2004; Ch'ng and Dieudonne 2007; Oberdorfer et al. 2009; Tan et al. 2009; Schwenk et al. 2014). On magnetic resonance imaging (MRI), the lesions of PML IRIS may show contrast enhancement and mass effect (Chapter 4, Figures 4.10c and 4.10d).

Both paradoxical and unmasking forms of CNS IRIS typically present within approximately 3 months of starting ART. In five paediatric cases of CNS TB IRIS, all five developed new neurological signs within 12 days of starting ART (van Toorn et al. 2012; Kalk et al. 2013). The time from ART initiation to presentation with neurological deterioration in three children reported with PML IRIS varied between 12 and 28 days but may be longer in cases of unmasking PML IRIS (Nuttall et al. 2004; Ch'ng and Dieudonne 2007; Oberdorfer et al. 2009; Schwenk et al. 2014). A child with CNS varicella zoster IRIS presented with acute onset right hemiplegia, facial palsy, and dysphasia 4 weeks after starting ART (Iro et al. 2013).

CNS IRIS occurring in the absence of an opportunistic infection among adult patients has been described as presenting with features of encephalitis or demyelination including headache, nausea, hearing impairment, weakness, impaired speech, disorientation, ataxia, and ischaemic events (Teo et al. 2007; Lindzen et al. 2008; Johnson and Nath 2011; Gray et al. 2013).

DIAGNOSIS AND DIFFERENTIAL DIAGNOSIS

There is no simple investigation that is able to exclude or confirm the diagnosis of CNS IRIS. Therefore, the diagnosis relies on recognition of typical clinical features with or without new or deteriorating neuroradiological findings occurring in a temporal relationship to the initiation of ART (Boulware, Callens, and Pahwa 2008). In addition, there may or may not be evidence of a virological or immunological response to ART (e.g. decrease in plasma HIV-1 RNA by >1 $\log_{10}$ value) and there must be exclusion of other causes of neurological and/or radiological deterioration to make a diagnosis of CNS IRIS (Boulware, Callens, and Pahwa 2008).

Alternative causes of neurological deterioration include infections not previously associated with CNS IRIS (e.g. acute bacterial meningitis), treatment failure (e.g. antiretroviral or other antimicrobial drug resistance), poor adherence to ART or other antimicrobial therapy, and adverse drug reactions (Boulware, Callens, and Pahwa 2008).

The criteria used to diagnose CNS IRIS are context specific and dependent on the availability of the resources that are required to confirm certain diagnoses (e.g. PML) and exclude other causes of CNS deterioration (e.g. antimicrobial drug resistance) in an HIV-infected patient who has recently initiated ART. There may also be limited availability of sensitive neuroimaging modalities (e.g. MRI) in resource-constrained settings.

A clinical case definition for the diagnosis of paradoxical CNS TB IRIS among adult patients in resource-constrained settings has been developed by the International Network for the Study of HIV-associated IRIS (INSHI) and incorporates the following criteria: (1) diagnosis of neuroTB with initial response to anti-TB treatment; (2) recurrence or new onset of TB disease manifestations within 24 weeks of anti-TB treatment; and (3) exclusion of alternative explanations for clinical deterioration (such as anti-TB drug resistance, poor adherence, drug toxicity or reaction, or an additional infection) (Meintjes et al. 2008). The INSHI case definition identifies TB IRIS with reasonable accuracy (Stek et al. 2021).

A similar set of clinical criteria focusing on infectious or inflammatory features has been developed for the diagnosis of paradoxical TB IRIS, including CNS TB IRIS, in children (Boulware, Callens, and Pahwa 2008). Additional features that may support a diagnosis of CNS TB IRIS include conversion of the tuberculin skin test from negative to positive during ART, TB treatment at the time of a suspected IRIS event, and manifestations of TB IRIS at other organ sites (e.g. worsening or new infiltrates on chest radiographs, mediastinal lymphadenopathy, fever) although the clinical utility of these features for identifying children at risk of developing CNS IRIS has not been studied (Boulware, Callens, and Pahwa 2008; van Toorn et al. 2012).

The diagnosis of CNS cryptococcal IRIS may be complicated by the presence of raised intracranial pressure, difficulties with adherence to antifungal medication, and resistance to antifungal medication.

CSF is frequently negative on fungal culture in the setting of IRIS but may remain culture positive despite effective therapy for up to 2 months after induction therapy. This phenomenon may even occur in the absence of antifungal resistance; however, it may not be possible to diagnose antifungal drug resistance in resource-constrained settings. In addition, paradoxical IRIS events may occur a year or longer after ART initiation (Govender et al. 2013).

The diagnosis of PML and PML IRIS is based on clinical and neuroradiological features and is confirmed by detection of John Cunningham virus DNA in the CSF or viral proteins on brain biopsy. The radiological modality of choice for diagnosis is MRI and lesions are typically asymmetrical involving the frontal and parieto-occipital white matter. Contrast enhancement of the demyelinating lesions is more commonly found in PML IRIS compared to non-IRIS PML cases (Tan et al. 2009). Among adults, the sensitivity of John Cunningham virus polymerase chain reaction has been found to be lower in patients receiving ART than in those not on ART (Marzocchetti et al. 2005). The majority of paediatric case reports have been John Cunningham virus DNA polymerase chain reaction positive (Nuttall et al. 2004; Ch'ng and Dieudonne 2007; Oberdorfer et al. 2009; Schwenk et al. 2014).

Residual HIV replication within the CNS despite reduction in HIV viral load in peripheral blood may contribute to chronic inflammation in the CNS and may be difficult to distinguish from CNS IRIS (Gray et al. 2013; Johnson and Nath 2014). There is limited evidence from adult studies that reduction in the CNS HIV viral load by using ART regimens with higher levels of CNS penetration may improve the neurological status of patients but paediatric evidence is lacking (Chan and Brew 2014; Johnson and Nath 2014).

MANAGEMENT

Corticosteroids, other immune modulators, and occasionally temporary interruption of ART are the treatment modalities most often used in CNS IRIS. Potential or proven infectious agents, including drug-resistant pathogens, must be diagnosed and treated with appropriate antimicrobial therapy as the use of anti-inflammatory or immunosuppressive agents in the presence of an untreated infection is dangerous. Active management of raised intracranial pressure, including repeat lumbar punctures for hydrocephalus if present, is frequently necessary.

There are no randomised controlled trials evaluating treatment of CNS IRIS in children, and current treatment strategies are based on case reports, anecdotal evidence, and extrapolation from adult studies. A randomised placebo-controlled trial of prednisone for paradoxical TB IRIS amongst adults reduced the time to recovery and the duration of hospitalisation; however, patients with CNS TB IRIS were excluded from the study (Meintjes et al. 2010). Paediatric case reports of both paradoxical and unmasking forms of CNS TB IRIS describe the use of corticosteroids in various sequences and for different durations on an individual patient basis. Medications and doses used include oral prednisone (usually 2mg/kg/day), intravenous dexamethasone (usually 0.4mg/kg/day), and intravenous methylprednisolone (10mg/kg/day for 3 days) (van Toorn et al. 2012; Kalk et al. 2013; Viel-Theriault et al. 2016).

Thalidomide is an agent with potent anti-inflammatory properties as a result of selective inhibition of tumour necrosis factor alpha secretion by monocytes and macrophages (van Toorn et al. 2012). A randomised, placebo-controlled trial investigating the use of thalidomide in children with severe TBM was stopped early as a result of frequent adverse events in the treatment arm (Schoeman et al. 2004). Subsequent studies in children, including HIV-infected children on ART with CNS TB IRIS, using lower doses than in the early terminated trial (2–5mg/kg/day), have shown benefit in the resolution of chronic TB mass lesions (abscesses and tuberculomas) in some cases (van Toorn et al. 2015; Viel-Theriault et al. 2016). The optimal duration of thalidomide therapy in complicated CNS TB is unknown but case reports suggest therapy should continue until resolution of cerebral oedema has been achieved (van Toorn et al. 2015; Viel-Theriault et al. 2016). Mycophenolate mofetil, another immunosuppressant agent with an inhibitory effect on active T-cell proliferation, has also been used in CNS TB IRIS (van Toorn et al. 2012).

Corticosteroids have been used in persistent or life-threatening CNS cryptococcal IRIS, but a double-blind, randomised placebo-controlled trial investigating the use of adjunctive dexamethasone in adults with HIV-associated cryptococcal meningitis was stopped prematurely after showing that dexamethasone did not reduce mortality and was associated with more adverse events and disability than placebo (Boulware et al. 2010; Bahr et al. 2013; Beardsley et al. 2016). Other agents used include hydroxychloroquine, adalimumab, and thalidomide as alternatives to corticosteroids (Sitapati et al. 2010; Narayanan, Banerjee, and Holt 2011; Brunel et al. 2012). The difficulty in excluding antifungal drug resistance has led some guidelines to recommend intensification of antifungal therapy by switching patients receiving fluconazole maintenance treatment back to a repeat of induction therapy with amphotericin B combined with fluconazole until fungal culture results are available (Bahr et al. 2013).

In PML IRIS, the use of corticosteroids did not improve mortality in a retrospective study in adults and there is no clinical trial evidence to support their use (Tan et al. 2009). Since there is no specific therapy that is effective in treating John Cunningham virus, corticosteroid-induced immunosuppression may be deleterious and should probably be reserved for cases with cerebral oedema.

In adult patients who develop autoimmune responses to CNS antigens, therapies that block lymphocyte trafficking into the CNS, such as natalizumab, have been used; however, this is untested in children (Johnson and Nath 2014).

OUTCOME

The outcome of CNS IRIS is generally much worse than with non-CNS IRIS. The mortality rate associated with CNS IRIS in adult cohorts is up to 30% but varies by underlying infection and other individual risk factors (Pepper et al. 2009; Tan et al. 2009; Boulware et al. 2010; Agarwal et al. 2012). In many of the paediatric CNS IRIS case reports, significant neurodisability or death occurred despite treatment interventions (Nuttall et al. 2004; Ch'ng and Dieudonne 2007; Zampoli, Kilborn, and Eley 2007; Oberdorfer et al. 2009; van Toorn et al. 2012; Iro et al. 2013; Kalk et al. 2013; Schwenk et al. 2014; Hassan, Cotton, and Rabie 2015). One of the main factors related to the poor outcome is thought to be the development of inflammation within the brain leading to swelling and compression of vital structures. In some cases, this leads to brain herniation and death.

In a recent report describing three children with paradoxical CNS TB IRIS and one child with unmasking of CNS tuberculomas following ART initiation, one of the children with paradoxical CNS TB IRIS died and the other three survived. The children who survived required prolonged hospitalisation and one child had residual mild hemiplegia. The child who died was a 10-year-old female who started ART 3 weeks after starting treatment for TBM (including prednisone 2mg/kg/day) but she showed progressive deterioration 7 days after starting ART despite changing to high-dose intravenous dexamethasone and including thalidomide (2mg/kg/day) in her treatment regimen. Details of the neurocognitive outcome of the three survivors were not provided (van Toorn et al. 2012).

Among 19 cases of PML in HIV-infected patients aged 6 to 22 years at diagnosis of PML, 12 (63%) died mostly within 2 to 6 months of diagnosis, four (21%) had persistent neurological disability (hemiparesis, cerebellar dysfunction, dystonia), in three (16%) children the outcome was not reported or the child was lost to follow-up, and one (5%) child showed progressive improvement (Oberdorfer et al. 2009). Despite the availability of ART, the lack of effective antimicrobial therapy directed against John Cunningham virus has resulted in a persistently poor prognosis. Risk factors associated with survival in adults include the John

Cunningham virus viral load in the CSF, a CD4+ lymphocyte count greater than 100 cells/mm^3, contrast enhancement on radiographic imaging, evidence of recovery in neurological function, and the presence of John Cunningham virus-specific cytotoxic T-cells (Hassan, Cotton, and Rabie 2015). However, these factors have not been adequately evaluated in children (Hassan, Cotton, and Rabie 2015).

An 11-year-old female with CNS varicella-zoster IRIS presenting with cerebral infarction and vasculopathy 1 month after starting ART, responded to treatment with a 3-week course of acyclovir while continuing ART; however, she was left with a mild hemiplegia (Meintjes et al. 2008).

PREVENTION

The strongest predictor of developing CNS IRIS in adult studies is a low nadir CD4+ lymphocyte count, suggesting that early initiation of ART will reduce the incidence of IRIS (Espinosa et al. 2010; Grant et al. 2010). Most reported cases of CNS IRIS among children have been in adolescents, the majority of whom had advanced immunosuppression at the time of starting ART (van Toorn et al. 2012; Iro et al. 2013; Schwenk et al. 2014). World Health Organization (WHO) guidelines recommend ART initiation for all HIV-infected individuals regardless of CD4+ lymphocyte count, but widespread implementation of HIV testing and ART remains challenging in many settings (WHO 2015). Effective prevention of mother-to-child transmission programmess have achieved vertical transmission rates of less than 5%, making the elimination of paediatric HIV infection potentially attainable (Goga et al. 2015). Interruption of clinical services, including HIV and TB screening and diagnosis as well as provision of ART and TB treatment, due to COVID-19 restrictions, put patients at increased risk of IRIS as a result of HIV and TB disease progression and transmission due to delays in diagnosis and treatment initiation (Jewell et al. 2020; Dorward et al. 2021).

In anti-TB treatment, the addition of corticosteroids, usually in the form of prednisone dosed at 2 to 4mg/kg/day for 4 weeks and then tapered over 2 weeks, improved survival and reduced morbidity in TBM and is recommended by the WHO in all cases of TBM in children (Schoeman et al. 1997; WHO 2014). However, there are insufficient data on the effectiveness of corticosteroids in preventing paradoxical CNS TB IRIS in HIV-infected children with TB involving the CNS. Case reports describing paradoxical CNS TB IRIS in children include cases that developed IRIS despite corticosteroid treatment being started at the same time as anti-TB therapy (van Toorn et al. 2012; Kalk et al. 2013). A randomised placebo-controlled trial of prednisone initiated at the same time as ART and continued for 4 weeks for the prevention of paradoxical TB IRIS in high-risk adult patients but excluding those with neurological TB found that prednisone resulted in a lower incidence of TB-IRIS than placebo and did not increase the risk of severe infections or cancers (Meintjes et al. 2018).

Delaying the initiation of ART in severely immunosuppressed individuals known to have opportunistic infections involving the CNS has been shown to reduce the incidence of paradoxical IRIS in adult studies (Torok et al. 2011; Boulware et al. 2014). South African guidelines recommend deferring ART for 4 to 8 weeks after initiation of treatment of TB at a neurological site (TBM or tuberculoma) or cryptococcal meningitis treatment initiation, although there are insufficient data supporting this in children (Republic of South Africa Department of Health 2019). There are few published data about the timing of ART initiation in patients with CNS drug-resistant TB and HIV. It is reasonable, at this stage, to use the same guidelines utilised in treating patients with drug-susceptible CNS TB and HIV (Wilson, Nilsen, and Marks 2020).

Prevention of unmasking CNS IRS is more challenging. However, screening for the presence of latent or subclinical opportunistic infections in HIV-infected individuals, particularly those with more advanced immunosuppression, followed by prophylaxis or pre-emptive treatment has the potential to reduce the number of patients with unmasking IRIS following ART initiation.

TB preventive treatment (TPT), directed at preventing progression from latent TB infection to active TB disease, is recommended by the WHO for a wider spectrum of at-risk populations in updated 2020 guidelines. Recommendations for TPT now include infants (<12 months of age) living with HIV infection who are in contact with a person with TB and who are unlikely to have active TB disease on an appropriate clinical evaluation. They also include children who are 12 years of age and older into adolescence. TPT is recommended for adults living with HIV infection who are not considered to have active TB disease on an appropriate clinical evaluation, but live in a setting with high TB transmission. The approach for these at-risk adults is regardless of known contact with a person with TB, and inclusive of those on ART, pregnant females, and those who have previously been treated for TB, irrespective of the degree of immunosuppression or availability of latent TB infection testing. TPT options applicable to different age groups and taking into account drug–drug interactions with other medications including ART and the availability of appropriate formulations for children, include 6 or 9 months of daily isoniazid, or a 3-month regimen of weekly rifapentine plus isoniazid, or a 3-month regimen of daily isoniazid plus rifampicin (WHO 2020). More widespread implementation of TPT has the potential to reduce rates of unmasking TB IRIS, including CNS TB IRIS.

Pre-ART serum cryptococcal antigen (CrAg) screening of patients with low CD4 T-cell counts (<100 cells/mm^3) and pre-emptive fluconazole therapy for adult patients who test CrAg positive is a public health strategy that has been shown to significantly reduce the number of unmasking cryptococcal meningitis cases (Meya et al. 2010; Longley et al. 2016; Greene et al. 2021). There are insufficient data to recommend routine CrAg screening and pre-emptive treatment for HIV-infected children in whom cryptococcal meningitis is much less common than in adults (Meiring et al. 2012).

RESEARCH PRIORITIES

The true incidence of CNS IRIS among children is not known and epidemiological studies of children are required. Screening strategies for occult/clinically inapparent CNS infections among immunosuppressed children and the institution of appropriate antimicrobial therapy before ART initiation, as has been used for cryptococcal infection amongst adult patients, also warrant further research in children. Case reports, case series, and observational or cohort studies are important in attempting to further refine clinical case definitions for CNS IRIS applicable to children in resource-constrained settings. Research leading to improved understanding of IRIS pathogenesis and metabolic signatures predisposing to and associated with the inflammatory manifestations of ART-induced IRIS is underway (Pei et al. 2021). The optimal use of corticosteroids and other immunomodulatory drugs (including thalidomide and mycophenolate mofetil) in children and adults at increased risk of developing CNS IRIS or with established CNS IRIS is unknown and warrants further evaluation.

The recognition of a chronic form of T-cell encephalitis in adult patients without evidence of CNS infections other than HIV itself is yet to be explored among HIV-infected children. The role of new experimental therapeutic modalities, including the use of drugs such as natalizumab that block T-cell entry into the CNS and HIV Tat protein antagonists, remains to be elucidated.

REFERENCES

Agarwal U, Kumar A, Behera D, French MA, Price P (2012) Tuberculosis associated immune reconstitution inflammatory syndrome in patients infected with HIV: Meningitis a potentially life threatening manifestation. *AIDS Res Ther,* 9(1): 17. doi: 10.1186/1742-6405-9-17.

Bahr N, Boulware D, Marais S, Scriven J, Wilkinson R, Meintjes G (2013) Central nervous system immune reconstitution inflammatory syndrome. *Curr Infect Dis Rep*, 15(6): 583–593. doi: 10.1007/s11908-013-0378-5.

Barber D, Andrade B, Sereti I, Sher A (2012) Immune reconstitution inflammatory syndrome: The trouble with immunity when you had none. *Nature Rev Microbiol*, 10(2): 150–156. doi: 10.1038/nrmicro2712.

Beardsley J, Wolbers M, Kibengo FM et al. (2016) Adjunctive dexamethasone in HIV-associated cryptococcal meningitis. *N Engl J Med*, 374(6): 542–554. doi: 10.1056/NEJMoa1509024.

Bicanic T, Meintjes G, Rebe K et al. (2009) Immune reconstitution inflammatory syndrome in HIV-associated cryptococcal meningitis: A prospective study. *J Acquir Immune Defic Syndr,* 51: 130–134. doi: 10.1097/QAI.0b013e3181a56f2e.

B-Lajoie M, Drouin O, Bartlett G et al. (2016) Incidence and prevalence of opportunistic and other infections and the impact of antiretroviral therapy among HIV-infected children in low- and middle-income countries: A systematic review and meta-analysis. *Clin Infect Dis*, 62(12): 1586–1594. doi: 10.1093/cid/ciw139.

Bong CN, Yu JK, Chiang HC et al. (2007) Risk factors for early mortality in children on adult fixed-dose combination antiretroviral treatment in a central hospital in Malawi. *AIDS,* 21: 1805–1810. doi: 10.1097/QAD.0b013e3282c3a9e4.

Boulware D, Callens S, Pahwa S (2008) Pediatric HIV immune reconstitution inflammatory syndrome. *Curr Opin HIV AIDS*, 3(4): 461–467. doi: 10.1097/COH.0b013e3282fe9693.

Boulware DR, Meya DB, Bergemann TL et al. (2010) Clinical features and serum biomarkers in HIV immune reconstitution inflammatory syndrome after cryptococcal meningitis: A prospective cohort study. *Plos Med*, 7(12): e1000384. http://dx.doi.org/10.1371/journal.pmed.1000384.

Boulware DR, Meya DB, Muzoora C et al. (2014) Timing of antiretroviral therapy after diagnosis of cryptococcal meningitis. *N Engl J Med*, 370: 2487–2498. doi: 10.1056/NEJMoa1312884.

Brunel AS, Reynes J, Tuaillon E et al. (2012) Thalidomide for steroid-dependent immune reconstitution inflammatory syndromes during AIDS. *AIDS*, 26(16): 2110–2111. doi: 10.1097/QAD.0b013e328358daea.

Chan P, Brew BJ (2014) HIV associated neurocognitive disorders in the modern antiviral treatment era: Prevalence, characteristics, biomarkers, and effects of treatment. *Curr HIV/AIDS Rep*, 11: 317–324. doi: 10.1007/s11904-014-0221-0.

Ch'ng T, Dieudonne A (2007) Immune reconstitution inflammatory syndrome associated with progressive multifocal leukoencephalopathy in a perinatally acquired human immunodeficiency virus-infected young adult. *Pediatr Infect Dis J*, 26(11): 1068–1070. doi: 10.1097/inf.0b013e31812e62fa.

Dorward J, Khubone T, Gate K et al. (2021) The impact of the COVID-19 lockdown on HIV care in 65 South African primary care clinics: An interrupted time series analysis. *Lancet HIV*, 8(3): e158–e165. https://doi.org/10.1016/S2352-3018(20) 30359-3.

Espinosa E, Ormsby CE, Vega-Barrientos RS et al. (2010) Risk factors for immune reconstitution inflammatory syndrome under combination antiretroviral therapy can be aetiology-specific. *Int J STD AIDS*, 21: 573–579. doi: 10.1258/ijsa.2010.010135.

Frattaroli P, Chueng TA, Abaribe O, Ayoade F (2021) Immune reconstitution inflammatory syndrome with recurrent paradoxical cerebellar HIV-associated progressive multifocal leukoencephalopathy. *Pathogens*, 10(7) (June 28): 813. doi: 10.3390/pathogens10070813; PMID: 34203265; PMCID: PMC8308763.

Gibb DM, Newberry A, Klein N, de Rossi A, Grosch-Woerner I, Babiker A (2000) Immune repopulation after HAART in previously untreated HIV-1-infected children. Paediatric European Network for Treatment of AIDS (PENTA) Steering Committee. *Lancet*, 355(9212) (April 1): 1331–1332.

Gkentzi D, Tebruegge M, Tudor-Williams G et al. (2014) Incidence, spectrum and outcome of immune reconstitution syndrome in HIV-infected children following initiation of antiretroviral therapy. *Pediatr Infect Dis J*, 33(9): 953–958. doi: 10.1097/INF.0000000000000331.

Goga AE, Dinh TH, Jackson DJ et al. (2015) First population-level effectiveness evaluation of a national programme to prevent HIV transmission from mother to child, South Africa. *J Epidemiol Community Health*, 69: 240–248. doi: 10.1136/jech-2014-204535.

Govender NP, Meintjes G, Bicanic T et al. (Southern African HIV Clinicians Society) (2013) Guideline for the prevention, diagnosis and management of cryptococcal meningitis among HIV-infected persons: 2013 update. *S Afr J HIV Med*, 14(2): 76–86. doi: 10.7196/SAJHIVMED.930; last accessed 4 September 2016.

Grant PM, Komarow L, Andersen J et al. (2010) Risk factor analyses for immune reconstitution inflammatory syndrome in a randomized study of early vs. deferred ART during an opportunistic infection. *PLoS One*, 5: e11416. doi: 10.1371/journal.pone.0011416.

Gray F, Lescure FX, Adle-Biassette H et al. (2013) Encephalitis with infiltration by CD8+ lymphocytes in HIV patients receiving combination antiretroviral treatment. *Brain Pathol*, 23: 525–533. doi: 10.1111/bpa.12038.

Greene G, Lawrence DS, Jordan A, Chiller T, Jarvis JN (2021) Cryptococcal meningitis: A review of cryptococcal antigen screening programs in Africa. *Expert Rev Anti Infect Ther*, 19(2): 233–244. doi: 10.1080/14787210.2020.1785871; Epub 2020 Jul 14.PMID: 32567406.

Haddow L, Colebunders R, Meintjes G et al. (2010) Cryptococcal immune reconstitution inflammatory syndrome in HIV-1-infected individuals: Proposed clinical case definitions. *Lancet Infect Dis*, 10(11): 791–802. doi: 10.1016/S1473-3099(10)70170-5.

Hassan H, Cotton M, Rabie H (2015) Complicated and protracted cryptococcal disease in HIV-infected children. *Pediatr Infect Dis J*, 34(1): 62–65. doi: 10.1097/INF.0000000000000480.

Iro M, Kirkham F, Macdonald J, Tebruegge M, Faust S, Patel S (2013) Varicella zoster virus central nervous system immune reconstitution inflammatory syndrome presenting in a child. *Pediatr Infect Dis J*, 32: 1283–1284. doi: 10.1097/inf.0b013e31829aa4fc.

Jewell BL, Mudimu E, Stover J et al. (2020) HIV modelling consortium: Potential effects of disruption to HIV programmes in sub-Saharan Africa caused by COVID-19: Results from multiple mathematical models. *Lancet HIV*, 7(9): e629–e640. https:// doi.org/10.1016/S2352-3018(20)30211-3.

Johnson T, Nath A (2011) Immune reconstitution inflammatory syndrome and the central nervous system. *Curr Opin Neurol*, 24: 284–290. doi: 10.1097/WCO.0b013e328346be57.

Johnson T, Nath A (2014) New insights into immune reconstitution inflammatory syndrome of the central nervous system. *Curr Opin HIV AIDS*, 9(6): 572–578. doi: 10.1097/COH.0000000000000107.

Kalk E, Technau K, Hendson W, Coovadia A (2013) Paradoxical mycobacterium tuberculosis meningitis immune reconstitution inflammatory syndrome in an HIV-infected child. *Pediatr Infect Dis J*, 32(2): 157–162. doi: 10.1097/INF.0b013e31827031aa.

Kestens L, Seddiki N, Bohjanen PR (2008) Immunopathogenesis of immune reconstitution disease in HIV patients responding to antiretroviral therapy. *Curr Opin HIV AIDS*, 3: 419–424. doi: 10.1097/COH.0b013e328302ebbb.

Lawn SD, Torok ME, Wood R (2011) Optimum time to start antiretroviral therapy during HIV-associated opportunistic infections. *Curr Opin Infect Dis*, 24: 34–42. doi: 10.1097/QCO.0b013e3283420f76.

Lindzen E, Jewells V, Bouldin T, Speer D, Royal W 3rd, Markovic-Plese S (2008) Progressive tumefactive inflammatory central nervous system demyelinating disease in an acquired immunodeficiency syndrome patient treated with highly active antiretroviral therapy. *J Neurovirol*, 14: 569–573. doi: 10.1080/13550280802304753.

Link-Gelles R, Moultrie H, Sawry S, Murdoch D, Van Rie A (2014) Tuberculosis immune reconstitution inflammatory syndrome in children initiating antiretroviral therapy for HIV infection: A systematic literature review. *Pediatr Infect Dis J*, 33(5): 499–503. doi: 10.1097/INF.0000000000000142.

Lipman M, Breen R (2006) Immune reconstitution inflammatory syndrome in HIV. *Curr Opin Infect Dis*, 19: 20–25. https://doi.org/10.1016/j.ijid.2009.05.016.

Longley N, Jarvis JN, Meintjes G et al. (2016) Cryptococcal antigen screening in patients initiating ART in South Africa: A prospective cohort study. *Clin Infect Dis*, 62(5) (Mar 1): 581–587. doi: 10.1093/cid/civ936; Epub 2015 Nov 12.PMID: 26565007.

Marais S, Lai R, Wilkinson K, Meintjes G, O'Garra A, Wilkinson R (2017) Inflammasome activation underlies central nervous system deterioration in HIV-associated tuberculosis. *J Infect Dis*, 215(5): 677–686. doi: 10.1093/infdis/jiw561.

Marzocchetti A, Di Giambenedetto S, Cingolani A, Ammassari A, Cauda R, De Luca A (2005) Reduced rate of diagnostic positive detection of JC virus DNA in cerebrospinal fluid in cases of suspected progressive multifocal leukoencephalopathy in the era of potent antiretroviral therapy. *J Clin Microbiol*, 43(8): 4175–4177. doi: 10.1128/JCM.43.8.4175-4177.2005.

McCombe JA, Auer RN, Maingat FG, Houston S, Gill MJ, Power C (2009) Neurologic immune reconstitution inflammatory syndrome in HIV/AIDS: Outcome and epidemiology. *Neurol*, 72: 835–841. doi: 10.1212/01.wnl.0000343854.80344.69.

Meintjes G, Lawn S, Scano F et al. (2008) Tuberculosis-associated immune reconstitution inflammatory syndrome: Case definitions for use in resource-limited settings. *Lancet Infect Dis*, 8(8): 516–523. doi: 10.1016/S1473-3099(08)70184-1.

Meintjes G, Wilkinson RJ, Morroni C et al. (2010) Randomized placebo-controlled trial of prednisone for paradoxical tuberculosis-associated immune reconstitution inflammatory syndrome. *AIDS*, 24: 2381–2390. doi: 10.1097/QAD.0b013e32833dfc68.

Meintjes G, Stek C, Blumenthal L et al. (2018) Prednisone for the prevention of paradoxical tuberculosis-associated IRIS. *N Engl J Med*, 379: 1915–1925. doi: 10.1056/NEJMoa1800762.

Meiring ST, Quan VC, Cohen C et al. (2012) A comparison of cases of paediatric-onset and adult-onset cryptococcosis detected through population-based surveillance, 2005–2007. *AIDS*, 26: 2307–2314. doi: 10.1097/QAD.0b013e3283570567.

Meya DB, Manabe YC, Castelnuovo B et al. (2010) Cost-effectiveness of serum cryptococcal antigen screening to prevent deaths among HIV-infected persons with a CD4+ cell count ≤100 cells/μL who start HIV therapy in resource-limited settings. *Clin Infect Dis*, 51(4): 448–455. doi: 10.1086/655143.

Meya DB, Manabe YC, Boulware DR, Janoff EN (2016) The immunopathogenesis of cryptococcal immune reconstitution inflammatory syndrome: Understanding a conundrum. *Curr Opin Infect Dis*, 29(1): 10–22. doi: 10.1097/QCO.0000000000000224; PMID: 26658650; PMCID: PMC4689618.

Narayanan S, Banerjee C, Holt PA (2011) Cryptococcal immune reconstitution syndrome during steroid withdrawal with hydroxychloroquine. *Internat J Infect Dis*, 15: 70–73. doi: 10.1016/j.ijid.2010.09.006

Nath A, Clements JE (2011) Eradication of HIV from the brain: Reasons for pause. *AIDS*, 25: 577–580. doi: 10.1097/QAD.0b013e3283437d2f.

Navis A, Siddiqi O, Chishimba L, Zimba S, Morgello S, Birbeck GL (2020) Immune reconstitution inflammatory syndrome in the central nervous system: Limitations for diagnosis in resource-limited settings *J Neurol Sci*, 416: 117042. doi: 10.1016/j.jns.2020.17042; Epub 2020 Jul 16.PMID: 32712429.

Nuttall J, Wilmshurst J, Ndondo A et al. (2004) Progressive multifocal leukoencephlopathy after initiation of highly active antiretroviral therapy in a child with advanced human immunodeficiency virus infection: A case of immune reconstitution inflammation syndrome. *Pediatr Infect Dis J*, 23(7): 683–685. doi: 10.1097/01.inf.0000130954.41818.07.

Oberdorfer P, Washington C, Katanyuwong K, Jittamala P (2009) Progressive multifocal leukoencephalopathy in HIV-infected children: A case report and literature review. *Int J Pediatr*, 1–6. doi: 10.1155/2009/348507.

Orikiiriza J, Bakeera-Kitaka S, Musiime V, Mworozi EA, Mugyenyi P, Boulware DR (2010) The clinical pattern, prevalence, and factors associated with immune reconstitution inflammatory syndrome in Ugandan children. *AIDS*, 24(13): 2009–2017. doi: 10.1097/QAD.0b013e32833b260a.

Pei L, Fukutani KF, Tibúrcio R et al. (2021) Plasma metabolomics reveals dysregulated metabolic signatures in HIV-associated immune reconstitution inflammatory syndrome. *Front Immunol*, 12: 693074. doi: 10.3389/fimmu.2021.693074; PMID: 34211479; PMCID: PMC8239348.

Pepper DJ, Marais S, Maartens G et al. (2009) Neurologic manifestations of paradoxical tuberculosis-associated immune reconstitution inflammatory syndrome: A case series. *Clin Infect Dis*, 48: e96–e107. doi: 10.1086/598988.

Price P, Murdoch DM, Agarwal U, Lewin SR, Elliott JH, French MA (2009) Immune restoration diseases reflect diverse immunopathological mechanisms. *Clin Microbiol Rev*, 22: 651–663. doi: 10.1128/CMR.00015-09.

Puthanakit T, Oberdorfer P, Akarathum N, Wannarit P, Sirisanthana T, Sirisanthana V (2006) Immune reconstitution syndrome after highly active antiretroviral therapy in human immunodeficiency virus-infected Thai children. *Pediatr Infect Dis J*, 25(1): 53–58. doi: 10.1097/01.inf.0000195618.55453.9a.

Puthanakit T, Aurpibul L, Oberdorfer P et al. (2007) Hospitalization and mortality among HIV-infected children after receiving highly active antiretroviral therapy. *Clin Infect Dis*, 44: 599–604. doi: 10.1086/510489.

Republic of South Africa Department of Health (2019) ART clinical guidelines for the management of HIV in adults, pregnancy, adolescents, children, infants and neonates [homepage on the internet]. [October 2019; updated March 2020; cited 29 November 2021]. Available from: https://www.knowledgehub.org.za/system/files/elibdownloads/2020-05/2019%20ART%20Guideline%2028042020%20 pdf.pdf.

Riveiro-Barciela M, Falcó V, Burgos J et al. (2013) Neurological opportunistic infections and neurological immune reconstitution syndrome: Impact of one decade of highly active antiretroviral treatment in a tertiary hospital. *HIV Med*, 14: 21–30. doi: 10.1111/j.1468-1293.2012.01033.x.

Schoeman JF, Van Zyl LE, Laubscher JA, Donald PR (1997) Effect of corticosteroids on intracranial pressure, computed tomographic findings, and clinical outcome in young children with tuberculous meningitis. *Pediatrics*, 99: 226–231. doi: 10.1542/peds.99.2.226.

Schoeman JF, Springer P, van Rensburg AJ et al. (2004) Adjunctive thalidomide therapy for childhood tuberculous meningitis: Results of a randomized study. *J Child Neurol*, 19: 250–257. doi: 10.1177/088307380401900402.

Schwenk H, Ramirez-Avila L, Sheu S et al. (2014) Progressive multifocal leukoencephalopathy in pediatric patients. *Pediatr Infect Dis J*, 33(4): e99–e105. doi: 10.1097/INF.0000000000000237.

Seddiki N, Sasson SC, Santner-Nanan B et al. (2009) Proliferation of weakly suppressive regulatory CD4+ T cells is associated with over-active CD4+ T-cell responses in HIV-positive patients with mycobacterial immune restoration disease. *Eur J Immunol*, 39: 391–403. doi: 10.1002/eji.200838630.

Shelburne SA, Visnegarwala F, Darcourt J et al. (2005) Incidence and risk factors for immune reconstitution inflammatory syndrome during highly active antiretroviral therapy. *AIDS*, 19: 399–406. doi: 10.1097/01.aids.0000161769.06158.8a.

Sitapati AM, Kao CL, Cachay ER, Masoumi H, Wallis RS, Mathews WC (2010) Treatment of HIV-related inflammatory cerebral cryptococcoma with adalimumab. *Clin Infect Dis*, 50: e7–e10. doi: 10.1086/649553.

Smith K, Kuhn L, Coovadia A et al. (2009) Immune reconstitution inflammatory syndrome among HIV-infected South African infants initiating antiretroviral therapy. *AIDS*, 23: 1097–1107. doi: 10.1097/QAD.0b013e32832afefc.

Speicher DJ, Sehu MM, Johnson NW, Shaw DR (2013) Successful treatment of an HIV-positive patient with unmasking Kaposi's sarcoma immune reconstitution inflammatory syndrome. *J Clin Virol*, 57(3): 282–285. doi: 10.1016/j.jcv.2013.03.005; Epub 2013 Apr 8. PMID: 23578530.

Stek C, Buyze J, Menten J et al. (2021) Diagnostic accuracy of the INSHI consensus case definition for the diagnosis of paradoxical tuberculosis-IRIS. *J Acquir Immune Defic Syndr*, 86(5): 587–592. doi: 10.1097/QAI.0000000000002606.

Tadokera R, Meintjes G, Skolimowska KH et al. (2011) Hypercytokinaemia accompanies HIV-tuberculosis immune reconstitution inflammatory syndrome. *Eur Respir J*, 37: 1248–1259. doi: 10.1183/09031936.00091010.

Tan HY, Yong YK, Shankar EM et al. (2016) Aberrant inflammasome activation characterizes tuberculosis-associated immune reconstitution inflammatory syndrome. *J Immunol*, 196: 4052–4063. doi: 10.4049/jimmunol.1502203.

Tan K, Roda R, Ostrow L, McArthur J, Nath A (2009) PML-IRIS in patients with HIV infection: Clinical manifestations and treatment with steroids. *Neurol*, 72: 1458–1464. doi: 10.1212/01.wnl.0000343510.08643.74.

Teo EC, Azwra A, Jones RL, Gazzard BG, Nelson M (2007) Guillain-Barré syndrome following immune reconstitution after antiretroviral therapy for primary HIV infection. .*J HIV Ther*, 12(3): 62–63. PMID: 17962793.

Torok M, Yen N, Chau T et al. (2011) Timing of initiation of antiretroviral therapy in human immunodeficiency virus (HIV)-associated tuberculous meningitis. *Clin Infect Dis*, 52(11): 1374–1383. doi: 10.1093/cid/cir230.

UNICEF (2019) Children, HIV and AIDS: Global snapshot 2019. Available at: https://data.unicef.org/resources/children-hiv-aids-global-snapshot/. Accessed 22 November 2021.

van Toorn R, Rabie H, Dramowski A, Schoeman J (2012) Neurological manifestations of TB-IRIS: A report of 4 children. *Eur J Paediatr Neurol*, 16(6): 676–682. doi: 10.1016/j.ejpn.2012.04.005.

van Toorn R, du Plessis AM, Schaaf HS, Buys H, Hewlett RH, Schoeman JF (2015) Clinicoradiologic response of neurologic tuberculous mass lesions in children treated with thalidomide. *Pediatr Infect Dis J*, 34, 214–218. doi: 10.1097/INF.0000000000000539.

Viel-Thériault I, Thibeault R, Boucher FD, Drolet JP (2016) Thalidomide in refractory tuberculomas and pseudoabscesses. *Pediatric Infectious Disease Journal*, 35(11): 1262–1264. doi: 10.1097/INF.0000000000001285.

Walker NF, Opondo C, Meintjes G et al. (2020) Invariant natural killer T-cell dynamics in human immunodeficiency virus-associated tuberculosis. *Clin Infect Dis*, 70(9): 1865–1874. doi: 10.1093/cid/ciz501; PMID: 31190065; PMCID: PMC7156773.

Wang ME, Castillo ME, Montano SM, Zunt JR (2009) Immune reconstitution inflammatory syndrome in human immunodeficiency virus-infected children in Peru. *Pediatr Infect Dis J*, 28: 900–903. doi: 10.1097/INF.0b013e-3181a4b7fa

Weld ED, Dooley KE (2018) State-of-the-art review of HIV-TB coinfection in special populations. *Clin Pharmacol Ther*, 104(6): 1098–1109. doi: 10.1002/cpt.1221; Epub 2018 Oct 26. PMID: 30137652.

WHO (2014) *Guidance for National Tuberculosis Programmes on the Management of Tuberculosis in Children. Second Edition*. Geneva, Switzerland: World Health Organization. Available at: http://apps.who.int/medicinedocs/documents/s21535en/s21535en.pdf; last accessed 27 July 2017.

WHO (2015) Policy brief: Consolidated guidelines on the use of antiretroviral drugs for treating and preventing HIV infection: What's new. Geneva: Switzerland: World Health Organization. Available at: https://apps.who.int/iris/handle/10665/198064; last accessed 27 July 2017.

WHO (2020) *WHO Consolidated Guidelines on Tuberculosis. Module 1: Prevention. Tuberculosis Preventive Treatment*. Geneva: World Health Organization. Available at: https://www.who.int/publications/i/item/9789240001503; last accessed 6 December 2021.

Wilson JW, Nilsen DM, Marks SM (2020) Multidrug-resistant tuberculosis in patients with human immunodeficiency virus. Management considerations within high-resourced settings. *Ann Am Thorac Soc*, 17(1): 16–23. doi: 10.1513/AnnalsATS.201902-185CME; PMID: 31365831; PMCID: PMC6938532.

Zampoli M, Kilborn T, Eley B (2007) Tuberculosis during early antiretroviral induced immune reconstitution in HIV-infected children. *Int J Tuberc Lung Dis*, 11: 417–423.

CHAPTER 11

The Effect of HIV Infection on Neurodevelopment, from Birth to 3 Years

Louisa R Mudawarima, Alliya Mohamed, and Kirsten A Donald

INTRODUCTION

The human brain grows rapidly in the early years, reaching 90% of its adult volume by 6 years of age (Stiles and Jernigan 2010). Vital skills are learned during these first years in all domains, laying the foundation for further skill acquisition and learning. This functional skill acquisition is underpinned by a range of neurobiological processes including neurogenesis, growth of axons and dendrites, synaptogenesis, pruning, and myelination (Grantham-McGregor et al. 2007). Insults during this critical period may fundamentally affect future development and maturation. This chapter focuses on the first 3 years of postnatal life.

There is increasing recognition that, despite acceptance of the genetic map as being foundational to neurological and developmental potential, the growth and interconnection of neurons and how they are used and disused is also significantly influenced by the individual's experiences. Infancy is a time with both opportunity for supporting optimal brain development, as well as a period of maximal vulnerability to insult (Huttenlocher and Dabholkar 1997; Huttenlocher 1999; Thompson and Nelson 2001). Child development and physical growth are optimal in an environment where physical needs such as nutrition and shelter, emotional needs such as secure attachment, and cognitive needs such as appropriate stimulation, are met. Lack of such an environment, or the presence of adverse circumstances, may not only affect the immediate development of a child but also its long-term potential (Grantham-McGregor et al. 2007). Factors that have been identified as having a negative impact on optimal child development can be broadly characterised as prenatal or postnatal. Multiple factors can be considered at any particular time period, as well as longitudinally, and relationships between these factors remain a complex challenge for paediatric neuro-analysis. Major risk factors that have been shown to prevent the achievement of the optimal developmental potential in resource-poor countries include iron deficiency, stunting, substance abuse, lack of access to a stimulating early childhood experience, and chronic illnesses, including human immunodeficiency virus (HIV). Maternal depression, societal violence and institutionalisation are additional risk factors for loss of developmental potential (Walker et al. 2007; Lo, Das, and Horton 2017; Daelmans et al. 2017; Sania et al. 2019).

Typical child development is a sequential process for skills acquisition. Beginning in utero, this process is continuous, and is closely tied to the rate of maturation of the central nervous system (CNS). The four developmental domains that are typically included in assessments of very young children include gross motor function, fine motor function, language, and psychosocial skills. Children attain various milestones in each domain at different rates, and each child has a different developmental trajectory. Despite this individual variation, there are age windows during which most children reach a particular milestone, or acquire a core developmental skill. Many studies of attention, literacy, and numeracy have shown that successful school outcomes are laid down in early childhood and infancy. Children growing up in adverse, or deprived environments, are more likely to have negative experiences in comparison to their peers growing up in supportive and stimulating environments. A study from South Africa found that it was common for HIV-infected mothers to be separated from their offspring in the first 4 years following delivery and this was associated with poorer maternal immunological outcomes, thus emphasising the vulnerability of this population (Mogoba et al. 2021). There is now direct neurobiological evidence to support the view that the preschool period is the foundation for a successful school experience and outcome, thereby supporting advocacy efforts to provide services, such as integrated early intervention programmes for this population (Lipina and Posner 2012; Hermida et al. 2019).

HIV encephalopathy (HIVE) is the most common primary HIV-related CNS complication and occurs when there is early invasion of the foetal or infant brain by the virus, usually after vertically-acquired HIV (see Chapter 5). Children with HIV, in comparison to those who are not infected, are reported to have significantly poorer performance in both motor and cognitive development. This is exacerbated in the presence of additional, frequently comorbid factors such as malnutrition, adverse living conditions, and other illnesses (Walker et al. 2007; Wu et al. 2018). The use of antiretroviral therapy (ART) has dramatically reduced the prevalence of HIVE globally; beyond this, starting antiretroviral treatment early results in improved neurodevelopmental outcomes compared to delayed initiation (Laughton et al. 2012, 2013).

The effect of HIV on neurodevelopment and behaviour is variable, and it is affected by comorbidities and other well-described developmental risk factors. This makes it difficult to isolate the outcomes as purely secondary to HIV disease, and it illustrates how multiple factors, individually or in combination, can impact children with HIV. HIV infection itself also directly affects growth, nutrition, metabolism, as well as the nervous system. The effects of HIV are accentuated by the previously mentioned associated illnesses, as well as the developmental risk factors, through the complex relationships present during the development of the foetus, infant, and toddler. The issues with caregiver stress, illness, and death are also applicable to the HIV-exposed uninfected (HEU) child (Walker et al. 2011), a group dealt with more fully in Chapter 15.

Great improvements in the care and treatment of HIV have developed over the last decade, leading to HIV now being considered a chronic disease rather than a deadly one. Between 2011 and 2012, there were 1.6 million more people on ART but this number had risen to 28.7 million people in 2021 (UNAIDS 2021). However, ART coverage in HIV-infected children has always lagged behind coverage for infected adults. Despite the treatment gap, there is a huge population of children who are living with HIV, including those on a now more widely accessible treatment. The focus has moved from primarily physical health to prioritising the optimal cognitive and developmental outcomes of children living with this condition.

EFFECT OF HIV INFECTION ON NEURODEVELOPMENT IN THE FIRST 3 YEARS

In this section, we will focus on the effects of HIV on overall development in the first 3 years of life, as well as its effects on specific domains of early development. A summary of published reports of developmental outcomes in HIV-infected children in the first 3 years of life is presented in Table 11A.1 in the Appendix at the end of this chapter.

General Considerations

A detailed description of the pathophysiology of HIV and its effects on the CNS is presented in Chapter 2 of this book. However, it is important to remember that vertical infection with HIV may be devastating to the CNS because it occurs when the brain is rapidly growing and maturing, making it particularly sensitive to external influences.

There has been research exploring the impact of HIV on neurodevelopment from the early stages of the HIV epidemic, including a recognition of the deleterious neurodevelopmental impact of infection on infants and young children (Belman et al. 1985; Diamond 1989; Diamond et al. 1990). In the pre-ART era, HIV was often devastating in the first few years of life, with HIVE being a frequent AIDS-defining condition in this population (WHO 2007). Children with HIVE were noted to have gross motor deficits. Many were classified as having bilateral lower limb spasticity and significant developmental delays across all domains. It is important to highlight the full range of effects that HIV infection can have on the immature CNS. Without ART, 50% to 90% of HIV-infected children are reported to have some form of CNS involvement (Kovacs 2009). Compared to adults, infants and children tend to have earlier manifestations of disease and a more rapid disease progression. Furthermore, the immune system in children is immature compared to adults, and children are also at higher risk of developing invasive opportunistic infections (Kovacs 2009; Palacio, Álvarez, and Muñoz-Fernández 2012).

Global Development

THE EFFECT OF HIV ON NEURODEVELOPMENT BEFORE ANTIRETROVIRAL THERAPY

As a result of the successful global roll-out of ART, data regarding how HIV affects development without treatment are mostly from the period before the year 2000. Despite these global public health successes, treatment coverage for children with HIV has continued to lag behind that of adults, and the developmental consequences of no or late treatment, still manifest (WHO 2013).

Evidence from early in the HIV pandemic indicates that early HIV infection has a negative effect on development, and several studies from low-resource settings support this conclusion (see Table 11A.1). Data from these first studies included reports from a cohort of HIV-infected mothers in Haiti, collected from 1986 to 1991, demonstrating a developmental lag in HIV-infected infants when compared to those who were uninfected at age 2 years (Gay et al. 1995). In Rwanda, a prospective study conducted in this pre-ART era revealed that, at all observation points over the period of the study, HIV-exposed infected (HEI) infants were significantly more likely to have overall neurodevelopmental impairments. Gross motor delay was found at all ages while fine motor delay was seen at 6 and 12 months of age. Language performance initially showed no difference between infected and uninfected infants, but deficits were apparent by 2 years old, and social development was also noted to be delayed from 6 months of age onwards (Msellati et al. 1993).

Similar findings were described from cohorts in the Democratic Republic of Congo where assessments done at 3, 6, 9, 12, and 18 months of age demonstrated that children who were HEI performed significantly worse on overall development when compared to other groups (Boivin et al. 1995). Another pre-ART study, from Uganda, found that HIV-infected participants had a significantly higher probability of impaired development at 12 months than the HIV-uninfected comparison groups, with this effect becoming more prominent over time (Drotar et al. 1997). Assessment of children from Brazil, a middle-income country, using the Denver Developmental Screening Test and the Clinical Adaptive Test and Clinical Linguistic and Auditory Milestone Scale (CAT/CLAMS) showed a significantly lower performance by the HIV-infected children on the CAT/CLAMS at all ages until 36 months old (Bruck et al. 2001).

Because of the global epidemiological profile of the HIV epidemic, relatively less evidence is available from well-resourced countries. Diamond and colleagues reported that HIV-infected infants in an American foster care system early in the pandemic had a higher risk of developmental impairments, as assessed on the Bayley Scales of Infant Development (BSID) and the Wechsler Preschool and Primary Scale of Intelligence (WPPSI), in a comparison of HIV-exposed groups (Diamond et al. 1990). Another study from the USA looked at the natural progression of perinatal HIV infection in the 1990s and examined the effect of HIV infection on neurodevelopment using the BSID. This showed a decline in the scores of HIV-infected children in both indices, mental development index (MDI) and psychomotor development index (PDI), over time, from the first assessment at around 3 months to 24 months.

More recently, despite the greater accessibility of ART, the problem of the severe end of the HIV–CNS spectrum has re-emerged, including HIVE with developmental delay, as well as abnormal neurological findings. In a Mozambiquan cohort investigating hospitalised infants with newly diagnosed HIV, 67% (18 out of 27) had developmental delay at assessment and 27% met the full presumed HIVE diagnostic criteria (Chaúque et al. 2021).

In summary, without access to ART, HIV-infected children are significantly more likely to have an abnormal developmental profile and trajectory, with lower performance on standard developmental assessments, when compared to their unexposed peer controls. These findings were consistent across economic contexts and study setting. Of particular note, from this early work, is that few studies addressed relevant contextual issues that could also have affected the developmental performance of participants. The use of different tools and at different ages in this older literature, means that direct comparison of findings across studies remains challenging.

HIV Infection and Development in the Presence of Antiretroviral Monotherapy

Before multidrug ART regimens were widely available, individual antiretroviral drugs were used in the treatment of HIV infection. A US cohort study, which focused on a population of pregnant women who were at risk of contracting HIV infection, monitored the outcomes of 65 children born to these women. These children were stratified into HEI, HEU, and HUU (HIV-unexposed uninfected). The infants were assessed at 4, 9, 12, 18, and 24 months using the BSID. Clinical AIDS developed in 3 of the 18 HEI children, and 11 of the 18 HEI children were started on azidothymidine (AZT) monotherapy, but the basis for AZT initiation was not detailed. Although there were no differences between groups when assessed at 4 months old, by 12 months the HEI children had lower scores on the MDI than the HEU and HUU groups. At 18 and 24 months, MDI scores for the HEI group were consistently the lowest. The PDI results showed a similar trend, as the three groups had equivalent initial scores, but they developed statistically significant differences at 12 months with the HEI group scoring the lowest. At the end of the study, only children with diagnosed HIV infection were considered severely developmentally delayed on the PDI. Higher HIV viral loads were associated with an increased risk of developing severe cognitive and motor delays. The effects of AZT were not factored into the study design, and only four participants had assessments conducted before and after initiating the medication (Pollack et al. 1996). Another study, looking specifically at the effect of AZT on neurodevelopmental functioning, included a wide age range of from 2 months to 12 years, showing no difference in neurodevelopmental functioning after 6 and 12 months of treatment (Nozyce et al. 1994).

There is currently little research on the impact of antiretroviral monotherapy on infant and toddler neurodevelopment. Existing studies have included children up to 3 years old who received monotherapy, but these studies did not specifically measure the effect of monotherapy on childhood development.

Given the current availability of better treatment options, antiretroviral monotherapy is not recommended to improve HIV-related developmental deficits.

THE NEURODEVELOPMENT OF CHILDREN WITH HIV INFECTION TREATED WITH MULTIDRUG ANTIRETROVIRAL THERAPY

The utilisation of multiple drug ART ushered in a new era in the management of HIV infection. ART implementation has reduced the incidence of HIVE but there is evidence that HIV-associated developmental impairments can still occur in infancy and early childhood despite early ART initiation, although these data are less consistent (Van Rie et al. 2007). This is in part explained by the rapidly changing global guidelines for treatment of HIV in children over the first two decades of the new millennium.

One of the earliest studies to investigate developmental outcomes of children with HIV treated with combination ART, is by Foster and colleagues from the UK. This case review of 62 HIV-infected children who developed HIV before 3 years of age found only a proportion of these children had access to ART, as it was formerly reserved for children with an AIDS-defining condition. All children were assessed using either the BSID or the Griffiths Mental Development Scale (GMDS). In terms of general HIV disease progression, of the 62 participants, half were either mildly symptomatic or asymptomatic (Centers for Disease Control and Prevention group N, A, or B) and half had severe disease (Centers for Disease Control and Prevention group C). The children in group C all received treatment with either antiretroviral monotherapy, dual therapy preceding ART, or ART as an initial treatment. In group C, 14 children (22.5%) had abnormal neurological signs, with 12 children (19.3%) having spastic diplegia and two children (3.2%) having quadriplegia. All 62 children had lower PDI and MDI scores than the general population. In the MDI, expressive and verbal items had lower scores than perceptual or visual items, while the PDI showed an overall delay in acquiring motor skills. There was a statistically significant difference between those with more severe disease in group C, compared to those in groups N, A, or B, with those in group C scoring significantly lower than the other groups on both the MDI and the PDI. Although a proportion of the children in this study were on ART, there were no comments on age at ART initiation, virological suppression status, or the difference in outcome of those with treatment compared to those without (Foster et al. 2006).

One of the first studies to investigate the impact of early ART initiation in children who were HEI was reported by Laughton and colleagues from South Africa (Laughton et al. 2012). This trial investigated the neurodevelopmental outcomes of 115 HIV-infected infants who received early ART initiation (<3 months old) compared to those whose ART-initiation was deferred. HIV-uninfected infants (HEU and HUU) were also included in this study. The results suggested that HIV-infected children receiving early ART did better on the GMDS general and locomotor scores compared to those who deferred ART. At 11 months old, HIV-infected children performed similarly to children without HIV in all subscales except the locomotor subscale. The mean age for initiating ART was 8.4 weeks in the early ART arm and 31.4 weeks in the deferred ART arm. The study found that there was little neurodevelopmental difference between HEI infants receiving early ART and HIV-uninfected children. This was one of the seminal studies that provided evidence for the value of early HIV testing and early initiation of ART to reduce risk for neurodevelopmental delay and morbidity in HIV-infected infants (Laughton et al. 2012).

In Kenya, a subsequent, prospective study investigated developmental outcomes of infants commenced on ART before 5 months old using questions adapted from the Denver Developmental Screening Test. Of the 99 infants recruited, the majority were severely immunocompromised. The median age at neck control was 4.3 months, and later neck control was associated with a lack of inclusion in the prevention of mother-to-child transmission (PMTCT) programme, a weight-for-age Z-score (WAZ) of less than −2, and a height-for-age Z-score (HAZ) of less than −2. The median age at independent walking was 16.1 months, and median age at monosyllabic speech was 16.6 months. Later acquisition of both milestones was associated with pre-ART hospitalisation, pre-ART WHO stage III/IV, an infant CD4+ count of less than 1500 cells, and a pre-ART WAZ of less than −2 and a HAZ of less than −2. Later speech acquisition was also associated with a maternal CD4+ count of less than 200. Those on lopinavir/ritonavir were less likely to be hospitalised pre-ART and they had earlier speech when compared to infants on a nevirapine-containing regime. After the initiation of ART, CD4+ a percentage of less than 20% at 6 months of age was associated with later unassisted walking and monosyllabic speech milestones. Higher viral loads were also associated with later monosyllabic speech development. Low body weight, stunting, or wasting were associated with later achievement of independent walking. Low body weight and stunting were also correlated with later monosyllabic speech development. Treatment in this cohort resulted in reduced delay in early motor and language acquisition. However, children whose viral suppression was inadequate performed worse compared to those whose HIV was well controlled (Benki-Nugent et al. 2015). A cohort study by the same group used the Malawi Developmental Assessment Tool to assess children at 2 to 4 weeks and 6 months after ART initiation. Lower baseline scores were associated with clinically and virologically more severe disease, poorer nutritional status, anthropometric measures, and preterm delivery. At the 6-month time point there was measured improvement in the gross motor and fine motor domains, which was not seen in the language and social subscales. Higher weight gain was associated with greater improvement in developmental indices (Gómez et al. 2018).

Although there is often documented improvement of neurological findings, this is not always complete, as found by a group in South Africa (Innes et al. 2020). This is hypothesised to be due partly to the nervous system being a potential reservoir site for HIV as well as the low blood–brain permeability of many antiretroviral agents. In order to mitigate these effects and improve motor and cognitive development, new technologies using several nanotechnological modalities are being developed to transport existing antiretroviral agents across the blood–brain barrier (Nabi et al. 2021). In vitro and in vivo testing in animal models of atazanavir transport across the blood–brain barrier using a lipid-carrier nanotechnology are promising (Khan et al. 2020). In addition, using modern innovative design strategies, the pace of development of new antiretroviral agents with tailored properties in the areas of bioavailability has accelerated, with the agents in different stages of testing (Zhuang et al. 2020). The partial or lack of reversal of neurological symptoms in children who are started on ART remains a concern, despite some gains in the development of improved ART drug delivery systems. In the meantime, the widely supported strategy, currently being applied, remains for active HIV screening after birth, followed by treatment on diagnosis, for infants with vertical HIV infection.

Overall, current evidence suggests that HIV-infected children on ART have better developmental outcomes than HIV-infected children without treatment. Prompt initial treatment is also associated with better developmental outcomes when compared to deferred treatment initiation. The expansion of national programmes providing HIV-infected children with ART should be encouraged to both reduce unequal treatment availability and to optimise the developmental outcomes of these children. Novel agents and delivery mechanisms may also improve the effectiveness of ART.

Individual Developmental Domains

To understand the specific ways in which HIV affects both development and the areas of potential development, this section details the evidence of HIV's effects on specific developmental domains.

Motor Development

Before the introduction of ART, HIV-infected children often experienced poorer physical development and significantly poorer gross motor development when compared to their HIV-uninfected peers

(Boivin et al. 1995). Haitian children living with HIV in the late 1980s to the early 1990s, prior to ART roll-out, without ART were found to have significant impairment on the BSID performance scale. This effect remained throughout the duration of the study, but was stable over time. HIV-infected children also had a higher chance of having severe delay on this performance scale when compared to their HIV-uninfected peers (29% vs 0% respectively) (Gay et al. 1995).

In a group of untreated Rwandan children, an initial difference in fine motor function between the HIV-infected and the HIV-uninfected children was reported at 6 months and 12 months old, although these differences did not persist past infancy (Msellati et al. 1993). Conversely a study on ART-naïve children from Uganda reported early, persistent motor developmental deficits, with HEI children having a 30% chance of an abnormal PDI score on the BSID, compared to 11% for HEU and 5% for HUU at 12 months. This difference became more prominent at 24 months (Drotar et al. 1997). Similarly, a US study concluded that HEI children identified as having motor delays in infancy would continue to have persistent poor motor performance after the age of 17 months (Chase et al. 1995). Pollack and colleagues (Pollack et al. 1996) demonstrated that, by the time all the children in their cohort study turned 12 months old, severe motor developmental delays were only seen in the HIV-infected children, even after initiation of AZT monotherapy in 11 out of 18 HEI children. All the groups demonstrated slight improvement in their scores between 18 and 24 months, but in the HEI this may have partially been due to the death of the most affected participants (Pollack et al. 1996). In Nigeria, Obiagwu (2019) also found motor delay using clinical screening.

The current evidence from cohort studies, which used data from both resource-rich and resource-poor settings, suggests that HIV-infected children without ART are at high risk of developing motor deficits. Both gross and fine motor skills are negatively impacted in this population. Motor skills seem to be the most prominent developmental domain clearly impacted by HIV infection in children – encouragingly, there is some evidence that these effects can be reduced by ART implementation. Ongoing research is investigating if HIV-induced developmental delay can be reversed by initiating ART. If so, this would show ART to be a particularly effective protocol in mitigating negative outcomes in HIV-infected children.

LANGUAGE DEVELOPMENT

One of the earliest studies on language development in HIV-infected children showed no significant initial differences in language development between HIV-infected and HIV-uninfected children when assessed at 6 months of age. However, at 24 months of age, these HIV-infected children scored significantly lower on a 3-question language test that assessed both expressive and receptive language skills. This suggests that HIV infection negatively impacts language acquisition skills as children develop (Msellati et al. 1993). Other studies also found that HIV had detrimental effects on language development, with Wolters et al. (1997) describing greater impact on expressive language compared to receptive language. An early study from the Democratic Republic of Congo (DRC) showed that 85% of HEI children were delayed in developing expressive language, and 77% demonstrated receptive language delays when compared to the HIV-uninfected children (Van Rie et al. 2008). Later assessment of this same cohort showed an improvement in mean scores with HEI children demonstrating the greatest improvement.

Motor function improvement in HEI children was statistically significant but improvements in areas contributing to cognitive function, including language, were not. Despite improvements in the HEI children, a gap between the scores of the HIV-infected and HIV-uninfected persisted throughout the study, and the HIV-uninfected children consistently performed better (Van Rie et al. 2009).

In a South African study of ART-naïve HEI children with low CD4+ counts between the ages of 18 and 30 months, 82.5% showed language delays on the BSID-II compared to the Bayley global norming sample (Baillieu and Potterton 2008). These children were all from low socioeconomic backgrounds, and there were no uninfected control groups to address contextual or cultural factors potentially impacting performance on this tool. Another study performed at a similar time compared HEI children, HEU children, and untested community controls in rural Kenya. Differences between HEI children and community controls were not evident between 8 and 15 months but, by 16 to 30 months, language performance between the groups was found to be different. Total language scores, language production, grammatical complexity, and the ability to combine words, were worse in the HEI group (Alcock et al. 2016). A proportion of HIV-infected children have also been described as having impaired hearing, often due to repeated ear infections, which remains an important secondary cause of language impairment in HEI children (Christopher et al. 2013; Donald et al. 2015).

HIV infection has detrimental effects on language development in infancy and early childhood. These deficits have been shown to manifest in expressive language, receptive language, and nonverbal communication. Significant difference between HIV-infected and uninfected children do not appear in infancy but become clearer as these children reach toddlerhood during the period when there is typically the greatest increase in expressive language acquisition. These differences might be partially attributable to adverse emotional, health, and economic circumstances.

Cognitive Development

HIV-uninfected children, regardless of exposure status, consistently out-perform their HEI counterparts in cognitive function tests. In a Ugandan study, Drotar et al. (1997) found no significant differences in information processing ability between the HEI, HEU, and HUU children. Participants were tested using the Fagan test of infant intelligence at 6, 9, and 12 months. In the BSID MDI, variance analysis found significant difference between the HEI group and the two HIV-uninfected groups when at tested at 6, 18, and 24 months old. HIV-infected children were significantly more likely to have a low MDI score at the age of 12 months: 26% for HIV-infected children versus 6% for HIV-uninfected. By 24 months, 35% of the children in the HEI group versus 10% of the children in the HIV-uninfected groups had low MDI scores (Drotar et al. 1997).

Using the BSID assessment, HEI children from a low- and middle-income community in Haiti showed higher likelihood (21%) of having severe delays on the BSID MDI, when compared to the HEU cohort. The HEI children also showed a lag in the acquisition rate of skills that scored on the mental development index compared to HIV-uninfected children, and this gap between them and grew over time (Gay et al. 1995). A US study using the BSID showed that while early MDI scores assessed between 4 and 17 months of age were comparable, scores were delayed in the HEI cohort compared to the HEU group at a second assessment between 17 and 30 months (Chase et al. 1995).

Imaging Findings and Correlates with Cognitive Development

In the South African-based Children with HIV Early Antiretroviral (CHER) trial, HEI children had increased volume in some subcortical grey matter areas that was attributed to a commencement of ART after 12 weeks. The corpus callosum was smaller in all HEI children regardless of the time of ART initiation. These findings were so despite a viral load suppression rate of 93% (less than 399 RNA copies per ml) in this population (Randall et al. 2017). Abnormalities in cortical gyri and subcortical grey matter were detected in this group at 7 years of age (Nwosu et al. 2018).

Neurodevelopmental assessments have been utilised to determine functional deficits in HIV-positive children. Where cognitive decline is ongoing, white matter damage has been hypothesised as a possible pathway. Using diffusion tension imaging (DTI) as a method of assessing white matter damage and tract injury, Ackermann et al. (2020) compared neurodevelopmental assessments – including GMDS and Beery-Buktenica tests – against DTI parameters in abnormal white matter. Study participants were derived from the CHER trial. Ventral (occipitotemporal) and dorsal (occipitoparietal) visual pathways exhibited abnormalities in HEI children at age 5 years despite early ART initiation. These pathways are essential for visuo-spatial perception, suggesting that DTI may be more sensitive than neurodevelopmental assessment tests in determining this difference. Further research is required to determine the pathophysiology of differential visuo-spatial damage (Ackermann et al. 2020).

Nwosu and colleagues (2021) carried out another study embedded in the CHER trial to determine whether early ART initiation and ART interruptions affect brain cortical thickness and cortical folding as determined by local gyrification indices. This study utilised T1-weighted high-resolution structural magnetic resonance imaging at age 5 years. Group comparisons of HEI and unexposed controls for cortical thickness and local gyrification indices over the whole brain were performed, adjusting for age and sex. HEI children had thicker cortices than unexposed children in bilateral frontal and temporal regions, but lower gyrification in the superior frontal region at this age. Within the HEI group, children whose treatment was interrupted had thinner cortical thickness in the left lateral occipital region and lower gyrification in bilateral parietal regions compared to those with continuous treatment. These results further support evidence that early ART initiation and avoidance of ART interruption are important for neurological development (Nwosu et al. 2021).

Functional imaging approaches, including magnetic resonance spectroscopy, have been used to examine metabolic changes in select brain regions (basal ganglia, midfrontal grey matter and peritrigonal white matter) in children with ART-induced viral suppression (Graham et al. 2020). Children with HEI had higher inflammatory factor scores than children without HIV, suggested by higher combined concentrations of total choline in the three regions of interest. These findings may indicate a simultaneous inflammatory response across the brain, in both grey and white matter (Graham et al. 2020).

The Effect of Timing of Infection on Developmental Outcomes

HIV can be transmitted before birth, at delivery, and during the breastfeeding period. There are a few studies that have specifically investigated the relative impact of infection during these different time periods. According to the limited evidence available, earlier HIV infection is correlated with poorer developmental outcomes. For example, an early study conducted in Tanzania, addressed this question. Children with confirmed HIV infection in the first 21 days of life were assumed to have been infected antenatally and had lower scores on the BSID in both PDI and MDI compared to uninfected infants. While infants who were infected after 21 days of age also scored lower in these indices, this was not as severe as in the earlier-infected group. Overall, for each additional month of HIV infection among the early-infected group, there was a 1.1-point decrease in the MDI and a 1.4-point decrease in the PDI compared to the uninfected children. The children who were HIV infected by day 21 had an almost 15 times higher risk of MDI delay compared to uninfected children, while those infected after the first 21 days had approximately three times higher risk (McGrath et al. 2006).

The effects of ART on development in children with earlier infection needs further investigation. HIV impacts neurodevelopment regardless of the timing of infection, highlighting the importance of ongoing prevention strategies for vertically-transmitted HIV.

EARLY CHILDHOOD DEVELOPMENT INTERVENTIONS IN THE CONTEXT OF HIV

To what extent can early nurturing and environment play a role in improving neurodevelopmental outcomes for HEI children? In a qualitative study from a community in western Kenya, involving health-care providers and caregivers of children, both identified environmental risks to optimal developmental outcomes, including poor nutrition, lack of stimulation and neglect in the home, as well as harsh disciplinary measures in the home (McHenry et al. 2018). Indeed, studies have shown that general interventions that improve the quality of life, health, and access to clean water and sanitation facilities may also have a positive impact on their neurodevelopment. In a study based in a rural district in Zimbabwe, families assigned to intervention with supplemental feeding and education, combined with water sanitation and hygiene, showed significant improvement in neurodevelopmental outcomes compared to standard levels of care (Chandna et al. 2020). Interestingly, the aforementioned Kenyan study also revealed that both health-care workers and caregivers still held the belief that, if children were compliant on ART, they could be expected to follow a typical developmental trajectory.

Another series of studies, based in Uganda, has shown that early childhood development training of caregivers has been found to enhance the development of both HEU and HEI children (Boivin et al. 2013; Bass et al. 2016; Boivin et al. 2020; Ikekwere et al. 2021). These reports were in the context of a broader study of children aged 18 months to 5 years that was designed to assess the effectiveness of the Mediational Intervention for Sensitizing Caregivers (MISC). The MISC was designed to be a year-long, biweekly, community-based nutrition and parent support programme for caregivers of HIV-exposed and HIV-infected children. Children in the MISC arm had greater gains in visual reception scale and memory testing post intervention. This benefit has been replicated in a later study in the same area after the wider roll out of ART: in children in the age range 2 to 3 years of age who had confirmed HIV infection, MISC had a positive effect on receptive language at the 1-year point, although the effect was attenuated on long-term follow up at 24 months of age compared with controls (Bass et al. 2016).

The Latency and Early Neonatal Provision of Antiretroviral Drugs (LEOPARD) trial in South Africa further demonstrated the efficacy of a year-long, home-based developmental stimulation programme from birth (Strehlau et al. 2021). Follow-up after 1 year reported benefits for cognitive and language development compared to the observation group.

Broader support for health and the social environment at early developmental stages may also help. A group from Zimbabwe has been assessing whether a savings-and-lending scheme to improve household economic status and facilitation of access to care and HIV treatment will improve developmental outcomes measured using the Mullen Scales of Early Learning (MSEL) (Chingono et al. 2018). This follows a study in Malawi, which also reported on integrated models of support, where caregivers who received an early childhood development intervention were also more likely to take up other psychosocial support services at the facility and perceived that their children had better development (Dovel et al. 2021). The importance of alleviating psychosocial stress is further underlined by a South African study which found that developmental scores could be partially attributed to maternal depression (Nöthling, Laughton, and Seedat 2021).

Beyond the fundamental development domains, other aspects of learning, including emerging executive function, have also been addressed by the Ugandan research group. The domain of attention was not specifically evaluated in earlier studies and this study aimed to look at whether attention improves with MISC intervention, evaluated using the Early Childhood Vigilance Test, a culturally appropriate tool to measure attention in children 2 to 4 years of age. The study had the same two intervention groups, one that received biweekly MISC intervention over the course of 1 year while the other received biweekly sessions on nutrition, hygiene, and health care. Children in both groups improved from baseline to 6 and 12 months, as would be expected. The children in the MISC arm performed better on the Early Childhood Vigilance Test at 6 months than the control group, but this did not persist to 12 months. A subsequent randomised control trial comparing the same interventions at the same site with new cohorts of children 2 to 3 years of age showed that the caregivers in the MISC arm showed significantly improved caregiving quality but not better child cognitive outcomes. MISC-group caregivers also scored better in activities of daily child caregiving, which may have resulted in the language benefits (Ikekwere et al. 2021). This suggests that there is a need for further investigation into interventions that can improve attention and concentration in the context of HIV infection as well as sustain the interaction that children receive from their caregivers as this is a potential mechanism.

SUMMARY

HIV is a neurotrophic virus that is devastating to the CNS, in particular when vertically transmitted, acting on a child's brain when it is growing and maturing rapidly. Compared to adults, infants and children tend to manifest disease symptoms earlier, with a more rapid disease progression. Furthermore, children's immature immune systems put them at higher risk of developing invasive, opportunistic infections. Without access to ART, HIV-infected children are significantly more likely to have an abnormal developmental profile and trajectory, with lower performance on standard developmental assessments, when compared to their unexposed peers. These findings are consistent across economic contexts and study settings.

The advent of ART has greatly modified the natural progression of HIV infection, showing improvements in neurodevelopmental outcomes in children when early, optimal treatment is applied. However, despite early diagnosis and ART-initiation, HIV-infected neonates, infants, and toddlers can still deviate from typical developmental trajectories, putting them at elevated risk of poor cognitive, motor, and language development. And ART coverage in HIV-infected children has always lagged behind coverage for infected adults. Given the huge population of children now living with HIV, the focus has moved from primarily physical health care to additionally prioritising the optimal cognitive and developmental outcomes of children living with this condition.

It is increasingly recognised that children develop best in an environment where basic physical, emotional, and cognitive needs are met, for example, nutrition and shelter, secure attachment, appropriate stimulation. Widely prevalent risk factors preventing optimal development, such as iron deficiency, substance abuse, maternal depression, lack of access to a stimulating early childhood experience, and chronic illnesses, including HIV, are particularly important in resource-limited countries. These factors need to be identified and relevant interventions be supported and managed in an integrated manner to be effective.

Medical management plans should carefully monitor HEI children and implement early intervention strategies to reduce the risk of developmental delays. Early, effective ART interventions that utilise home-based caregiver interventions may have positive effects on HEI children's development, and these interventions could be explored for their potential for wider feasibility and scalability.

The improved developmental outcomes that accompany early ART highlight the importance of prioritising strategies for early HIV detection and intervention, such as developmental screening and monitoring. Finally, early child stimulation and caregiver psychosocial support – key components of a comprehensive care strategy for HIV-infected children – may promote not only survival of the child but also the child's ability to thrive in later life.

REFERENCES

Ackermann C, Andronikou S, Saleh MG et al. (2020) Diffusion tensor imaging point to ongoing functional impairment in HIV-infected children at age 5, undetectable using standard neurodevelopmental assessments. *AIDS Research and Therapy*, 17: 1–15.

Alcock K, Abubakar A, Newton CR, Holding P (2016) The effects of prenatal HIV exposure on language functioning in Kenyan children: Establishing an evaluative framework. *BMC Research Notes*, 9(1): 463.

Baillieu N, Potterton J (2008) The extent of delay of language, motor, and cognitive development in HIV-positive infants. *Journal of Neurologic Physical Therapy* 32(3): 118–121.

Bass JK, Nakasujja N, Familiar-Lopez I et al. (2016) Association of caregiver quality of care with neurocognitive outcomes in HIV-affected children aged 2–5 years in Uganda. *AIDS Care*, 28: 76–83.

Belman AL, Ultmann MH, Horoupian D et al. (1985) Neurological complications in infants and children with acquired immune deficiency syndrome. *Annals of Neurology*, 18(5): 560–566.

Benki-Nugent S, Eshelman C, Wamalwa D et al. (2015) Correlates of age at attainment of developmental milestones in HIV-infected infants receiving early antiretroviral therapy. *The Pediatric Infectious Disease Journal*, 34(1): 55.

Boivin MJ, Green SD, Davies AG et al. (1995) A preliminary evaluation of the cognitive and motor effects on pediatric HIV infection in Zairian children. *Health Psychology*, 14(1): 13.

Boivin MJ, Bangirana P, Nakasujja N et al. (2013) A year-long caregiver training program improves cognition in preschool Ugandan children with human immunodeficiency virus. *The Journal of Pediatrics*, 163(5): 1409–1416. e1401–e1405.

Boivin MJ, Augustinavicius JL, Familiar-Lopez I et al. (2020) Early childhood development caregiver training and neurocognition of HIV-exposed Ugandan siblings. *Journal of Developmental & Behavioral Pediatrics*, 41(3): 221–229.

Bruck I, Tahan TT, Cruz CR et al. (2001) Developmental milestones of vertically HIV infected and seroreverters children: Follow up of 83 children. *Arquivos De Neuro-Psiquiatria*, 59(3-B): 691–695.

Chandna J, Ntozini R, Evans C et al. (2020) Effects of improved complementary feeding and improved water, sanitation and hygiene on early child development among HIV-exposed children: Substudy of a cluster randomised trial in rural Zimbabwe. *BMJ Glob Health*, 5(1): e001718.

Chase C, Vibbert N, Pelton SI, Coulter DL, Cabral H (1995) Early neurodevelopmental growth in children with vertically transmitted human immunodeficiency virus infection. *Archives Of Pediatrics & Adolescent Medicine*, 149(8): 850–855.

Chaúque S, Mohole J, Zucula H et al. (2021) HIV encephalopathy in ART-naïve, hospitalized infants in Mozambique. *J Trop Pediatr*, 67(6): fmab 106. doi: 10.1093/tropej/fmab106.

Chingono R, Mebrahtu H, Mupambireyi Z et al. (2018) Evaluating the effectiveness of a multi-component intervention on early childhood development in paediatric HIV care and treatment programmes: A randomised controlled trial. *BMC Pediatr*, 18(1): 222.

Christopher N, Edward T, Sabrina B-K, Agnes N (2013) The prevalence of hearing impairment in 6 months–5 years HIV/AIDS-positive patients attending paediatric infectious disease clinic at Mulago Hospital. *Int J Pediatr Otorhinolaryngol*, 77(2): 262–265.

Daelmans B, Darmstadt GL, Lombardi J et al. (2017) Early childhood development: The foundation of sustainable development. *The Lancet*, 389(10064): 9–11.

Diamond GW (1989) Developmental problems in children with HIV infection. *Mental Retardation*, 27(4): 213–217.

Diamond GW, Gurdin P, Wiznia AA et al. (1990) Effects of congenital HIV infection on neurodevelopmental status of babies in foster care. *Developmental Medicine & Child Neurology*, 32(11): 999–1004.

Donald KA, Walker KG, Kilborn T et al. (2015) HIV encephalopathy: Pediatric case series description and insights from the clinic coalface. *AIDS Research and Therapy*, 12(1): 2.

Dovel K, Kalande P, Udedi E et al. (2021) Integrated early childhood development services improve mothers' experiences with prevention of mother to child transmission (PMTCT) programs in Malawi: A qualitative study. *BMC Health Serv Res*, 21(1): 348.

Drotar D, Olness K, Wiznitzer M et al. (1997) Neurodevelopmental outcomes of Ugandan infants with human immunodeficiency virus type 1 infection. *Pediatrics*, 100(1): e5.

Foster C, Biggs R, Melvin D, Walters M, Tudor-Williams G, Lyall E (2006) Neurodevelopmental outcomes in children with HIV infection under 3 years of age. *Developmental Medicine & Child Neurology*, 48(8): 677–682.

Gay CL, Armstrong FD, Cohen D et al. (1995) The effects of HIV on cognitive and motor development in children born to HIV-seropositive women with no reported drug use: Birth to 24 months. *Pediatrics*, 96(6): 1078–1082.

Gómez LA, Crowell CS, Njuguna I et al. (2018) Improved neurodevelopment after initiation of antiretroviral therapy in human immunodeficiency virus-infected children. *Pediatr Infect Dis J*, 37(9): 916–922.

Graham AS, Holmes MJ, Little F et al. (2020) MRS suggests multi-regional inflammation and white matter axonal damage at 11 years following perinatal HIV infection. *NeuroImage: Clinical*, 28: 102505.

Grantham-McGregor S, Cheung YB, Cueto S et al. (2007) Developmental potential in the first 5 years for children in developing countries. *The Lancet*, 369(9555): 60–70.

Hermida MJ, Shalom DE, Segretin MS et al. (2019) Risks for child cognitive development in rural contexts. *Frontiers in Psychology*, 9: 2735.

Huttenlocher PR, Dabholkar AS (1997) Regional differences in synaptogenesis in human cerebral cortex. *Journal of Comparative Neurology*, 387(2): 167–178.

Huttenlocher PR (1999) Synaptogenesis in human cerebral cortex and the concept of critical periods. The role of early experience in infant development. In: Fox NA, Leavitt LA, Warhol JG, editors, *The Role of Early Experience in Infant Development.* Calverton, NY: Johnson & Johnson Pediatric Institute, pp. 15–28.

Ikekwere J, Ucheagwu V, Familiar-Lopez I et al. (2021) Attention test improvements from a cluster randomized controlled trial of caregiver training for HIV-exposed/uninfected Ugandan preschool children. *The Journal of Pediatrics*, (August): 226–232. doi: 10.1016/j.jpeds.2021.03.064.

Innes S, Laughton B, van Toorn R et al. (2020) Recovery of HIV encephalopathy in perinatally infected children on antiretroviral therapy. *Dev Med Child Neurol*, 62(11): 1309–1316.

Khan SA, Rehman S, Nabi B et al. (2020) Boosting the brain delivery of atazanavir through nanostructured lipid carrier-cased approach for mitigating neuroAIDS. *Pharmaceutics*, 12(11): 1059.

Kovacs A (2009) Early immune activation predicts central nervous system disease in HIV-infected infants: Implications for early treatment. *Clinical Infectious Diseases*, 48(3): 347–349.

Laughton B, Cornell M, Grove D et al. (2012) Early antiretroviral therapy improves neurodevelopmental outcomes in infants. *AIDS (London, England)*, 26(13): 1685.

Laughton B, Cornell M, Boivin M, van Rie A (2013) Neurodevelopment in perinatally HIV-infected children: A concern for adolescence. *Journal of the International AIDS Society*, 16: 18603–18603.

Lipina SJ, Posner MI (2012) The impact of poverty on the development of brain networks. *Frontiers in Human Neuroscience*, 6: 238.

Lo S, Das P, Horton R (2017) A good start in life will ensure a sustainable future for all. *The Lancet*, 389(10064): 8–9.

McGrath N, Fawzi WW, Bellinger D et al. (2006) The timing of mother-to-child transmission of human immunodeficiency virus infection and the neurodevelopment of children in Tanzania. *The Pediatric Infectious Disease Journal*, 25(1): 47–52.

McHenry MS, Oyungu E, McAteer CI et al. (2018) Early childhood development in children born to HIV-infected mothers: Perspectives from Kenyan clinical providers and caregivers. *Global Pediatric Health*, 5: 2333794X18811795.

Mogoba P, Phillips TK, le Roux S et al. (2021) Mother–child separation among women living with HIV and their children in the first four years postpartum in South Africa. *Trop Med Int Health*, 26(2): 173–183.

Msellati P, Lepage P, Hitimana DG, Van Goethem C, Van de Perre P, Dabis F (1993) Neurodevelopmental testing of children born to human immunodeficiency virus type 1 seropositive and seronegative mothers: A prospective cohort study in Kigali, Rwanda. *Pediatrics*, 92(6): 843–848.

Nabi B, Rehman S, Pottoo FH, Baboota S, Ali J (2021) Directing the antiretroviral drugs to the brain reservoir: A nanoformulation approach for NeuroAIDS. *Current Drug Metabolism*, 22(4): 280–286.

Nöthling J, Laughton B, Seedat S (2021) Maternal depression and infant social withdrawal as predictors of behaviour and development in vertically HIV-infected children at 3.5 years. *Paediatr Int Child Health*, 41(4): 268–277.

Nozyce M, Hoberman M, Arpadi S et al. (1994) A 12-month study of the effects of oral zidovudine on neurodevelopmental functioning in a cohort of vertically HIV-infected inner-city children. *AIDS (London, England)*, 8(5): 635–639.

Nwosu EC, Robertson FC, Holmes MJ et al. (2018) Altered brain morphometry in 7-year old HIV-infected children on early ART. *Metabolic Brain Disease*, 33(2): 523–535.

Nwosu EC, Holmes MJ, Cotton MF et al. (2021) Cortical structural changes related to early antiretroviral therapy (ART) interruption in perinatally HIV-infected children at 5 years of age. *IBRO Neuroscience Reports*, 10: 161–170.

Obiagwu PN (2019) Gross motor developmental delay in human immunodeficiency virus-infected children under 2 years of age. *Ann Afr Med*, 18(4): 185–190.

Palacio M, Álvarez S, Muñoz-Fernández M (2012) HIV-1 infection and neurocognitive impairment in the current era. *Reviews in Medical Virology*, 22(1): 33–45.

Pollack H, Kuchuk A, Cowan L et al. (1996) Neurodevelopment, growth, and viral load in HIV-infected infants. *Brain, Behavior, and Immunity*, 10(3): 298–312.

Randall SR, Warton CM, Holmes MJ et al. (2017) Larger subcortical gray matter structures and smaller corpora callosa at age 5 years in HIV infected children on early ART. *Frontiers in Neuroanatomy*, 11: 95.

Sania A, Sudfeld CR, Danaei G et al. (2019) Early life risk factors of motor, cognitive and language development: A pooled analysis of studies from low-/middle-income countries. *BMJ Open*, 9(10): e026449.

Stiles J, Jernigan TL (2010) The basics of brain development. *Neuropsychology Review*, 20(4): 327–348.

Strehlau R, Burke M, van Aswegen T, Kuhn L, Potterton J (2021) Neurodevelopment in early treated HIV-infected infants participating in a developmental stimulation programme compared with controls. *Child Care Health Dev*, 47(2): 154–162.

Thompson RA, Nelson CA (2001) Developmental science and the media: Early brain development. *American Psychologist*, 56(1): 5.

UNAIDS (2021) Fact Sheet 2022.

Van Rie A, Harrington PR, Dow A, Robertson K (2007) Neurologic and neurodevelopmental manifestations of pediatric HIV/AIDS: A global perspective. *European Journal of Paediatric Neurology*, 11(1): 1–9.

Van Rie A, Mupuala A, Dow A (2008) Impact of the HIV/AIDS epidemic on the neurodevelopment of preschool-aged children in Kinshasa, Democratic Republic of the Congo. *Pediatrics*, 122(1): e123–128.

Van Rie A, Dow A, Mupuala A, Stewart P (2009) Neurodevelopmental trajectory of HIV-infected children accessing care in Kinshasa, Democratic Republic of Congo. *JAIDS Journal of Acquired Immune Deficiency Syndromes*, 52(5): 636–642.

Walker SP, Wachs TD, Gardner JM et al. (2007) Child development: Risk factors for adverse outcomes in developing countries. *The Lancet*, 369(9556): 145–157.

Walker SP, Wachs TD, Grantham-McGregor S et al. (2011) Inequality in early childhood: Risk and protective factors for early child development. *The Lancet*, 378(9799): 1325–1338.

WHO (2007) *WHO Case Definitions of HIV for Surveillance and Revised Clinical Staging and Immunological Classification of HIV-related Disease in Adults and Children*. Geneva: World Health Organization.

WHO (2013) *Global Update on HIV Treatment 2013: Results, Impact and Opportunities*. WHO Report in partnership with UNICEF and UNAIDS. Geneva: World Health Organization.

Wolters PL, Brouwers P, Civitello L, Moss HA (1997) Receptive and expressive language function of children with symptomatic HIV infection and relationship with disease parameters: A longitudinal 24-month follow-up study. *AIDS*, 11(9): 1135–1144.

Wu J, Li J, Li Y et al. (2018) Neurodevelopmental outcomes in young children born to HIV-positive mothers in rural Yunnan, China. *Pediatr Int*, 60(7): 618–625.

Zhuang C, Pannecouque C, De Clercq E, Chen F (2020) Development of non-nucleoside reverse transcriptase inhibitors (NNRTIs): Our past twenty years. *Acta Pharmaceutica Sinica B*, 10(6): 961–978.

APPENDIX

Table 11A.1 Neurodevelopmental studies of HIV-infected children from birth to 3 years of age.

Study, Location	Study type	Number of participants	Groups studied	Age group	Developmental tools and area of development	Exposure to ARVs and other exposures	Developmental findings and other significant findings	Proportion with developmental delay
Smith et al. (2000), USA	Cohort	114	All HIV exposed. Compared those with early and late infection	4–18 months	BSID All, motor	Zidovudine but variable	All HIV-infected infants had poorer outcomes. Those with earlier infections fared worse. Motor was worst affected. There is also an increasing separation with age in both psychomotor and mental developmental indices	Not listed
Foster et al. (2006), UK	Cohort clinic based	62	HIV infected	Under 3 years (7–33 months)	Bayley and GMDS All	Depended on clinical stage	More severe HIV disease associated with worse developmental outcomes. Lower verbal scores than the general population. Overall growth reduction in HIV infected	11/50 = 22% on the Bayley tool
Bagenda et al. (2006), Uganda	Case–control study subset from a cohort	28	HIV infected, HEU, HIV unexposed	6–12 years	K-ABC and WRAT-3 All mainly cognitive	Zero ARV exposure	Older children who had previously been found to have higher incidence of developmental abnormalities as infants may not be destined to remain on the same trajectory if they survive beyond the toddler years. They found less cognitive abnormalities	No difference in psychometric status when compared to HIV unexposed children
Potterton et al. (2010), South Africa	Randomised controlled trial. Unblinded	122	122 HIV infected	18 months (SD: 8.1)	BSID All	Depended on clinical stage. By 12-month follow up 86% of cases and controls were on ART	A home stimulation programme can improve cognitive and motor outcome but there are still significant delays in HIV-positive children vs the normed mean of the BSID. A simple programme may be very helpful	Not described

Table 11A.1	Continued						
Study, Location	**Study type**	**Number of participants**	**Groups studied**	**Age group**	**Developmental tools and area of development**	**Exposure to ARVs and other exposures**	**Developmental findings and other significant findings**	**Proportion with developmental delay**
Boivin et al. (2010), Uganda	Descriptive	102	HIV infected	6–12 years	KABC-2, TOVA, BOT, and HOME All	ARV naïve but started on ARV as per Uganda National Guidelines after diagnosis	Children with HIV-subtype A demonstrated poorer neurocognitive performance compared to subtype D in this cross-sectional study	Neurocognitive impairment was described as a score >2SD below mean for HIV-infected children. Seven of 37 subtype A infected children (19%), four of 24 subtype D infected children (17%), and one out of one subtype C infected child (100%)
Kandawasvika et al. (2011), Zimbabwe	Cohort study 593 HIV infected, HEU, HIV unexposed	593	HIV infected, HEU, HIV unexposed	6 weeks to 12 months	BINS (screener) All	Nevirapine at delivery	A majority had low risk. 9.4% had a high risk screen at any time. Rate of impairment double in HIV-infected vs non-infected. Outcome affected by head circumference. A screening programme that is easy to administer may help to pick up children with developmental risks	17% of children who screened positive for high risk of neurodevelopmental delay were HIV positive, 9% were sero-exposed uninfected, and 9% were unexposed. 5% had unknown status
Valcour et al. (2012), Thailand	Case–control data subset from cohort study	20	HIV-infected	Adult	Nil-imaging study using magnetic resonance spectroscopy N/A	ARV naïve	HIV is detected in the CSF as early as 8 days post infection. Positive correlation with plasma levels but much less. 28% have evidence of CSF inflammation in the acute infection. Clade differences may influence CNS virulence	Not determined

(Continued)

Table 11A.1 Continued

Study, Location	Study type	Number of participants	Groups studied	Age group	Developmental tools and area of development	Exposure to ARVs and other exposures	Developmental findings and other significant findings	Proportion with developmental delay
Ruel et al. (2012), Uganda	Case–control	199	93 HIV infected vs 106 HIV uninfected	6–12 years	KABC-2, TOVA, BOT-2 Cognitive and motor	ART naïve	Children with HIV did worse on tests for attention and planning than controls despite having normal CD4 counts. This is regardless of clinical stage 1 or 2. HIV RNA level was associated with poorer cognitive and motor functioning	Not stated
Hutchings and Potterton (2014), Zimbabwe	Cross-sectional	60	32 HEU, 28 HEI	Infants between 6 weeks and 12 months of age	Bayley-III All	31 (96.88%) HEU infants received ARV prophylaxis compared to only 16 (57.14%) HEI infants	Children with HIV were significantly more likely to have delays than children with HIV exposure but not infection. There were significant differences in the cognitive, language, and motor areas. The majority of mothers were able to correctly predict developmental delay in their children	64.29% HEI infants showed cognitive delay, 60.7% had language delay, and 53.6% had motor delay compared to 3.1%, 12.5%, and 0% respectively in the HEU group
Springer et al. (2012), South Africa	Cross-sectional 37 participants: 17 HEU, 20 HUU	37	17 HEU, 20 HUU	<18 months, median age 11months (IQR 10–14 months)	GMDS All	PMTCT	Looked at 17–19 months old and compared the development of HEU and HUU groups using GMDS. There was no difference in the general quotient of the GMDS. The HEU infants scored lower on the personal social scale	Not mentioned
Tyor et al. (2013), Uganda, Botswana, Zambia, Ethiopia, South Africa, India, China	Review article		HIV-infected	Adult	N/A	Some exposed, some not exposed	Some clades of HIV such as b, c, and a, are associated with a higher risk of developing neurological complications	Approximately 50% of the roughly 34 million PLHIV despite cART

Table 11A.1	Continued						
Study, Location	Study type	Number of participants	Groups studied	Age group	Developmental tools and area of development	Exposure to ARVs and other exposures	Developmental findings and other significant findings	Proportion with developmental delay
Laughton et al. (2013), Netherlands, USA, Canada, Thailand, Cambodia, Uganda, South Africa	Review article		HIV-infected vs HIV-uninfected	Adolescents	KABC, KABC-2, SON-R, WASI, WISC-R, WISC-III, WISC-IV All	ART naive in the Uganda and South African studies. All other studies had ART initiated at different ages	There may be continued concerns for development extending to adolescence and even beyond. 25% had mental health problems, 20% had hearing impairment in high-resource settings vs 38% in low-resource settings, 42% with a learning disability, 27–33% receiving special education, 15% having repeated two or more grades and 51% having failed at least one grade	
Benki-Nugent et al. (2015), Kenya	Cohort	165	73 HIV infected and 92 HUU	1.1–4.9 months at enrollment	Screening tool adapted from DDST. Full neck control, walking, talking	All PMTCT	Infants were severely immunocompromised at enrollment. Also high rates of wasting, stunting. Median age at neck control was 4.3 months. Later neck control associated with lack of PMTCT; WAZ <–2, HAZ <–2. Median age at walking was 16.1 months, median age at speech was 16.6 months. Later walking and speech were associated with pre-ART hospitalisation, pre-ART WHO stage III/IV, an infant CD4 count of <1500 cells, pre-ART WAZ <–2 and HAZ <–2. Later speech was associated with a maternal CD4 count of <200. Those on lopinavir/ritonavir were less likely to be hospitalised pre-ART and had earlier speech compared to infants on a nevirapine containing regime	

(Continued)

Table 11A.1 Continued

Study, Location	Study type	Number of participants	Groups studied	Age group	Developmental tools and area of development	Exposure to ARVs and other exposures	Developmental findings and other significant findings	Proportion with developmental delay
							The effect of the response to ART on development: if the CD4% was less than 20% at 6 months, this was associated with later walking and speech. Higher viral loads were also associated with later speech. Underweight, stunting, or wasting were associated with later walking, and underweight or stunting with later speech. Those children with later attainment of neck control had later walking but not talking especially if the age at neck control was more than 4 months WAZ, HAZ, WHZ, and HCZ scores were significantly less in HIV infected vs HIV uninfected unexposed	

Table 11A.1 Continued

Study, Location	Study type	Number of participants	Groups studied	Age group	Developmental tools and area of development	Exposure to ARVs and other exposures	Developmental findings and other significant findings	Proportion with developmental delay
Strehlau et al. (2016), South Africa	Cohort	195	HEI before and after ART	0–24 months	ASQ All	HAART	Pre-treatment, the worst affected domain was the gross motor; children with a WAZ <–2 below the mean or WHO stage 3 or 4 disease were more likely to fail in each of the ASQ domains pre-ART. There was a significant reduction in the number of participants failing assessments after viral suppression. However, there was only a slight improvement in the communication domain post viral suppression. If there was a WAZ <–2 when achieving viral suppression the participant was more likely to fail fine motor and problem solving domains. There were no other factors associated with failing a domain at viral suppression. There was no association with poverty, parental employment, or having other family members with HIV. However, the ASQ is not normed in South African children. And there were still some persistent abnormalities	Compared with pre-ART, better outcomes were reported at time of viral suppression with a lower proportion of children failing the gross motor (31.5% vs 13%, $p = 0.0002$), fine motor (21.3% vs 10.2%, $p = 0.017$), problem solving (26.9% vs 9.3%, $p = 0.0003$), and personal–social (19.6% vs 7.4%, $p = 0.019$) domains. However, there was no change in the communication domain (14.8% vs 12.0%, $p = 0.6072$)

(*Continued*)

Table 11A.1 Continued

Study, Location	Study type	Number of participants	Groups studied	Age group	Developmental tools and area of development	Exposure to ARVs and other exposures	Developmental findings and other significant findings	Proportion with developmental delay
Van Rie, Mupuala, and Dow (2008), Democratic Republic of Congo	Case–control	160	35 HIV infected, 35 HEU, 90 HU	18–72 months	BSID-II, PDMS, SON-R, Rossetti Infant-Toddler language scale. Mental development index and psychomotor development index (18–29 months), language (up to 36 months), motor	ART naïve or less than one week exposure	Mental development – severe delay in 60% HI, 40% HEU, 24.4% HU; moderate delay in 25.7% HI, 31.4% HEU, and 26.7% HU. Severe motor delay in 28.6% HI, 14.3% HEU, 0% HU; and mild motor delay in 40% HI and 14.3% HEU vs 7.8% HU. Language comprehension delay 76.9% HI, 10.5% HEU, 12.9% HU. Language expression delay in 84.6% HI, 47.4% HEU, 12.9% HU. Significantly higher number of the HI group were maternal orphans than in the other groups. HI had significantly higher rates of stunting and low WAZ. Inadequate income was much lower in HU	
Van Rie et al. (2009), Democratic Republic of Congo	Prospective cohort	160	35 HI, 35 HEU, 90 HU	18–71 months at time of enrollment with 6- and 12-month follow up	BSID II, PDMS, SON-R (abbreviated) Motor and mental development	6 and 12 months post-ART initiation for the HI Nil	There was a statistically significant difference in cognitive and motor development between the HI and other groups at all time points. There was initially a significant difference between HI and HEU but this was no longer present at the 6-month assessment for cognitive development and the 12-month assessment for motor development. Stunting more frequent among HIV infected and HIV exposed	

Table 11A.1 Continued

Study, Location	Study type	Number of participants	Groups studied	Age group	Developmental tools and area of development	Exposure to ARVs and other exposures	Developmental findings and other significant findings	Proportion with developmental delay
Boivin et al. (2013), Uganda	Randomised controlled trial	120	60 to intervention arm, 60 to standard care HI	16 months to 5 years	MSEL, CBCL, COAT, HSCL-25, HOME, OMI General, behaviour, memory	Children were put on ART using WHO criteria. MISC was given to caregivers biweekly	Intervention group scored higher on all MSEL measures and there were greater gains over time in the intervention group	Other tools: HOME, OMI, HSCL
Ackermann et al. (2014), South Africa	Randomised controlled trial	88	44 children; 10 on deferred treatment and 34 on early treatment HI	<5 years	GMDS, MRI, CDC growth charts Brain structure and volume	All exposed, PMTCT received	Ventral (occipitotemporal) and dorsal (occipitoparietal) visual pathways exhibited abnormalities in HIV-positive children at age 5 years despite early ART initiation	For those with WMSA, significantly fewer (36%) had declining head growth as an indication for neuroimaging referral vs 64% without WMSA ($p = 0.01$). There was no difference in the frequency of developmental delay, increased muscle tone, or pathological tendon reflexes as a reason for referral between the children with or without WMSA

(Continued)

Table 11A.1 Continued

Study, Location	Study type	Number of participants	Groups studied	Age group	Developmental tools and area of development	Exposure to ARVs and other exposures	Developmental findings and other significant findings	Proportion with developmental delay
Bass et al. (2017), Uganda	Cluster randomised trial	130	18 geographic clusters with 112 children participating. HI	2–4 years	MSEL, ECVT, BRIEF, COAT, HOME, OMI Development, behaviour, memory, executive function, maternal anxiety and depression	ART in 67% of the intervention arm and 58% of the standard of care arm	MISC improved receptive language significantly and the effect persisted at 1 year. Improved caregiver mental health. Caregiver mental health and functioning at baseline were explored post hoc as potential moderators of intervention effects on child outcomes	
Randall et al. (2017), South Africa	Prospective cohort	61	43 HIV infected and 18 uninfected (12 HEU + 6HU)	Follow up of children initiated on ART before or after 12 weeks	MRI Brain structure volume	HI on ART	HI children had increased volume in some subcortical grey matter areas. The corpus callosum was smaller in all HI children	The largest volume difference between HI and HU children was observed in the corpus callosum, with the corpus callosum of HIV-positive children being on average 24% smaller at 5 years of age
Boivin et al. (2018), Multisite	Randomised controlled trial	611	211 HI, 183 HEU, 182 HU	Children 5–11 years of age	KABC-II, BOT-2, BRIEF, TOVA Memory, visual-spatial processing and problem solving, learning, planning, and motor development	All on early ART initiation	Delayed cognitive development still detectable at school age regardless of age at ART initiation	Not mentioned

Table 11A.1 Continued

Study, Location	Study type	Number of participants	Groups studied	Age group	Developmental tools and area of development	Exposure to ARVs and other exposures	Developmental findings and other significant findings	Proportion with developmental delay
McHenry et al. (2018), Kenya	Qualitative: in-depth interviews and focus group discussions	N/A	N/A	N/A	N/A Health worker and caregiver perceptions	N/A N/A	Caregivers and health care providers had differences in their understanding of growth, with caregivers perceiving growth as development. Both groups recognised the importance of nutrition and the home environment in ECD. There was an assumption that ART adherence would lead to typical development	N/A
Nwosu et al. (2018), South Africa	Randomised controlled trial	102	60 HIV positive and 42 HU	7 years	MRI, KABC-II Brain structure and volume	All ART exposed. 45 at ≤12weeks; and 15 at >12 weeks of age	Abnormalities in the gyral pattern and increased thickness. Volume changes in subcortical grey matter was apparent at 7 years of age in HI HIV-positive children had lower gyrification than uninfected controls in large bilateral medial parietal and right temporal regions	Not stated
Sania et al. (2019), 8 studies Asia; 7 sub-Saharan Africa; 5 Latin America; 1 Europe	Meta-analyses	20882 children from 21 studies	Studies that assessed at least one domain of child development in at least 100 children	<7 years of age	BSID-I, BSID-II, Bayley-III, and ASQ Cognitive, motor, and language outcomes. Socio-emotional outcomes were not measured	Yes, where mentioned in primary study. Parental education, gestational age, clean water and sanitation, breastfeeding, HIV status	Children of mothers with secondary schooling had higher cognitive scores compared with children whose mothers had primary education. Preterm birth was associated with reductions in cognitive, and motor scores. Higher attained maternal education was associated with improved cognitive, motor, and language development scores. Normal birth weight and appropriate gestational age had higher cognitive and motor scores	Not stated

(*Continued*)

Table 11A.1 Continued

Study, Location	Study type	Number of participants	Groups studied	Age group	Developmental tools and area of development	Exposure to ARVs and other exposures	Developmental findings and other significant findings	Proportion with developmental delay
Ackermann et al. (2020), South Africa	CHER trial	49	38 HI and 11 (9 HEU + 2 HU)	<7 years of age	Diffusion tension imaging compared to GMDS and Beery–Buktenica tests. Visual, motor, spatial	All 38 HI on early ART	Diffusion tensor imaging studies may detect abnormalities that are not readily picked up on standard developmental testing	Not stated
Boivin et al. (2020), Uganda	Cluster randomised control trial	216	Siblings of target 2- to 3-year-old children in MISC intervention	5–12 years	KABC, BRIEF-Parents, ADHD-RS-IV, MISC, or UCOBAC intervention tool. Neurocognitive	All the 2–3-year-old siblings were on ARVs	MISC training resulted in some short-term neurocognitive benefits for school-aged siblings but these differences were not sustained at 1-year follow-up	Not stated

Abbreviations: ADHD-RS-IV: ADHD Rating Scale, Fourth Edition; ART: antiretroviral therapy; ARV, antiretroviral; ASQ, Ages & Stages Questionnaire; Bayley-III, Bayley Scales of Infant and Toddler Development, Third Edition; BINS: Bayley Infant Neurodevelopmental Screener; BOT-2: Bruninks–Oseretsky Test of Motor Proficiency, Second Edition; BRIEF: Behavior Rating Inventory of Executive Function; BSID: Bayley Scales of Infant Development; CBCL: Child Behavior Checklist; CDC: Centers for Disease Control and Prevention; CHER Trial: Children with HIV Early Antiretroviral Trial; COAT: Color-Object Association Test; CNS: central nervous system; CSF: cerebrospinal fluid; DDST: Denver Developmental Screening Test; ECSP: Early Childhood Screening Profiles; ECVT: Early Childhood Vigilance Test; GMDS: Griffiths Mental Developmental Scales; HAZ: height-for-age z-score; HCZ: head circumference-for-age z-score; HEI: HIV exposed, infected; HEU: HIV exposed, uninfected; HI: HIV-infected; HOME: Caldwell Home Observation for Measurement of Environment; HSCL-25: Hopkins Symptom Checklist-25; HU: HIV-uninfected; HUU: HIV unexposed, uninfected; IQR: interquartile range; KABC: Kaufman Assessment Battery for Children; Mac Arthur CDI: Mac Arthur Bates Communication Development Inventories; MDI: mental developmental index; MSEL: Mullen Scales of Early Learning; OMI: Observing Mediational Interactions; PDI: psychomotor developmental index; PDMS: Peabody Developmental Motor Scales; PLHIV: people living with HIV; PMTCT: prevention of mother-to-child transmission; SON-R: Snijders–Oomen Nonverbal Intelligence Test for Children and Adolescents, Abridged Edition; TOVA: Test Of Variables of Attention; UCOBAC: Uganda Community Based Association for Women and Children's Welfare; WASI: Wechsler Abbreviated Scale of Intelligence; WAZ: weight-for-age z-score; WHO: World Health Organization; WHZ: weight-for-height z-score; WISC-R: Wechsler Intelligence Scale for Children, Revised Edition; WISC: Wechsler Intelligence Scale for Children; WPPSI: Wechsler Preschool and Primary Scale of Intelligence; WRAT-3: Wide Range Achievement Test, Third Edition.

REFERENCES FOR TABLE 11A.1

Ackermann CS, Andronikou B, Laughton M et al. (2014) White matter signal abnormalities in children with suspected HIV-related neurologic disease on early combination antiretroviral therapy. *The Pediatric Infectious Disease Journal*, 33(8): e207–12.

Ackermann CS, Andronikou MG, Saleh M et al. (2020) Diffusion tensor imaging point to ongoing functional impairment in HIV-infected children at age 5, undetectable using standard neurodevelopmental assessments. *AIDS Research and Therapy*, 17: 1–15.

Bagenda DA, Nassali I, Kalyesubula B et al. (2006) Health, neurologic, and cognitive status of HIV-infected, long-surviving, and antiretroviral-naive Ugandan children. *Pediatrics*, 117(3): 729–740.

Bass JK, Opoka R, Familiar I et al. (2017) Randomized controlled trial of caregiver training for HIV-infected child neurodevelopment and caregiver well-being. *AIDS (London, England)*, 31(13): 1877–1883.

Benki-Nugent SC, Eshelman D, Wamalwa A et al. (2015) Correlates of age at attainment of developmental milestones in HIV-infected infants receiving early antiretroviral therapy. *The Pediatric Infectious Disease Journal*, 34(1): 55.

Boivin MJ, Augustinavicius JL, Familiar-Lopez I et al. (2020) Early childhood development caregiver training and neurocognition of HIV-exposed Ugandan siblings. *Journal of Developmental & Behavioral Pediatrics*, 41(3): 221–229.

Boivin MJ, Bangirana P, Nakasujja N et al. (2013) A year-long caregiver training program improves cognition in preschool Ugandan children with human immunodeficiency virus. *The Journal of Pediatrics*, 163(5): 1409–1416.e1–5.

Boivin MJ, Barlow-Mosha L, Chernoff MC et al. (2018) Neuropsychological performance in African children with HIV enrolled in a multi-site anti-retroviral clinical trial. *AIDS (London, England)*, 32(2): 189.

Boivin MJ, Ruel TD, Boal HE et al. (2010) HIV-subtype A is associated with poorer neuropsychological performance compared to subtype D in ART-naïve Ugandan children. *AIDS (London, England)*, 24(8): 1163.

Foster CJ, Biggs RL, Melvin D, Walters MD, Tudor-Williams G, Lyall EG (2006) Neurodevelopmental outcomes in children with HIV infection under 3 years of age. *Developmental Medicine & Child Neurology*, 48(8): 677–682.

Hutchings J, Potterton J (2014) Developmental delay in HIV-exposed infants in Harare, Zimbabwe. *Vulnerable Children and Youth Studies*, 9(1): 43–55.

Kandawasvika GQ, Ogundipe E, Gumbo FZ, Kurewa EN, Mapingure MP, Stray-Pedersen B (2011) Neurodevelopmental impairment among infants born to mothers infected with human immunodeficiency virus and uninfected mothers from three peri urban primary care clinics in Harare, Zimbabwe. *Developmental Medicine & Child Neurology*, 53(11): 1046–1052.

Laughton B, Cornell M, Boivin M, Van Rie A (2013) Neurodevelopment in perinatally HIV-infected children: a concern for adolescence. *Journal of the International AIDS Society*, 16: 18603.

McHenry MS, Oyungu E, McAteer CI et al. (2018) Early childhood development in children born to HIV-infected mothers: perspectives from Kenyan clinical providers and caregivers. *Global Pediatric Health*, 5: 2333794X18811795.

Nwosu EC, Robertson FC, Holmes MJ et al. (2018) Altered brain morphometry in 7-year old HIV-infected children on early ART. *Metabolic Brain Disease*, 33(2): 523–535.

Potterton J, Stewart A, Cooper P, Becker P (2010) The effect of a basic home stimulation programme on the development of young children infected with HIV. *Developmental Medicine & Child Neurology*, 52(6): 547–551.

Randall SR, Warton CMR, Holmes MJ et al. (2017) Larger subcortical gray matter structures and smaller corpora callosa at age 5 years in HIV infected children on early ART. *Frontiers in Neuroanatomy*, 11: 95.

Ruel TD, Boivin MJ, Boal HE et al. (2012) Neurocognitive and motor deficits in HIV-infected Ugandan children with high CD4 cell counts. *Clinical Infectious Diseases*, 54(7): 1001–1009.

Sania A, Sudfeld CR, Danaei G et al. (2019) Early life risk factors of motor, cognitive and language development: a pooled analysis of studies from low/middle-income countries. *BMJ Open*, 9(10): e026449.

Smith R, Malee K, Charurat M et al. (2000) Timing of perinatal human immunodeficiency virus type 1 infection and rate of neurodevelopment. *The Pediatric Infectious Disease Journal*, 19(9): 862–871.

Springer P, Laughton B, Tomlinson M, Harvey J, Esser M (2012) Neurodevelopmental status of HIV-exposed but uninfected children: A pilot study. *South African Journal of Child Health*, 6(2): 51–55.

Strehlau R, Kuhn L, Abrams EJ, Coovadia A (2016) HIV associated neurodevelopmental delay: Prevalence, predictors and persistence in relation to antiretroviral therapy initiation and viral suppression. *Child: Care, Health and Development*, 42(6): 881–889.

Tyor W, Fritz-French C, Nath A (2013) Effect of HIV clade differences on the onset and severity of HIV-associated neurocognitive disorders. *Journal of Neurovirology*, 19(6): 515–522.

Valcour V, Chalermchai T, Sailasuta N et al. (2012) Central nervous system viral invasion and inflammation during acute HIV infection. *Journal of Infectious Diseases*, 206(2): 275–282.

Van Rie A, Dow A, Mupuala A, Stewart P (2009) Neurodevelopmental trajectory of HIV-infected children accessing care in Kinshasa, Democratic Republic of Congo. *JAIDS Journal of Acquired Immune Deficiency Syndromes*, 52(5): 636–642.

Van Rie A, Mupuala A, Dow A (2008) Impact of the HIV/AIDS epidemic on the neurodevelopment of preschool-aged children in Kinshasa, Democratic Republic of the Congo. *Pediatrics*, 122(1): e123–e128.

CHAPTER 12

Neurodevelopmental and Mental Health Outcomes of HIV in School-age Children

Adam Mabrouk, Derrick Ssewanyana, and Amina Abubakar

INTRODUCTION

Human immunodeficiency virus (HIV)/AIDS remains a major public health problem globally, with about 38 million people living with HIV worldwide (UNAIDS 2020). Of these, 1.7 million are children below 15 years of age. Although significant progress has been made in preventing HIV infections in children through the prevention of mother-to-child transmission programmes, the burden of the disease is still measurably high and disproportionately greater in low-resource settings, especially sub-Saharan Africa (SSA). In 2018, for example, about 160 000 new infections were reported in children aged 0 to 14 years, with SSA accounting for almost 90% of these new infections (Wang et al. 2016; UNAIDS 2020). Notwithstanding, the survival of children living with HIV has greatly improved following improved access to combined antiretroviral therapy (cART), and, more than ever, many perinatally HIV-infected (PHIV+) children are aging into adolescence and young adulthood (Montaner et al. 2014; Davies, Gibb, and Turkova 2016).

School age (6–12 years) is a fundamental development stage during which significant physical, cognitive, behavioural, and mental development take place (National Research Council 1984). However, early infection with HIV is known to alter the course of this unique growth and neurodevelopmental stage. Compared to HIV-negative children, poor growth patterns such as stunting and malnourishment have been reported among PHIV+ children living in low- and middle-income countries (Sherr et al. 2018). Similarly, suboptimal brain development has been observed in both PHIV+ children (including those with early combined antiretroviral therapy initiation and the virally suppressed) and perinatally HIV-exposed uninfected (HEU) children in South Africa (Jankiewicz et al. 2017; Hoare et al. 2018). Suboptimal brain development among HIV-infected and HEU children is plausibly linked to direct adverse effects of the HIV virus on the central nervous system and toxicity from prolonged exposure to HIV medication (Thompson et al. 2005; Shah et al. 2016). Indeed, PHIV+ children exhibit a range of neurocognitive impairments including executive dysfunction (Koekkoek et al. 2008; Linn et al. 2015), diminished general neurocognitive ability (Fundaro et al. 1998; Louw et al. 2016), poor motor functioning (Parks and Danoff 1999; Linn et al. 2015), and behavioural problems (Havens et al. 1994; Kalembo et al. 2019).

The objective of this chapter is to summarise the available evidence on neurocognitive and mental health outcomes among children aged 6 to 12 years in the context of HIV. A rapid review of the literature using the search terms mental health, mental disorders, cognition, cognitive function, neurocognitive, neurodevelopment, child, children, school-age, and HIV was conducted for studies published between 1994 and 2022. The retrieved references from the database were first screened by title and abstract, followed by a full text review. Only articles focused on mental health and cognitive development among HIV-infected children aged 6 to 12 years (school age) were included. A narrative summary of the findings is presented in both text and tabular formats in the proceeding sections of this chapter.

THE IMPACT OF HIV ON BRAIN STRUCTURE AND FUNCTION

HIV-infected children are at an increased risk of altered brain development compared to their HIV-negative counterparts. This is partly attributable to the neurotropic nature of the HIV virus (Kovalevich and Langford 2012). Both structural and functional abnormalities such as lower functional connectivity, lower white matter and grey matter volumes, altered white matter micro-structures, and increased cortical thickness have been observed among HIV-infected school-age children (Blanchette et al. 2002; Hoare et al. 2015; Jankiewicz et al. 2017; Toich et al. 2017; Yadav et al. 2017; Nwosu et al. 2018; Yadav et al. 2018). Jankiewicz and colleagues carried out a follow-up study of 7-year-old children among a cohort of virally suppressed PHIV+ children initially scanned at age 5 years in Cape Town, South Africa (Ackermann et al. 2016). Compared to the controls within this cohort, lower fractional anisotropy and higher mean diffusivity were observed among HIV-infected children with early ART initiation. Additionally, the white matter alteration observed among HIV-infected children at age 5 years was still visible at age 7 years (Jankiewicz et al. 2017). This observation may suggest that early structural brain damage is persistent among HIV-infected school-going children, even among those initiated on ART. Similarly, diffusion tensor imaging comparing 75 HIV-positive and 30 HIV-negative school-going children in South Africa revealed damage to neuronal microstructure among HIV-infected children, as indicated by increased mean diffusivity and decreased fractional anisotropy (Hoare et al. 2015). The brain magnetic resonance imaging (MRI) study has shown significantly altered brain structures (fractional anisotropy and mean diffusivity) and poor cognitive functions among PHIV+ compared to HIV-exposed uninfected (HEU) and HIV-unexposed uninfected (HUU) children in India (Yadav et al. 2020). Notably, significantly reduced fractional anisotropy and altered mean diffusivity in multiple brain sites, and impaired cognitive functions, were observed among HIV-negative children born to HIV-infected mothers. This finding supports the evidence that exposure to HIV and ART has deleterious effects even in the absence of HIV infection among school-going children (Yadav et al. 2020). However, HIV-infected children with late ART initiation have more impaired brain functionality and significantly altered brain structures such as reduced brain volume compared to those with early ART initiation (Heany et al. 2020).

Several studies have revealed that structural brain damage is significantly associated with behavioural and cognitive dysfunction (Hoare et al. 2015, 2018; Yadav et al. 2018; Dean et al. 2020). In one of the recent neurocognitive and neuroimaging studies conducted among PHIV+ South African children with more than 6 months of ART medication, lower white matter and grey matter volumes were found among PHIV+ children with cognitive disorders compared to PHIV+ children without cognitive disorders such as executive dysfunction and poor visuo-spatial ability (Hoare et al. 2020). Similarly, cognitive impairments have been attributed to altered brain functionality among HIV-infected school-age children (Yadav et al. 2018). In a study involving school-age children in India (49 HIV infected, 23 controls), Yadav et al. reported significantly reduced amplitudes of low-frequency fluctuations and functional connectivity in several brain regions associated with the different domains of cognitive function. The functional and structural brain abnormality positively correlated with cognitive impairment, suggesting that cognitive impairment among school-going children living with HIV may be as result of functional and brain abnormalities (Yadav et al. 2018).

THE IMPACT OF HIV ON GENERAL COGNITION

Several studies have linked HIV infection to diminished cognitive functioning in school-age children of 6 to 12 years. Table 12.1 is a summary of studies on the general cognitive ability in children aged 6 to 12 years, listed by year of publication. Notwithstanding the methodological differences in these studies, the evidence on the impact of HIV on general cognitive ability in children aged 6 to 12 years is mixed, with some studies reporting significantly lower cognitive function in this group (Fundaro et al. 1998; Ruel et al. 2012; Boyede et al. 2013; Linn et al. 2015; Louw et al. 2016; Weber et al. 2017; Boivin et al. 2018; Musindo et al. 2018; Sherr et al. 2018; Boivin et al. 2020; Familiar et al. 2020; van Wyhe et al. 2021), while others reported non-significant differences in cognitive scores (Blanchette et al. 2002; Bagenda et al. 2006; Kandawasvika et al. 2015; Bangirana et al. 2017; Brahmbhatt et al. 2017). In a large cross-sectional study conducted across six sites in four SSA countries (Malawi, South Africa, Uganda, and Zimbabwe), significantly lower mean cognitive scores as measured by the Kaufman Assessment Battery for Children, Second Edition were observed among PHIV+ children compared to both the HEU and HUU children (Boivin et al. 2018). There is also evidence indicating that, for PHIV+ children, there is no significant difference (mean difference: 0.20; 95% confidence intervals: –0.11, 0.50; p = 0.21) in mean cognitive scores between children with HIV subtype A and those with HIV subtype D (Bangirana et al. 2017).

Globally, improved accessibility and the use of antiretrovirals have been documented to significantly improve various HIV-related outcomes such as mortality and morbidity and to lower HIV transmission (Morison 2001; Kasamba et al. 2012; Montaner et al. 2014). However, some deficits in subtle cognitive outcomes persist regardless of early ART initiation and adherence. Indeed, significantly poor cognitive function has been observed in some populations of children on ART (Linn et al. 2015; Boivin et al. 2018; Musindo et al. 2018). Reports on the impact of the duration and timing of ART initiation among school-age children are mixed. Some studies report decreased impairments among those who initiated ART early (Weber et al. 2017; Heany et al. 2020), while others report no significant differences in cognitive function with regards to the time of ART initiation (Puthanakit et al. 2013; Linn et al. 2015; Musindo et al. 2018). For instance, there were no significant changes in the cognitive scores observed in Jamaican children with HIV encephalopathy during a 1-year period post-ART initiation (Walker et al. 2013). For virally suppressed school-age children on ART, there is no association between ART regimen type and cognitive outcomes. A Ugandan study reported that there was no significant difference in cognitive processing skills between virally suppressed children on protease inhibitors-based ART and non-protease inhibitors-based ART (Nalwanga et al. 2021).

Plausibly, broader health system and contextual factors such as quality of HIV care and treatment beyond mere ART prescription and adherence may have led to mixed results on the association between ART and cognitive outcomes. Other factors such as quality of nutrition, home stimulation, poverty, and quality of education among others may also have an impact on cognitive outcomes, yet often they may not be adequately assessed in various studies (Rice et al. 2012; Boivin et al. 2020; Mbewe et al. 2022).

THE IMPACT OF HIV ON MOTOR FUNCTION

Motor functioning is a set of skills involving the movement of muscles in the body and is broadly sub-divided into gross motor skills and fine motor skills. Gross motor skills involve the use of large muscles such as those in the arms and feet during movements such as running or jumping. Fine motor skills involve the use of smaller muscles during movements such as grasping an object or closing bolts and tightening nuts (Wells 2018).

Table. 12.1 Summary of studies on general cognitive outcomes among HIV-infected children aged 6–12 years.

Study	Country	Study design	Age in years or years: months (mean or range)	Sample size	Anti-retroviral use	Tool used	Key findings
Fundaro et al. (1998)	Italy	Case control	6–12	8 PHIV+, 8 HEU	Not reported	WISC	Significantly lower cognitive score among PHIV+ children (mean = 92.8 vs 104.9; $p < 0.007$)
Blanchette et al. (2002)	Canada	Cohort	9:10	14 PHIV+, 11 HIV-	Yes	WISC-R	No statistically significant difference in general cognitive ability between PHIV+ and HEU siblings
Bagenda et al. (2006)	Uganda	Cross-sectional	6–12	28 PHIV+, 42 HEU, 37 HUU	No	KABC	No significant differences in the cognitive scores between the three study groups
Koekkoek et al. (2008)	The Netherlands	Cross-sectional	9:6	22 PHIV+	Yes (90.9%)	SON-R	Mean IQ within the normal range for PHIV+
Boivin et al. (2010)	Uganda	Cohort	6–12	102 HIV+	ART-naïve	KABC-II	Children who had HIV subtype A demonstrated poorer neurocognitive performance compared those with HIV subtype D
Puthanakit et al. (2010)	Thailand	Cohort	6–12	39 PHIV+, 40 HEU, 42 HUU	Yes (87%)	WISC-III	Significantly lower cognitive ability in HIV infected and HEU compared to control ($p < 0.01$)
Ruel et al. (2012)	Uganda	Cohort	6–12	93 PHIV+, 106 HIV-	Yes	KABC-II	Poorer cognitive functions among HIV+ ART-naïve children compared to their uninfected counterparts, and it correlates with HIV plasma RNA levels
Boyede et al. (2013)	Nigeria	Cohort	9:10	69 PHIV+, 69 HIV-	Yes (56%)	RCPM	Lower RPM scores in HIV-infected children (mean 18.2 vs 27.2; $p < 0.0001$) compared to HIV-negative children
Walker et al. (2013)	Jamaica	Cross-sectional	7–10	30 HIV+	Yes	RCPM	Poor cognitive functions in children with HIV encephalopathy (median 13.0 vs 18.0; $p = 0.006$) compared to non-encephalopathy group
Ghate et al. (2015)	India	Cross-sectional	6–12	50 HIV+, 50 HIV-	Not reported	ICIT	No significant difference between the two groups
Kandawasvika et al. (2015)	Zimbabwe	Cross-sectional	6–8	32 PHIV+, 121 HEU, 153 HUU	Yes (30%)	MSCA	No significant difference between the three groups

Table. 12.1 (Continued)

Study	Country	Study design	Age in years or years: months (mean or range)	Sample size	Anti-retroviral use	Tool used	Key findings
Louw et al. (2016)	South Africa	Cross-sectional	10	78 PHIV+, 30 HUU	Yes (82%)	WISC	Poor cognitive functions among PHIV+ compared to HUU
Bangirana et al. (2017)	Uganda	Cohort	7:5	78 HIV+ (sub-type A), 27 HIV+ (sub-type D)	Yes	KABC-II	No significant differences in neurocognitive scores between children with HIV subtype A and subtype D
Brahmbhatt et al. (2017)	Uganda	Cohort	9:5	140 PHIV+, 204 HUU, 26 HEU	Yes (41%)	KABC-II	No significant difference in neurocognitive scores between the three study groups
Weber et al. (2017)	Germany	Cross-sectional	8:5	14 PHIV+	Yes	WISC-IV	Cognitive scores of PHIV+ within normal range
Boivin et al. (2018)	Zambia, Uganda, Malawi, Zimbabwe	Cohort	7:2	246 PHIV+, 183 HEU, 182 HUU	Yes	KABC-II	Significantly poor cognitive performance among PHIV+ compared to both HEU and HUU children ($p < 0.001$)
Musindo et al. (2018)	Kenya	Cross-sectional	11:5	90 PHIV+	Yes	KABC-II	60% had neurocognitive disorder
Sherr et al. (2018)	South Africa, Malawi	Cohort	8:11	135 PHIV+, 854 HIV-	Yes (92.5%)	WISC-IV	Significantly lower cognitive scores in HIV-infected children compared to their HIV-negative counterparts
Heany et al. (2020)	South Africa	Cohort	10:5	64 PHIV+, 20 HUU	Yes	MWM task	Poor cognitive function among PHIV+ compared to HUU
Familiar et al. (2020)	South Africa, Malawi, Zimbabwe, Uganda	Cohort	7:2	246 PHIV+, 185 HEU, 184 HUU	Yes	KABC-II	Significantly lower KABC score among HIV+ compared to both HEU and HUU children. No association between caregiver depression and neurocognitive scores
Boivin et al. (2020)	South Africa, Malawi, Zimbabwe, Uganda	Cohort	7:2	246 PHIV+, 185 HEU, 184 HUU	Yes	KABC-II	Significantly lower KABC score among virally suppressed HIV+ children with early ART initiation compared to both HEU and HUU children

(Continued)

Table. 12.1 (Continued)

Study	Country	Study design	Age in years or years: months (mean or range)	Sample size	Anti-retroviral use	Tool used	Key findings
Nalwanga et al. (2021)	Uganda	Cross-sectional	5–12	76 PHIV+	Yes	KABC-II	No significant differences in neurocognitive scores between virally suppressed children on protease-inhibitor-based and non-protease-inhibitor-based ART
van Wyhe et al. (2021)	South Africa	Cohort	7–9	69 PHIV+, 25 HEU, 32 HUU	Yes	KABC-II	Similar improvement in cognitive outcomes between HIV+, HEU, and HUU. Significantly lower cognitive scores among HIV+ group
Mbewe et al. (2022)	Zambia	Cohort	11:8	206 HIV+ 183 HEU	Yes	NIHTB-CB	Poor cognitive function among children living with HIV compared to HIV-negative children. Higher social economic status was associated with reduced risk of cognitive impairment in both groups, with similar effects in children with HIV and HEU groups

Abbreviations: HEU: HIV-exposed uninfected; HUU: HIV-unexposed uninfected; HIV+: HIV-positive children; HIV-: HIV-negative children; ICIT: Indian Child Intelligence Test; KABC: Kaufmann Assessment Battery for Children; MSCA: McCarthy Scales of Children's Abilities; MWM: Maintenance Working Memory; NIHTB-CB: National Institute of Health Toolbox-Cognition Battery; PHIV+: perinatally HIV-infected children; RCPM: Raven's Colored Progressive Matrices; RPM: Raven's Standard Progressive Matrices; SES: socioeconomic status; SON-R: Snidjers-Oomen nonverbal intelligence tests; WISC-R: Wechsler Intelligence Scale for Children.

Studies on motor functioning among HIV-infected school-age children have generally been comprised of small sample sizes with varied assessment measures. However, various studies from North America (Parks and Danoff 1999; Blanchette et al. 2002; Walker et al. 2013), Africa (Ruel et al. 2012; Bangirana et al. 2017; Boivin et al. 2020; Familiar et al. 2020), and Southeast Asia (Linn et al. 2015) generally suggest that the motor skills of HIV-infected children are more compromised in comparison to their HIV-uninfected counterparts. In one of the studies on the impact of HIV on motor function, Parks and Danoff (1999) administered the Bruininks-Oseretsky Test of Motor Proficiency to investigate whether performance scores (raw and standard) would change with HIV prognosis. A total of 34 HIV-infected children and pre-adolescents in Maryland in the USA were tested on the Bruininks-Oseretsky Test of Motor Proficiency at initial diagnosis of HIV infection and again over a 2-year period at 6-month intervals for a total of 5 test sessions. The study reported that the HIV-infected children performed significantly worse in both gross and fine motor functioning compared to normative means and that there seemed to be a greater level of impairment in the gross motor domain compared to the fine motor domain. Similar results have been reported among studies from low-income settings, both among the ART-naïve children and ART-initiated children (Ruel et al. 2012; Walker et al. 2013; Boivin et al. 2020). In a study conducted by Ruel et al. that involved 93 HIV-infected Ugandan children aged 6 to 12 years, the Bruininks-Oseretsky Test of Motor Proficiency, Second Edition, was administered to assess motor function. Ruel and colleagues reported that HIV-infected children generally performed worse in speed/agility ($p < 0.01$) and manual dexterity ($p < 0.001$) than the uninfected children (Ruel et al. 2012). The worse motor outcomes were associated with higher HIV/RNA levels and an advanced World Health Organization (WHO) clinical stage of HIV (Ruel et al. 2012). Among virally suppressed children receiving ART, protease inhibitors-based ART was associated with better gross and fine motor scores compared to non-protease inhibitors-based ART (Nalwanga et al. 2021).

Children's gross and fine motor skills at preschool age are significant predictors of motor functioning among school-going children living with HIV. In a Beninese cohort of children living with HIV, gross and fine motor skills at age 1 year as measured by a neurodevelopmental performance-based assessment tool (Mullen Scales of Early Learning) was a strong predictor of Bruininks-Oseretsky Test of Motor Proficiency, Second Edition scores during school age (Boivin et al. 2021). This finding underpins the importance of supporting early motor development in children living with HIV, as it defines the trajectories for motor skills during school age and adolescence. However, the impact of HIV on motor functioning in this age group does not seem to vary across the HIV subtypes (Boivin et al. 2010; Bangirana et al. 2017).

THE IMPACT OF HIV ON LANGUAGE DEVELOPMENT

Language development among children starts in early infancy and develops continually throughout childhood to adolescence, although the rate of development varies among individuals (Margaret 2020). Language impairment is one of the most commonly reported form of developmental impairment among PHIV+ school-age children. In a study involving 20 HIV-infected and 20 HIV-uninfected children in a children's home in India, Ravindran and colleagues reported a significantly lower mean score in the language domain (21.7 vs 30.3, $p < 0.01$) among HIV-infected children (Ravindran, Rani, and Priya 2014). Another study, conducted among 306 HIV-infected children and 162 HEU children in the USA, reported a comparable burden of language impairment (18.5 vs 17.4, $p = 0.57$) between the two groups (Rice et al. 2012). Some studies indicate that among HIV-infected children, expressive language is more impaired than receptive language (Wolters et al. 1995; Hoare et al. 2016). In a study that evaluated both receptive and expressive language impairment at baseline in 6- and 24-month-old HIV-infected children with normal hearing ability in the USA, a significantly higher burden of expressive language impairment was observed. Notably, there was an overall increase in the level of impairment of both expressive and receptive language abilities among this cohort of PHIV+ children during the 24-month follow-up period (Wolters et al. 1995). On the contrary, overall cognitive functions and brain abnormalities did not differ between the two groups at baseline and at 24 months (Wolters et al. 1995).

Besides HIV infection, other factors have been reported to influence language impairment among school-age children. Among HIV-infected school-age children in the USA, children whose caregivers were their biological parents were at a lower risk of language impairment, whereas being black and a caregiver's low education level were associated with an increased risk of language impairment (Rice et al. 2012).

THE IMPACT OF HIV ON MENTAL HEALTH OUTCOMES

Studies from various parts of the world suggest that school-going children living with HIV experience more mental health problems compared to their HIV-uninfected peers. However, some studies reported that there were no significant differences in the scores of school-going children living with HIV compared to their uninfected peers, as shown in Table 12.2. Studies using the Child Behavior Checklist (CBCL) have reported high rates of behavioural problems among HIV-infected children from low-income countries (ranging from 39.3–80.7%) (Grover, Pensi, and Banerjee 2007; Tadesse et al. 2012; Ruiseñor-Escudero et al. 2015). Studies examining the occurrence of emotional and behavioural problems in similar populations have reported mixed findings, with some reporting a higher burden among HIV-infected children (Havens et al. 1994; Grover, Pensi, and Banerjee 2007; Visser, Hecker, and Jordaan 2018; Hoare et al. 2020), while others did not observe differences in the burden of behavioural and emotional problems between HIV-infected children and their uninfected counterparts (Louw et al. 2016; Sherr et al. 2018). Compared to HIV-negative children, a higher proportion of HIV-infected children has behavioural problems as measured by the CBCL (Havens et al. 1994; Grover, Pensi, and Banerjee 2007; Visser, Hecker, and Jordaan 2018; Hoare et al. 2020). In one study conducted in South Africa, Visser and colleagues observed that perinatally PHIV+ children had higher somatic and affective problems, lower self-esteem, and higher levels of anxiety compared to their uninfected peers (Visser, Hecker, and Jordaan 2018). This study involved the collection of data from the HIV-infected children and their caregivers/mothers ($n = 54$), as well as from a comparison group of 113 HIV-uninfected children and their uninfected mothers. Caregivers completed the CBCL to assess children's mental health, whereas the children completed the Self-Description Questionnaire and the Revised Children's Manifest Anxiety Scale. The findings from the assessments, when controlled for age differences, indicated that HIV-infected children experienced significantly more somatic problems, physiological anxiety, and lower self-esteem than the HIV-uninfected children in the comparison group (Visser, Hecker, and Jordaan 2018). Similarly, a Dutch study reported that PHIV+ school-going children are at an increased risk of having behavioural and emotional difficulties with higher scores, particularly in emotional problems, hyperactivity, and problems with peers' subscales compared to Dutch normative data (van Opstal et al. 2021). Compared with their non-infected siblings, caregivers reported significantly more problems with peers for HIV-infected children. For their exposed and uninfected siblings, caregivers reported significantly more hyperactivity and conduct, emotional, and behavioural problems, when compared to Dutch normative data (van Opstal et al. 2021). The presence of increased mental health problems among siblings of HIV-infected school-going children underpins the impacts of other shared risks such as economic status, genetic predisposition, exposure to violence, and family history of drug and substance use on mental health.

Table 12.2 Summary of studies on mental health among HIV-infected children aged 6 to 12 years.

Study	Country	Study design	Age in years or years:months (mean or range)	Sample size	Anti-retroviral	Tool used	Key findings
Havens et al. (1994)	USA	Cross-sectional	6:10	26 PHIV+, 14 HEU, 20 HUU	Yes	DISC, CBCL, A pictorial interview on behaviour (Dominique)	Significantly higher anxiety problems among children living with HIV($p < 0.05$) compared to controls
Grover, Pensi, and Banerjee (2007)	India	Cohort	6–11	140 PHIV+, 301 HUU	Yes	CBCL	Higher proportion (80.7% vs 18.3%) of HIV-positive children had behavioural problems
Tadesse et al. (2012)	Ethiopia	Cross-sectional	9:7	318 PHIV+	Yes	CBCL, ASEBA	39.3% of HIV-infected children had behavioural and emotional problems
Ruiseñor-Escudero et al. (2015)	Uganda	Cross-sectional	8:11	144 PHIV+	Yes (56.9%)	CBCL	Higher mean CD8 activation percentage was associated with higher scores on the externalising Problems and Total Problems scales of the CBCL
Louw et al. (2016)	South Africa	Cross-sectional	10	78 PHIV+, 30 HUU	Yes (82%)	CBCL	No significant difference in total problem scores between PHIV+ and HUU
Kikuchi et al. (2017)	Rwanda	Cross-sectional	11:1	475I PHIV+	Yes	BDI-Y	22.1% of the children were depressed. Regimen type and caregiver depression were significantly associated with child's depression
Adefalu, et al. (2018)	Nigeria	Cross-sectional	9:2	196 PHIV+	Yes (82.1%)	CBQ	19.4% of PHIV+ children had psychiatric disorders
Sherr et al. (2018)	South Africa, Malawi	Cross-sectional	8:11	135 PHIV+, 854 HIV-	Yes (92.5%)	SDQ, TSCC, RSS, CDI	No significant difference in depressive symptoms, self-esteem, emotional and behavioural problems between the two groups
Visser, Hecker, and Jordaan (2018)	South Africa	Cross-sectional	6–12	54 PHIV+, 113 HIV-	Yes	CBCL, RCMAS	HIV-infected children had higher somatic (mean = 3.0 vs 2.0, $p = 0.006$), lower self-esteem (mean = 109.3 vs 113.6, $p = 0.036$), and higher anxiety (mean = 3.6 vs 2.5, $p = 0.007$)
Kalembo et al. (2019)	Malawi	Cross-sectional	6–12	429 HIV+	Yes	SDQ	31% of PHIV+ children had behavioral and emotional difficulties with higher scores in peer problem and emotional subscale

Table 12.2 (Continued)

Study	Country	Study design	Age in years or years:months (mean or range)	Sample size	Anti-retroviral	Tool used	Key findings
Familiar et al. (2020)	Uganda	Cohort	5–12	104 Severe malaria, 144 PHIV+	Yes (44.0%)	CBCL	Higher emotional and behavioural problems among children with severe malaria compared to those with HIV
Hoare et al. (2020)	South Africa	Cross-sectional	9–12	168 PHIV+, 43 HIV-	Yes	CBCL	PHIV+ children have lower functional competence ($p = 0.017$) compared to HIV-negative children
Namuli et al. (2021)	Uganda	Cross-sectional	11:7	271 HIV+	Yes	CDI, CBCL	Prevalence of suicidal ideation was 17%. Correlates of suicidal ideation include rule-breaking behaviour, familial/friends' death, depression, anxiety, and HIV wasting syndrome
van Opstal et al. (2021)	The Netherlands	Cross-sectional	9:11	43 PHIV+, 24 HEU siblings	Yes	SDQ	PHIV+ children have more behavioural and emotional difficulties with higher scores particularly in emotional problems, hyperactivity, and problems with peers' subscale compared to Dutch normative data. Compared with their non-infected siblings, caregivers reported significantly more problems with peers for HIV-infected children. For siblings, caregivers reported significantly more conduct problems compared to HIV-infected children

Abbreviations: ASEBA: Achenbach System of Empirically Based Assessment; BDI-Y: Beck Depression Inventory for Youth; CBCL: Children Behavior Checklist; CBQ: Child Behavioral Questionnaire; CDI: Child Depression Inventory; DISC: Diagnostic Interview for Children-Parent version; HEU: HIV exposed uninfected; HIV+: HIV-infected children; HIV-: HIV-negative children; HUU: HIV unexposed uninfected; RCMAS: Revised Children Manifest Anxiety Scale; RSS: Rosenberg Self-esteem Scale; SDQ: Self-Description Questionnaire; TSCC: Trauma Symptom Checklist for Children.

Most of the results indicated that school-going children living with HIV are more likely to experience greater mental health impairment as compared to their uninfected peers. However, the magnitude of mental health impairment may plausibly depend on differences in disease-related factors such as ART adherence and disease prognosis, the differences in contextual and home environment factors such as household poverty, sociocultural norms, and stigma, and variations in health-system related factors such as accessibility to quality care. Some study characteristics, such as the use of inadequate sample sizes or the lack of appropriate control groups, may also potentially explain the differences in reported mental health outcomes of HIV-infected children.

PATHWAYS TO POOR OUTCOMES

Poor neurodevelopmental and mental health outcomes among HIV-infected school-age children have been attributed to various factors, including both clinical factors, such as low CD4 levels, advanced WHO clinical stage, regimen type, high viral load, late ART initiation, and poor adherence (Martin et al. 2006; Hermetet-Lindsay et al. 2017; Kikuchi et al. 2017; Weber et al. 2017), and familial/psycho-social factors, such us caregiver unemployment, low level of caregiver education, caregiver depression, stigma, exposure to violence, low economic status, and maternal age (Boyede et al. 2013; Kandawasvika et al. 2015; Louw et al. 2016; Skeen et al. 2016; Gamarel et al. 2017; Besthorn et al 2018; Mbewe et al. 2022). This is an indication that, among school-age children, neurodevelopmental impairments following HIV infection are attributable to factors that can be beyond exposure to disease-related factors such as HIV infection/prognosis and exposure to ART. Besides, such factors are often a combination of clinical, psychosocial, and environmental factors. This accentuates the need for a holistic approach to examining and addressing the neurodevelopmental and health outcomes of HIV-infected children.

The impact of familial factors on the cognitive outcomes of HIV-infected school-going children is well documented. Generally, HIV-infected children and children from HIV-affected households are faced with several challenges, including stigmatisation, parental loss, violence, and poverty (Abubakar et al. 2016). Compared to HIV-negative children, HIV-infected and HEU children face an elevated risk of exposure to domestic and community violence, which is significantly associated with the development of depression, trauma, and behavioural problems (Skeen et al. 2016). Moreover, PHIV+ children with poor a caregiver–child relationship and those who lack adequate emotional support are more likely to have emotional and behavioural problems (Hermetet-Lindsay et al. 2017; Kalembo et al. 2019).

HIV-infected and HEU children may more often experience adverse childhood experiences such as the loss of their caregivers or living with sick caregivers. The death of parents following HIV infection or other causes leads to traumatic life experiences and renders many school-going children orphans, thus predisposing them to several life challenges (Lala 2014). Additionally, orphanhood has been linked to poor cognitive functions. For example, compared to children living with both biological parents, orphaned PHIV+ children are more likely to be cognitively impaired and depressed (Tadesse et al. 2012; Kandawasvika et al. 2015). Furthermore, lower cognitive scores among HIV-infected school-going children have been associated with low socioeconomic status (Tadesse et al. 2012; Boyede et al. 2013), lower parental education (Ajayi et al. 2017; Kalembo et al. 2019), parental unemployment (Kandawasvika et al. 2015), and single parenthood (Adefalu et al. 2018). This emphasises the potential negative impact of cumulative psychosocial risk factors that in many cases are a reality for HIV-infected children.

Several studies have reported a significant association between CD4 count (Martin et al. 2006), WHO clinical disease stage (Ruel et al. 2012), ART duration (Brahmbhatt et al. 2017), time of ART initiation (Puthanakit et al. 2013; Weber et al. 2017), and ART regimen type (Kikuchi et al. 2017) with cognitive function. However, the evidence in support of these findings is mixed for some of the factors. A study conducted among 370 school-age Ugandan children reported a significant association between early ART initiation, longer ART duration, and improved cognitive skills. Among PHIV+ children in this study, sequential processing skills were less impaired in children with a longer duration of ART (Brahmbhatt et al. 2017). Another study, involving 14 PHIV+ children in Germany, found that children who initiated ART within 12 months after birth, had better overall IQ scores measured on Wechsler Intelligence Scale for Children, Fourth Edition (Weber et al. 2017). A similar correlation between time of ART initiation and cognitive functions has been observed among PHIV+ children in the USA (Hermet-Lindsay et al. 2017). However, other studies have not found a significant association between ART and cognitive function among PHIV+ school-going children (Puthanakit et al. 2013; Musindo et al. 2018).

CONCLUSION

The adverse effects of HIV in school-age children are reflected in their day-to-day activities, including poor educational outcomes, poor physical functioning, and socio-emotional and behavioural problems. Despite the evidence for HIV's disastrous impact, various studies indicate that optimal ART initiation and adherence provide protective benefits against a host of the problems. Efforts to increase accessibility to ART are timely, especially in resource-poor settings like SSA where health-system challenges are still a major barrier. The risk factors for suboptimal neurodevelopment and mental health arise from multi-faceted levels such as family, community, and the individual (disease-specific factors). Therefore, there is a need for the application of a socio-ecological approach towards assessment of HIV's impacts on children's well-being as well as in designing interventions targeting children affected by HIV.

Current research also points to inherent challenges such as serious variation in sample sizes, the use of various measures that make comparability challenging, and the lack or use of inappropriate comparison groups. More rigorous, longitudinal studies, with a focus on diverse ecological factors are required, especially in low-resource settings like SSA, to better understand the impact of HIV and associated factors on the neurodevelopmental and mental health outcomes of school-going children.

REFERENCES

Abubakar A, Van de Vijver FJR, Fischer R et al. (2016) 'Everyone has a secret they keep close to their hearts': Challenges faced by adolescents living with HIV infection at the Kenyan coast. *BMC Public Health*, 16, 197. doi: 10.1186/s12889-016-2854-y.

Ackermann C, Andronikou S, Saleh MG et al. (2016) Early antiretroviral therapy in HIV-infected children is associated with diffuse white matter structural abnormality and corpus callosum sparing. *American Journal of Neuroradiology*, 37(12): 2363–2369.

Adefalu MO, Tunde-Ayinmode MF, Issa BA, Adefalu AA, Adepoju SA (2018) Psychiatric morbidity in children with HIV/AIDS at a tertiary health institution in north-central Nigeria. *J Trop Pediatr*, 64(1): 38–44. doi: 10.1093/tropej/fmx025.

Ajayi OR, Matthews G, Taylor M et al. (2017) Factors associated with the health and cognition of 6-year-old to 8-year-old children in KwaZulu-Natal, South Africa. *Trop Med Int Health*, 22(5): 631–637. doi: 10.1111/tmi.12866.

Bagenda D, Nassali A, Kalyesubula I et al. (2006) Health, neurologic, and cognitive status of HIV-infected, long-surviving, and antiretroviral-naive Ugandan children. *Pediatrics*, 117(3): 729–740.

Bangirana P, Ruel TD, Boivin MJ et al. (2017) Absence of neurocognitive disadvantage associated with paediatric HIV subtype A infection in children on antiretroviral therapy. *J Int AIDS Soc*, 20(2): e25015. doi: 10.1002/jia2.25015.

Besthorn F, Kalomo EN, Lightfoot E, Liao M (2018) The relationship between social support and anxiety amongst children living with HIV in rural northern Namibia. *Afr J AIDS Res*, 17(4): 293–300. doi: 10.2989/1608590 6.2018.1534748.

Blanchette N, Smith ML, King S, Fernandes-Penney A, Read S (2002) Cognitive development in school-age children with vertically transmitted HIV infection. *Dev Neuropsychol*, 21(3): 223–241.

Boivin MJ, Ruel TD, Boal HE et al. (2010) HIV-subtype A is associated with poorer neuropsychological performance compared to subtype D in ART-naïve Ugandan children. *Aids*, 24(8): 1163.

Boivin MJ, Barlow-Mosha L, Chernoff MC et al. (2018) Neuropsychological performance in African children with HIV enrolled in a multisite antiretroviral clinical trial. *Aids*, 32(2): 189–204. doi: 10.1097/qad.0000000000001683.

Boivin MJ, Chernoff M, Fairlie L et al. (2020) African multi-site 2-year neuropsychological study of school-age children perinatally infected, exposed, and unexposed to human immunodeficiency virus. *Clinical Infectious Diseases*, 71(7): e105–e114.

Boivin MJ, Zoumenou R, Sikorskii et al. (2021) Neurodevelopmental assessment at one year of age predicts neuropsychological performance at six years in a cohort of West African Children. *Child Neuropsychology*, 27(4): 548–571.

Boyede GO, Lesi FE, Ezeaka VC, Umeh CS (2013) Impact of sociodemographic factors on cognitive function in school-aged HIV-infected Nigerian children. *HIV AIDS (Auckl)*, 5: 145–152. doi: 10.2147/hiv.S43260.

Brahmbhatt H, Boivin M, Ssempijja V et al. (2017) Impact of HIV and antiretroviral therapy on neurocognitive outcomes among school-aged children. *J Acquir Immune Defic Syndr*, 75(1): 1–8. doi: 10.1097/qai.0000000000001305.

Davies MA, Gibb D, Turkova A (2016) Survival of HIV-1 vertically infected children. *Curr Opin HIV AIDS*, 11(5): 455–464. doi: 10.1097/coh.0000000000000303.

Dean O, Buda A, Adams HR et al. (2020) Brain magnetic resonance imaging findings associated with cognitive impairment in children and adolescents with human immunodeficiency virus in Zambia. *Pediatr Neurol*, 102: 28–35. doi: 10.1016/j.pediatrneurol.2019.08.014.

Familiar I, Chernoff M, Ruisenor-Escudero H et al. (2020) Association between caregiver depression symptoms and child executive functioning. Results from an observational study carried out in four sub-Saharan countries. *AIDS Care*, 32(4): 486–494.

Fundaro C, Miccinesi N, Baldieri NF, Genovese O, Rendeli C, Segni G (1998) Cognitive impairment in school-age children with asymptomatic HIV infection. *AIDS Patient Care STDS*, 12(2): 135–140.

Gamarel KE, Kuo C, Boyes ME, Cluver LD (2017) The dyadic effects of HIV stigma on the mental health of children and their parents in South Africa. *J HIV AIDS Soc Serv*, 16(4): 351–366. doi: 10.1080/15381501. 2017.1320619.

Ghate M, Narkhede H, Rahane G, Nirmalkar A, Gaikwad N, Kadam D (2015) Cognitive function among HIV infected children in Pune. *Indian J Pediatr*, 82(6): 515–518. doi: 10.1007/s12098-014-1629-7.

Grover G, Pensi T, Banerjee T (2007) Behavioural disorders in 6–11-year-old, HIV-infected Indian children. *Ann Trop Paediatr*, 27(3): 215–224. doi: 10.1179/146532807x220334.

Havens JF, Whitaker AH, Feldman JF, Ehrhardt AA (1994) Psychiatric morbidity in school-age children with congenital human immunodeficiency virus infection: A pilot study. *J Dev Behav Pediatr*, 15(3 Suppl): S18–S25.

Heany SJ, Phillips N, Brooks S et al. (2020) Neural correlates of maintenance working memory, as well as relevant structural qualities, are associated with earlier antiretroviral treatment initiation in vertically transmitted HIV. *J Neurovirol*, 26(1): 60–69. doi: 10.1007/s13365-019-00792-5.

Hermetet-Lindsay KD, Correia KF, Williams PL et al. (2017) Contributions of disease severity, psychosocial factors, and cognition to behavioral functioning in US youth perinatally exposed to HIV. *AIDS Behav*, 21(9): 2703–2715. doi: 10.1007/s10461-016-1508-5.

Hoare J, Fouche JP, Phillips N et al. (2015) White matter micro-structural changes in ART-naive and ART-treated children and adolescents infected with HIV in South Africa. *Aids*, 29(14): 1793–1801. doi: 10.1097/qad.0000000000000766.

Hoare J, Phillips N, Joska JA et al. (2016) Applying the HIV-associated neurocognitive disorder diagnostic criteria to HIV-infected youth. *Neurology*, 87(1): 86–93. doi: 10.1212/WNL.0000000000002669.

Hoare J, Fouche JP, Phillips N et al. (2018) Structural brain changes in perinatally HIV-infected young adolescents in South Africa. *Aids*, 32(18): 2707–2718. doi: 10.1097/qad.0000000000002024.

Hoare J, Myer L, Heany S et al. (2020) Cognition, structural brain changes, and systemic inflammation in adolescents living with HIV on antiretroviral therapy. *J Acquir Immune Defic Syndr*, 84(1): 114–121. doi: 10.1097/qai.0000000000002314.

Jankiewicz M, Holmes MJ, Taylor PA et al. (2017) White matter abnormalities in children with HIV infection and exposure. *Front Neuroanat*, 11: 88. doi: 10.3389/fnana.2017.00088.

Kalembo FW, Kendall GE, Ali M, Chimwaza AF (2019) Prevalence and factors associated with emotional and behavioural difficulties among children living with HIV in Malawi: A cross-sectional study. *BMC Psychiatry*, 19(1): 60. doi: 10.1186/s12888-019-2046-2.

Kandawasvika GQ, Kuona P, Chandiwana P et al. (2015) The burden and predictors of cognitive impairment among 6- to 8-year-old children infected and uninfected with HIV from Harare, Zimbabwe: A cross-sectional study. *Child Neuropsychol*, 21(1): 106–120. doi: 10.1080/09297049.2013.876493.

Kasamba I, Baisley K, Mayanja BN, Maher D, Grosskurth H (2012) The impact of antiretroviral treatment on mortality trends of HIV-positive adults in rural Uganda: A longitudinal population-based study, 1999–2009. *Tropical Medicine & International Health*, 17(8): e66–e73.

Kikuchi K, Poudel KC, Rwibasira JM et al. (2017) Caring for perinatally HIV-infected children: Call for mental care for the children and the caregivers. *AIDS Care*, 29(10): 1280–1286. doi: 10.1080/09540121.2017.1307917.

Koekkoek S, de Sonneville LM, Wolfs TF, Licht R, Geelen SP (2008) Neurocognitive function profile in HIV-infected school-age children. *Eur J Paediatr Neurol*, 12(4): 290–297. doi: 10.1016/j.ejpn.2007.09.002.

Kovalevich J, Langford D (2012) Neuronal toxicity in HIV CNS disease. *Future Virol*, 7(7): 687–698. doi: 10.2217/fvl.12.57.

Lala MM (2014) Orphans of the HIV epidemic: The challenges from toddlerhood to adolescence and beyond. *J Int AIDS Soc*, 17(4 Suppl 3): 19483. doi: 10.7448/ias.17.4.1948319483.

Linn K, Fay A, Meddles K et al. (2015) HIV-related cognitive impairment of orphans in Myanmar with vertically transmitted HIV taking antiretroviral therapy. *Pediatr Neurol*, 53(6): 485–490. e481. doi: 10.1016/j.pediatr-neurol.2015.08.004.

Louw KA, Ipser J, Phillips N, Hoare J (2016) Correlates of emotional and behavioural problems in children with perinatally acquired HIV in Cape Town, South Africa. *AIDS Care*, 28(7): 842–850. doi: 10.1080/09540121.2016.1140892.

Margaret A (2020) Language development. Retrieved from http://www.healthofchildren.com/L/Language-Development.html.

Martin SC, Wolters PL, Toledo-Tamula MA, Zeichner SL, Hazra R, Civitello L (2006) Cognitive functioning in school-aged children with vertically acquired HIV infection being treated with highly active antiretroviral therapy (HAART). *Dev Neuropsychol*, 30(2): 633–657. doi: 10.1207/s15326942dn3002_1.

Mbewe EG, Kabundula PP, Mwanza-Kabaghe S et al. (2022) Socioeconomic status and cognitive function in children with HIV: Evidence from the HIV-associated neurocognitive disorders in Zambia (HANDZ) study. *J Acquir Immune Defic Syndr*, 89(1): 56–63. doi: 10.1097/qai.0000000000002825.

Montaner JS, Lima VD, Harrigan PR et al. (2014) Expansion of HAART coverage is associated with sustained decreases in HIV/AIDS morbidity, mortality and HIV transmission: The 'HIV Treatment as Prevention' experience in a Canadian setting. *PLoS One*, 9(2).

Morison L (2001) The global epidemiology of HIV/AIDS. *British Medical Bulletin*, 58(1): 7–18.

Musindo O, Bangirana P, Kigamwa P, Okoth R, Kumar M (2018) Neurocognitive functioning of HIV positive children attending the comprehensive care clinic at Kenyatta national hospital: Exploring neurocognitive deficits and psychosocial risk factors. *AIDS Care*, 30(5): 618–622. doi: 10.1080/09540121.2018.1426829.

Nalwanga D, Musiime V, Bangirana P et al. (2021) Neurocognitive function among HIV-infected children on protease inhibitor-based versus non-protease inhibitor-based antiretroviral therapy in Uganda: A pilot study. *BMC Pediatr*, 21(1): 198. doi: 10.1186/s12887-021-02676-2.

Namuli JD, Nalugya JS, Bangirana P, Nakimuli-Mpungu E (2021) Prevalence and factors associated with suicidal ideation among children and adolescents attending a pediatric HIV clinic in Uganda. *Front Sociol*, 6: 656739. doi: 10.3389/fsoc.2021.656739.

National Research Council (1984) *Development During Middle Childhood: The Years from Six to Twelve*. Washington (DC): National Academies Press.

Nwosu EC, Robertson FC, Holmes MJ et al. (2018) Altered brain morphometry in 7-year old HIV-infected children on early ART. *Metab Brain Dis*, 33(2): 523–535. doi: 10.1007/s11011-017-0162-6.

Parks RA, Danoff JV (1999) Motor performance changes in children testing positive for HIV over 2 years. *Am J Occup Ther*, 53(5): 524–528. doi: 10.5014/ajot.53.5.524.

Puthanakit T, Aurpibul L, Louthrenoo O et al. (2010) Poor cognitive functioning of school-aged children in Thailand with perinatally acquired HIV infection taking antiretroviral therapy. *AIDS Patient Care STDS*, 24(3): 141–146. doi: 10.1089/apc.2009.0314.

Puthanakit T, Ananworanich J, Vonthanak S et al. (2013) Cognitive function and neurodevelopmental outcomes in HIV-infected children older than 1 year of age randomized to early versus deferred antiretroviral therapy: The PREDICT neurodevelopmental study. *Pediatr Infect Dis J*, 32(5): 501–508. doi: 10.1097/INF.0b013e-31827fb19d.

Ravindran OS, Rani MP, Priya G (2014) Cognitive deficits in HIV-infected children. *Indian J Psychol Med*, 36(3): 255–259. doi: 10.4103/0253-7176.135373.

Rice ML, Buchanan AL, Siberry GK et al. (2012) Language impairment in children perinatally infected with HIV compared to children who were HIV-exposed and uninfected. *J Dev Behav Pediatr*, 33(2): 112–123. doi: 10.1097/DBP.0b013e318241ed23.

Ruel TD, Boivin MJ, Boal HE et al. (2012) Neurocognitive and motor deficits in HIV-infected Ugandan children with high CD4 cell counts. *Clin Infect Dis*, 54(7): 1001–1009. doi: 10.1093/cid/cir1037.

Ruiseñor-Escudero H, Familiar I, Nakasujja N et al. (2015) Immunological correlates of behavioral problems in school-aged children living with HIV in Kayunga, Uganda. *Global Mental Health*, 2: e9.

Shah A, Gangwani MR, Chaudhari NS, Glazyrin A, Bhat HK, Kumar A (2016) Neurotoxicity in the post-HAART era: Caution for the antiretroviral therapeutics. *Neurotoxicity Research*, 30(4): 677–697.

Sherr L, Hensels IS, Tomlinson M, Skeen S, Macedo A (2018) Cognitive and physical development in HIV-positive children in South Africa and Malawi: A community-based follow-up comparison study. *Child Care Health Dev*, 44(1): 89–98. doi: 10.1111/cch.12533.

Skeen S, Macedo A, Tomlinson M, Hensels IS, Sherr L (2016) Exposure to violence and psychological well-being over time in children affected by HIV/AIDS in South Africa and Malawi. *AIDS Care*, 28(Suppl 1): 16–25. doi: 10.1080/09540121.2016.1146219.

Tadesse AW, Berhane Tsehay Y, Girma Belaineh B, Alemu YB (2012) Behavioral and emotional problems among children aged 6-14 years on highly active antiretroviral therapy in Addis Ababa: A cross-sectional study. *AIDS Care*, 24(11): 1359–1367. doi: 10.1080/09540121.2011.650677.

Thompson PM, Dutton RA, Hayashi KM et al. (2005) Thinning of the cerebral cortex visualized in HIV/AIDS reflects CD4+ T lymphocyte decline. *Proceedings of the National Academy of Sciences*, 102(43): 15647–15652.

Toich JTF, Taylor PA, Holmes MJ et al. (2017) Functional connectivity alterations between networks and associations with infant immune health within networks in HIV infected children on early treatment: A study at 7 years. *Front Hum Neurosci*, 11: 635. doi: 10.3389/fnhum.2017.00635.

UNAIDS (2020) Global HIV & AIDS statistics – 2019 Fact Sheet.

van Opstal SEM, Dogterom EJ, Wagener MN et al. (2021) Neuropsychological and psychosocial functioning of children with perinatal HIV-infection in The Netherlands. *Viruses*, 13(10). doi: 10.3390/v13101947.

van Wyhe KS, Laughton B, Cotton MF et al. (2021) Cognitive outcomes at ages seven and nine years in South African children from the children with HIV early antiretroviral (CHER) trial: A longitudinal investigation. *J Int AIDS Soc*, 24(7): e25734.

Visser MJ, Hecker HE, Jordaan J (2018) A comparative study of the psychological problems of HIV-infected and HIV-uninfected children in a South African sample. *AIDS Care*, 30(5): 596–603. doi: 10.1080/09540121.2017.1417530.

Walker SY, Pierre RB, Christie CD, Chang SM (2013) Neurocognitive function in HIV-positive children in a developing country. *Int J Infect Dis*, 17(10): e862–e867. doi: 10.1016/j.ijid.2013.02.014.

Wang H, Wolock TM, Carter A et al. (2016) Estimates of global, regional, and national incidence, prevalence, and mortality of HIV, 1980–2015: The Global Burden of Disease Study 2015. *The Lancet HIV*, 3(8): e361–e387.

Weber V, Radeloff D, Reimers B et al. (2017) Neurocognitive development in HIV-positive children is correlated with plasma viral loads in early childhood. *Medicine (Baltimore)*, 96(23): e6867. doi: 10.1097/md.0000000000006867.

Wells K (2018) *Encyclopedia of Children's Health: Infancy through Adolescence* [online].

Wolters PL, Brouwers P, Moss HA, Pizzo PA (1995) Differential receptive and expressive language functioning of children with symptomatic HIV disease and relation to CT scan brain abnormalities. *Pediatrics*, 95(1): 112–119.

Yadav SK, Gupta RK, Garg RK et al. (2017) Altered structural brain changes and neurocognitive performance in pediatric HIV. *Neuroimage Clin*, 14: 316–322. doi: 10.1016/j.nicl.2017.01.032.

Yadav SK, Gupta RK, Hashem S et al. (2018) Changes in resting-state functional brain activity are associated with waning cognitive functions in HIV-infected children. *Neuroimage Clin*, 20: 1204–1210. doi: 10.1016/j.nicl.2018.10.028.

Yadav SK, Gupta RK, Hashem S et al. (2020) Brain microstructural changes support cognitive deficits in HIV uninfected children born to HIV infected mothers. *Brain Behav Immun Health*, 2: 100039. doi: 10.1016/j.bbih.2020.100039.

Neurobehavioural Manifestations of HIV in Adolescence

Derrick Ssewanyana, Moses K Nyongesa, and Amina Abubakar

EPIDEMIOLOGICAL TRENDS IN HIV AMONG ADOLESCENTS

Adolescence, generally considered the time between 10 and 19 years of age, is a crucial developmental period. This period is characterised by increased autonomy and various psychosocial and biological changes (WHO 2014). At this stage, many teenagers begin exploring their sexuality and experimenting with psychoactive substances, which can predispose them to increased vulnerability (Idele et al. 2014; Bekker et al. 2015; de Andrade et al. 2017). Many adolescents currently experience extreme vulnerability in the aftermath of the coronavirus-19 (COVID-19) pandemic, which has led to extreme poverty, loss of opportunities, homelessness, dropping out of school, mental health problems, violence, and discrimination in many parts of the world (Guessoum et al. 2020; Bhatia et al. 2021). Nearly 90% of people between the ages of 10 and 24 years live in low- and middle-income countries (LMICs), where human immunodeficiency virus (HIV) infection remains prevalent. Less is known about HIV progression and AIDS development in adolescents than in other age groups, as research has predominately focused on infants and adults (Idele et al. 2014).

By 2020, an estimated 1.8 million adolescents were HIV infected, and 88% (1.5 million) of them lived in sub-Saharan Africa (SSA) (UNICEF 2021a). In the same period, 78 000 HIV-infected adolescents lived in South Asia, 58 000 in Eastern Asia, 40 000 in Latin America and the Caribbean, 15 000 in Eastern Europe and Central Asia, and 2300 in the Middle East and Northern Africa (UNAIDS 2021). Moreover, it is plausible that, due to low HIV-testing rates in the most affected regions, the HIV burden in this subpopulation is higher than current estimates, It is estimated that only 25% of females and 17% of males aged 15 to 19 in Eastern and Southern Africa had been tested and received their HIV test results in 2020 (UNICEF 2021a). Some of these cases can be attributed to HIV-positive children growing into adolescence but a significant portion is from adolescents who contract HIV during this period (Joint United Nations Programme on HIV/AIDS 2014; UNICEF 2016). Vertical transmission accounts for the majority of HIV-infected adolescents (WHO 2013). However, over the past 15 years, mother-to-child HIV transmission has reduced by 70%. The increase in health care and social services has helped boost the prevention of mother-to-child HIV transmission (UNAIDS 2016c).

Globally, adolescents accounted for 11% (about 150 000) of new HIV infections in 2020. Adolescent females accounted for the largest share (80%) of the new infections (UNICEF 2021a). The gender disparities in new HIV infections are most magnified in SSA, where newly HIV-infected adolescent females numbered nearly six times as many as males. However, in Eastern Asia and the Pacific region, more adolescent males than females (64% vs 34%) were newly infected with HIV (UNICEF 2021a). Similar trends have been reported previously. In 2013 almost 60% of new infections in adolescents were in females, 80% of whom lived in SSA (Joint United Nations Programme on HIV/AIDS 2014). HIV prevalence in 15 to 19-year-olds in Eastern and Southern African countries, including Botswana, Kenya, Lesotho, Uganda, Malawi, Rwanda, Mozambique, and Zimbabwe, was twice as likely in females as it was in males. The same ratio was found in other SSA countries, including Cameroon, Gabon, Guinea, and the Ivory Coast (Joint United Nations Programme on HIV/AIDS 2014). Females in these regions acquired HIV approximately 5 to 7 years earlier than their male counterparts (Joint United Nations Programme on HIV/AIDS 2014).

Adolescent females from these countries with HIV prevalence often endure exploitation and violence, lack access to sexual and reproductive health services, and lack comprehensive knowledge about sexually transmitted infections. These teenagers are thus at an elevated risk of acquiring HIV (Joint United Nations Programme on HIV/AIDS 2014). Studies performed in regions facing an HIV epidemic reported high rates of sexual exploitation, including rape through coercion, age and economic disparity within sexual relationships, and intimate partner violence. Adolescent females and young adult females from these regions were thus at higher risk of contracting HIV (Moore et al. 2007; Jewkes et al. 2010). Similarly, in Cambodia (Couture et al. 2011), Thailand (Lau 2008), and India (Joffres et al. 2008), sexual exploitation like child prostitution and child sex trafficking is linked with an elevated risk of contracting HIV. Despite these data, hesitancy remains regarding targeted HIV prevention and treatment in adolescents. This is attributed to the social consequences these adolescents might face – including stigma, marginalisation, and criminalisation – for receiving these services (Idele et al. 2014; UNAIDS 2016b).

Key Populations

A breakdown of the global HIV-infected population shows that 62% of this population comprises five key populations. Nearly a quarter (23%) of HIV-infected people are gay males and other males who have sex with males; 19% are clients of sex workers and sex partners of all key populations; 10% are people who inject drugs; 8% are sex workers; and 2% are transgender people (UNAIDS 2020).

Understanding the HIV burden and specific needs of adolescent key populations is complicated by disparate legal and ethical frameworks (i.e. criminalising or unclear regulations or ethical guidelines) in many parts of the world, especially in LMICs. These create numerous challenges related to adolescent consent to research participation and access to specific clinical services (Mustanski and Fisher 2016; Day et al. 2020). While adolescent-specific data are scarce, growing evidence indicates that young people (ages 10–24 years) who are transgender, sexually exploited (e.g. child prostitution or childhood marriage), use injectable drugs and who have sex with males experience heightened risks of contracting HIV (Joint United Nations Programme on HIV/AIDS 2014; Idele et al. 2014; Baggaley et al. 2015; Bekker et al. 2015). Findings from a national-level HIV surveillance conducted in 2009 to 2014 in the USA reported that 8% of transgender adolescents (13–19 years) were diagnosed with HIV (Clark et al. 2017). In the USA, males who have sex with males aged 13 to 24 years make up 80% of HIV diagnoses in this age bracket and make up 22% of new HIV diagnoses (CDC 2015). Studies among adolescent sex workers report a high prevalence of sexually transmitted infections, including HIV. For example, a 30% prevalence of sexually transmitted infections was found among adolescent female sex workers in China (Zhang et al. 2013), a 35% HIV prevalence among young female sex workers (18–24 years) from 14 sites in Zimbabwe (Napierala et al. 2018), and a 10% HIV prevalence among adolescent females and young adult females (14–24 years) who engaged in sex work in Mombasa,

Kenya (Becker et al. 2018). Evidence shows that close to 5.2% of intravenous drug users younger than 25 years of age are HIV positive (UNAIDS 2014). A Tanzanian study conducted among young people (17–25 years) who inject drugs reported that 12% of the males and 55% of the females were HIV seropositive (Atkinson et al. 2011).

NEUROCOGNITIVE OUTCOMES OF HIV-INFECTED ADOLESCENTS

The current body of research shows HIV's adverse effects on neurocognition in infected children, but little research has been carried out on neurocognition in HIV-positive adolescents. Due to long-term antiretroviral use and potential resulting neurotoxicity, survival bias, and the increased demands on cognitive function in adolescence, it cannot be assumed that adolescents experience neurocognitive outcomes similar to those that children do. Transitioning from adolescence to young adulthood requires adapting to more demanding social, academic, and individual responsibilities, which also places new demands on neurocognitive function (Robbins et al. 2020). Table 13.1 summarises some existing studies on HIV and neurocognition in adolescents, most of which were conducted in the USA. These studies present evidence of delay and impairment in cognitive function among perinatally HIV-infected (PHIV) adolescents.

Neurocognitive impairments are associated with structural changes in the brains of HIV-infected adolescents. HIV infects the brain early in development for perinatally infected adolescents, and research shows altered grey matter morphometry in this population (Lewis-de Los Angeles et al. 2017, 2020). In a study by Nichols and colleagues, grey matter reduction was pronounced in the anterior cingulate cortex, the right pallidum, the right occipital lobe, the inferior parietal lobe, and the bilateral cerebellum crus (Nichols et al. 2015). In another study from the USA, structural magnetic resonance imaging (MRI) and cognitive testing were carried out among 40 PHIV young people, who were compared to 334 typically developing, uninfected young people (Lewis-de Los Angeles et al. 2016). This study observed that both total and regional cortical grey matter brain volume of PHIV young people were reduced (2.8–5.1%) compared to HIV-unexposed and HIV-uninfected young people. A study from Zambia used regression models to evaluate the relationships between MRI findings and cognitive function (Mbewe et al. 2022). The study identified cerebrovascular disease in 7 of 34 participants with HIV compared with 0 of 17 controls (21% vs 0%, $p = 0.04$). The study also reported decreased total brain volumes ($1036cm^3$ vs $1162cm^3$, $p = 0.03$) and decreased cortical thickness in the right temporal lobes (3.12mm vs 3.29mm; $p = 0.01$) and right fusiform gyri (3.10mm vs 3.25mm; $p = 0.02$) of HIV-infected participants with cognitive impairment. Taken together these studies provide strong evidence that there is structural brain damage in a significant proportion of adolescents who are perinatally infected with HIV.

Various clinical characteristics of PHIV adolescents have been associated with more adverse neurocognitive outcomes. Studies indicate that late initiation of ARV drugs, a history of encephalopathy, low viral load, and a history of AIDS diagnosis were significantly associated with lower neurocognitive scores (Nichols et al. 2015, 2016; Van den Hof et al. 2020). Recent studies have expanded the range of clinical indicators studied to examine newer hypotheses. For instance, Shiau et al. (2021) examined the association of metabolic syndrome (MetS) and its components (abdominal obesity, elevated triglycerides, low high-density lipoprotein cholesterol, elevated blood pressure, and impaired fasting glycemia) with neurocognitive impairment among adolescents perinatally infected with HIV or HIV exposed uninfected adolescents. Among adolescents living with HIV, no associations were observed between MetS components and neurocognitive indices at baseline. However, over time, elevated baseline blood pressure was associated with a greater decrease in mean perceptual reasoning scores

Table 13.1 A summary of identified studies on neurocognitive outcomes in HIV-infected adolescents.

Study	Country	Year	Age (years)	Sample size	Key findings
Mbewe et al. (2022)	Zambia	2022	8–17	208 PHIV 208 PHEU	• Adolescents with HIV performed significantly worse on a composite measure of cognitive function (NPZ8 score −0.19 vs 0.22, $p < 0.001$) and were more likely to have cognitive impairment (33% vs 19%, $p = 0.001$). • Higher socioeconomic status was associated with a reduced risk of cognitive impairment (odds ratio 0.8, 95% confidence interval: 0.75–0.92, $p < 0.001$) in both groups.
Zielińska-Wieniawska et al. (2021)	Poland	2021	6–18	50 PHIV 24 PHEU 43 PHUU	• Results of the research indicate deterioration of executive functioning in the PHIV+ group associated with a longer duration of HIV neuroinfection and severity of infection before treatment.
Shiau et al. (2021)	USA	2021	10–19	350 PHIV 68 PHEU	• Elevated metabolic syndrome was associated with a higher risk of decreased performance in neurocognitive tests.
Robbins et al. (2020)	China	2020	15–29	206 PHIV 134 PHEU at baseline	• Few differences in the tests of perceptual speed, executive function, and working memory in this longitudinal study.
Patel et al. (2021)	Thailand	2020	10–20	59 PHIV 67 HEU 79 PHUU	• After controlling for demographic factors of age and household income, adolescents with PHIV had higher inattentive symptomatology and poorer neuropsychological test scores compared to uninfected controls.
Van den Hof et al. (2020)	The Netherlands	2020	Mean 21 years	21 PHIV 23 PHU	• Processing speed, working memory, learning ability, and visual-motor function trajectories were not statistically different between groups. • Executive function scores declined significantly over time for HIV-infected adolescents, while their IQ scores increased significantly over time.
Kerr et al. (2019)	Thailand	2019	10–17	231 PHIV 125 PHEU 138 PHU	• Most of the PHIV adolescents were virologically suppressed. • However, they still had higher impairment rates in executive functions and mental health.
Hermetet-Lindsay et al. (2017)	USA	2017	7–16 (mean 10 years 11 months)	231 PHIV 151 PHEU	• This study reported that both caregiver and child stress had a negative impact on behavioural function in both groups. • Among PHIV young people, disease factors adversely impacted cognitive function.
Lewis-de Los Angeles et al. (2016)	USA	2017	Mean 16 years 8 months	40 PHIV 334 PHU	• PHIV young people had reduced regional and total grey matter volumes compared with HIV-unexposed and -uninfected young people. • Poor cognitive performance correlated with reduced volume. • Reduced volume of grey matter was associated with a history of illness, non-viral immunosuppression, and substance abuse.

(Continued)

Table 13.1 Continued.

Study	Country	Year	Age (years)	Sample size	Key findings
Nichols et al. (2015)	USA	2016	9–19	173 PHIV 85 PHEU	• No significant HIV status group differences were found on executive function performance-based scores. • Poor executive functioning was attributed mainly to the timing and severity of diseases.
Nichols et al. (2016)	USA	2016	9–19	173 PHIV 85 PHEU	• Young people with PHIV, particularly those with CDC Class C diagnosis, showed poorer performance on some measures of learning and memory compared to PHEU young people. • Group differences in verbal memory were largely attributed to sociodemographic and clinical characteristics.
Ezeamama et al. (2016)	Uganda	2016	7–18	58 PHIV 55 PHEU 53 PHU	• PHIV infection was associated with significant global and domains-specific executive function deficit compared to PHU children.
Redmond et al. (2016)	USA	2016	1–15	212 PHIV 107 PHEU	• Both the PHIV and PHEU young people were at risk for persistent language impairment. • Family history of language delay was a risk factor for the persistence of language developmental delays.
Garvie et al. (2014)	USA	2014	7–16	295 PHIV 165 PHEU	• Both PHIV and PHEU groups demonstrated lower achievement than the normative sample. • Lower achievement was associated with prior encephalopathy and older age. • Non-HIV factors such as being male, lower caregiver IQ, and black ethnicity were associated with lower achievement, further emphasising the role of multiple biological and social risk factors.
Rice et al. (2012)	USA	2012	7–16 (median 12 years)	284 PHIV 234 PHEU	• Both PHIV and PHEU groups had high rates of language impairment at 40% compared to an expected rate of 16% in the US population.
Nachman et al. (2012)	USA and Puerto Rico	2012	6–17	319 HIV young people	• A lower nadir CD4 percentage was associated with lower quality of life, worse WISC-CR scores, and worse social functioning. • HIV illness severity markers were associated with the severity of some psychiatric symptoms and, notably, with cognitive, academic, and social functioning.
Smith et al. (2012)	USA	2012	7–16	88 PHIV/C 270 PHIV/NOC 200 PHEU	• All three groups had low mean scores. • Scores were significantly lower for young people with PHIV+/C. • Prior diagnosis for encephalopathy was correlated with poor cognitive scores.

Table 13.1 Continued.

Study	Country	Year	Age (years)	Sample size	Key findings
Puthanakit et al. (2010)	Thailand	2010	6–12	40 PHIV, 40 HIV affected, 42 control children	• HIV-infected children had lower cognitive function than HIV-affected and normal children. • Cognitive function was not improved after receiving ART.
Woods et al. (2004)	USA	2009	13–17	81 PHIV	• A history of AIDS diagnosis was associated with poorer neurocognitive performance and psychiatric impairment in adolescents.
Brackiss-Cott et al. (2009)	USA	2009	9–15	43 PHIV	• PHIV young people performed poorly, although their scores were similar to scores of uninfected young people living in the inner city.
Paramesparan et al. (2010)	UK	2010	Mean 18 years 10 months (range 17–23) Older adults >60	37 HIV infected	• The study found a higher rate of neurocognitive impairment in asymptomatic adolescents compared to adults >60 years old (67% vs 19%).
Koekkoeka et al. (2008)	The Netherlands	2007	6–17	22 PHIV	• Compared with age-appropriate norms, the mean IQ of the HIV-infected children was in the average range. • HIV-infected children performed poorer on several neuropsychological tests compared with age-appropriate norms. • Executive function (attentional flexibility, visuospatial working memory) and processing speed emerged as the most sensitive cognitive measures in relation to HIV disease. • Higher CD4 percentage at the initiation of HAART and longer treatment duration were associated with better working memory function and attentional control respectively.
Martin et al. (2006)	USA	2006	6–16	41 vertically infected children (treated with HAART)	• Children with HIV infection being treated with HAART typically score at the low end of the average range (low 90s) on a composite measure of cognitive functioning, with Full Scale IQ scores ranging from the mentally deficient to very superior classification.

Abbreviations: ART, antiretroviral therapy; CDC: Centers for Disease Control and Prevention; HAART: highly active antiretroviral therapy; HEU: HIV exposed uninfected; PHEU: perinatally HIV exposed uninfected; PHIV: perinatally HIV infected; PHIV/C: perinatally HIV infected/CDC Stage C; PHIV/NOC: perinatally HIV infected/Non-CDC Stage C; PHU: perinatally HIV unexposed; WISC-CR: Wechsler Intelligence Scale for Children Coding Recall.

(–4.3; 95% confidence interval: –8.8, 0.3) and ≥2 MetS components was associated with a greater decrease in mean processing speed scores (–5.1; 95% confidence interval: –9.4, –0.8). Among adolescents who were HIV exposed but uninfected, various components of MetS were associated with lowered neurocognitive scores longitudinally (Shiau et al. 2021). Studies to elucidate how modifying metabolic risk factors early in life may improve neurocognitive outcomes in this population are warranted.

Additionally, non-HIV related factors can explain many of the deficits seen in perinatally-infected adolescents. It has been reported that various psychosocial factors also influence the cognitive development of HIV-positive adolescents. In a study carried out in the USA involving 231 PHIV and 151 perinatally HIV exposed uninfected (PHEU) young people, home environment, psychosocial factors, and demographics played a role in neurocognitive outcomes (Hermetet-Lindsay et al. 2017). Recent evidence indicates that early childhood experiences may continue to influence neurocognitive functioning among adolescents. In a study from South Africa, the researchers examined the associations between adversity and neurocognitive functioning among adolescents (14–17 years) with PHIV (Santoro et al. 2021). These adolescents completed the Adverse Childhood Experiences scale and a tablet-based neurocognitive assessment. It was reported that the Adverse Childhood Experiences scores predicted performance on various neurocognitive tests, including those of processing speed and executive functioning. These studies provide evidence that early childhood experiences continue to negatively impact the outcomes of adolescents living with HIV.

Addressing impaired neurocognitive outcomes among adolescents living with HIV is essential since some preliminary reports indicate that cognitive impairment is associated with functional impairment. A study conducted among South African young people found a strong association between HIV-infected young people's functional impairment on the Child Behaviour Checklist, the Vineland Adaptive Behavior Scale, Second Edition, and repeated grades with a degree of cognitive impairment; and that when cognitive impairment was present, the young people had a higher risk of experiencing functional impairment as well (Phillips et al. 2021). Based on these findings, the authors proposed that simple screening questions on functional outcomes such as repeating of grades may be used to screen for potential cognitive impairments in adolescents and can be used to identify adolescents who need to be sent for in-depth assessments.

PSYCHIATRIC MORBIDITY AMONG HIV-INFECTED ADOLESCENTS

HIV-associated psychiatric morbidity among adolescents is generally under-researched compared to similar research among HIV-positive adults, regardless of the setting. Before 2010 Scharko (2006) identified only eight studies that quantified the prevalence of psychiatric disorders in HIV-infected adolescents using the fourth edition of the *Diagnostic and Statistical Manual of Mental Disorders* (DSM-IV) criteria. The author found a high prevalence of psychiatric problems among these adolescents: for instance, 28.6% for attention-deficit/hyperactivity disorder, 25% for depression, and 24.3% for anxiety. From 2010 onwards, research on psychiatric manifestations in HIV-infected adolescents has progressively increased across contexts (Mellins and Malee 2013; Vreeman et al. 2017; Too et al. 2021). In the first half of the last decade (2010–2015), studies reporting mental disorders among HIV-infected adolescents were mostly from high-income countries (HICs), largely the USA; very few studies were from LMICs. From the second half of the last decade through to the current decade, many studies reporting psychiatric disorders in HIV-infected adolescents are notably from LMICs, especially SSA. This increased effort may be due to the availability of a variety of validated mental health instruments for these contexts (Ali et al. 2016; Mughal et al. 2020) and to calls for prioritisation of mental health research in settings with a high HIV burden (Abas et al. 2014). Table 13.2 summarises data on the burden of psychiatric disorders among HIV-infected adolescents from select studies across contexts since 2010.

Table 13.2 A summary of select studies on the burden of psychiatric disorders among HIV-infected adolescents.

Study	Country	Age (range or mean) (years)	Sample size	Mental disorder(s)	Mental health measures used	Key finding (prevalence estimates unless otherwise stated)
Studies from high-income countries (HICs)						
Gadow et al. (2010)	USA (and Puerto Rico)	12–17	Total = 301 HIV+ = 196 HIV− = 105	– ADHD – ODD – Conduct disorder – Generalised anxiety disorder – Separation anxiety disorder – Social phobia – Major depressive episode – Dysthymic disorder – Somatisation disorder – Disturbing events – Any disorder	CASI-4R (CgR) YI-4R (self-report)	**HIV+** **HIV−** ADHD: 12.2% 12.5%[a] ODD: 4.1% 6.7%[a] Conduct disorder: 4.6% 8.6%[a] Generalised anxiety disorder: 0.5% 1.0%[a] Separation anxiety disorder:* 1.0% 5.7%[a] Social phobia: 0.5% 1.0%[a] Major depressive episode: 0.5% 1.9%[a] Dysthymic disorder: 0.0% 1.9%[a] Somatisation disorder: 11.7% 8.6%[a] Disturbing events: 24.0% 25.7%[a] Any disorder: 39.3% 39.1%[a]
Elkington et al. (2011)	USA	9–16	Total = 545 HIV+ = 196 HIV− = 349	– Internalising problems – Externalising problems – Depression – Anxiety	CBCL (CgR) CDI (self-reported) STAIC	**CBCL (cutoff score ≥ 63):** Total: 14.4% – Externalising problems: 16.1% – Internalising problems: 11.8% **CDI (cut-off score ≥ 13):** 16.7% STAIC scores, mean (SD): 33.8 (7.4)
Kapetanovic et al. (2011)	USA	13–24	197	– Mood disorders – ADHD – Disruptive disorders – Anxiety disorders – Adjustment disorders – Elimination disorders – Anxiety/depression due to medical condition – Schizoaffective disorder – Affective psychosis – Eating disorders	History from medical records	Mood disorders: 25% ADHD: 17% Disruptive disorders: 15% Anxiety disorders: 5% Adjustment disorders: 4% Elimination disorders: 2% Anxiety/depression due to medical condition: 0.005% Schizoaffective disorder: 0.005% Affective psychosis: 0.005% Eating disorders: 0.01%

(Continued)

Table 13.2 Continued

Study	Country	Age (range or mean) (years)	Sample size	Mental disorder(s)	Mental health measures used	Key finding (prevalence estimates unless otherwise stated)
Mellins et al. (2011)	USA (and Puerto Rico)	10–16	Total = 349 HIV+ = 238 HIV– = 111	– Behavioural and emotional problems	BASC-2	HIV+: 26% HIV–: 33%
Gadow et al. (2012)	USA (and Puerto Rico)	6–17	Total = 525 HIV+ = 296 HIV– = 229	– ADHD – Disruptive disorders – Anxiety – Depression	CASI (CgR)	HIV+ HIV– ADHD: 16% 15% Disruptive disorders: 11% 14% Anxiety: 4% 5% Depression: 4% 7%
Mellins et al. (2012)	USA	9–16	Total = 280 HIV+ = 166 HIV– = 114	– Anxiety – Mood disorders – Disruptive behaviours – ADHD – SUDs	DISC-IV	HIV+ HIV– Any disorder: 60.2% 57% Anxiety disorder: 48.2% 49.1% Mood disorder: 12.7% 4.4% Disruptive behaviour: 28.9% 27.2% ADHD: 21.8% 11.6% Any SUD: 1.8% 3.5%
Nachman et al. (2012)	USA (and Puerto Rico)	6–17	319	– ADHD – Disruptive behaviour – Depression – Anxiety – Any disorder	CASI-4R (CgR) YI-4R (self-report)	CASI YI-4R ADHD: 14% 10% Disruptive behaviour: 7% 12% Depression: 1% 14% Anxiety: 1% 10% Any disorder: 17% 26%
Kacanek et al. (2015)	USA (and Puerto Rico)	6–17	294	– ADHD – Disruptive behaviour – Depression – Anxiety – Any disorder	CASI-4R (CgR) YI-4R (self-report)	ADHD: 17%[b] Disruptive behaviour: 13%[b] Depression: 14%[b] Anxiety: 18%[b] Any disorder: 38%[b]
Mutumba et al. (2016a)	USA	9–16	Total = 325 PHIV = 196 PHEU = 129	– Internalising symptoms – Externalising symptoms	DISC-IV	**Internalising symptom score, mean (SD)** PHIV vs PHEU: 19.5 (12.6) vs 20.6 (14.0), $p > 0.05$ (t-test = 0.76) **Externalising symptom score, mean (SD)** PHIV vs PHEU: 14.8 (9.1) vs 14.4 (10.1), $p > 0.05$ (t-test = –0.37)

Table 13.2 Continued

Study	Country	Age (range or mean) (years)	Sample size	Mental disorder(s)	Mental health measures used	Key finding (prevalence estimates unless otherwise stated)
Le Prevost et al. (2018)	England	13–23	Total = 379 HIV+ = 283 HIV– = 96	– Depressive symptoms – Anxiety symptoms	HADS	**Moderate depressive symptoms** HIV+ : 5% HIV– : 0% **Moderate/severe anxiety symptoms** HIV+ :16% HIV– : 14%
Smith et al. (2019)	USA (and Puerto Rico)	10–22	Total = 551 PHIV = 355 PHEU = 196	– ADHD – Mood disorder – Anxiety disorder – Behavioural disorder – Trauma disorder – Autism spectrum disorder – Other disorders – Any disorder	History from medical records provided on the Diagnosis Report NPD interview (for current mental health diagnoses) BASC-2	PHIV PHEU ADHD: 21% 28%c Mood disorder: 12% 8%c Anxiety disorder: 4% 6%c Behavioural disorder: 3% 5%c Trauma disorder: 2% 1%c Autism spectrum disorder: 1% 2%c Other disorders:‡ 1% 2%c Any disorder: 31% 33%c
Kreniske et al. (2021)	USA	9–16	Total = 339 PHIV = 206 PHEU = 133	– Suicide attempt – Anxiety disorder – Mood disorder	DISC-IV DISC-2.3	**Attempted suicide:** Whole sample: 22% PHIV vs PHEU: 27% vs 16%, p = 0.019 **Anxiety disorder** Whole sample: 31% HIV+: 31% PHEU: 32% **Mood disorder** Whole sample: 3% HIV+: 3% PHEU: 2%

(Continued)

Table 13.2 Continued

Study	Country	Age (range or mean) (years)	Sample size	Mental disorder(s)	Mental health measures used	Key finding (prevalence estimates unless otherwise stated)
Studies from low- and middle-income countries						
Kamau et al. (2012)	Kenya	6–18	162	– Major depression – Social phobia – ADHD – ODD – Suicidality – Specific phobia – Bipolar disorders – Panic disorders – Conduct disorder – Agoraphobia – Dysthymia – Separation anxiety disorder – Psychotic disorders – PTSD	MINI-KID	Major depression: 17.3% Social phobia: 12.8% ADHD: 12.2% ODD: 12.2% Suicidality: 10.3% Specific phobia: 7.1% Bipolar disorders: 6.4% Panic disorders: 5.8% Conduct disorder: 4.5% Agoraphobia: 2.6% Dysthymia: 2.6% Separation anxiety disorder: 2.6% Psychotic disorders: 1.9% PTSD: 1.3%
Louthrenoo, Oberdorfer, and Sirisanthana (2014)	Thailand	11–18	Total = 106 HIV+ = 50 HIV– = 56	– Internalising problems – Externalising problems	YSR CBCL	**Total problems score, means (SD)** YSR HIV+ vs HIV–: 38.5 (20.7) vs 31.3 (20.1), $p = 0.07$ CBCL HIV+ vs HIV–: 32.0 (19.2) vs 30.3 (23.0), $p = 0.68$ **Internalising problems score, means (SD)** YSR HIV+ vs HIV–: 13.8 (8.0) vs 9.9 (7.9), $p = 0.02$ CBCL HIV+ vs HIV–: 11.3 (7.1) vs 9.3 (8.2), $p = 0.19$ **Externalising problems score, means (SD)** YSR HIV+ vs HIV–: 9.4 (5.9) vs 8.7 (6.3), $p = 0.56$ CBCL HIV+ vs HIV–: 7.4 (4.8) vs 8.6 (7.4), $p = 0.35$

Table13.2 Continued

Study	Country	Age (range or mean) (years)	Sample size	Mental disorder(s)	Mental health measures used	Key finding (prevalence estimates unless otherwise stated)
Betancourt et al. (2014)	Rwanda	10–17	Total = 683 HIV+ = 218 HIV– = 237 PHEU = 228	– Depression – Anxiety/internalising problems – Conduct disorders	CES-D YSR (internalising subscale) Locally developed scale for conduct disorders	**Depression:#** HIV affected: 1.68 (1.15–2.44) HIV unaffected: 1.32 (0.90–1.95) **YSR anxiety/internalising:#** HIV affected: 1.77 (1.14–2.75) HIV unaffected: 1.13 (0.71–1.81) **Conduct problems:#** HIV affected: 1.59 (1.04–2.45) HIV unaffected: 1.34 (0.86–2.10)
Dow et al. (2016)	Tanzania	12–24	182	– Depressive symptoms – Emotional and behavioural problems – PTSD	PHQ-9 SDQ UCLA-PTSD	Depressive symptoms: 12.1% Emotional/behavioural problems: 13.7% PTSD: 10%
Abubakar et al. (2017)	Kenya	Mean 14 years 4 months	Total = 130 PHIV = 44 HIV– = 33 PHEU = 53	– Depressive symptoms	BDI	**BDI scores, mean (SD)** PHIV vs HIV– 18.4 (8.3) vs 12.0 (7.9), $p < 0.001$ HIV– vs PHEU: 12.0 (7.9) vs 16.8 (7.3), $p = 0.007$
Bankole et al. (2017)	Nigeria	8–16	Total = 150 HIV+ = 75 HIV– = 75	– Major depression – Suicidality	MINI-KID	**Major depression:** HIV+ vs HIV–: 20% vs 6.7%, $p = 0.01$ **Suicidal ideation:** HIV+ vs HIV–: 16% vs 6.7%, $p = 0.07$ **Suicidal attempts:** HIV+ vs HIV–: 1.3% vs 0.0%, $p = 0.24$
Ashaba et al. (2018)	Uganda	13–17	224	– Major depression – Suicidality	MINI-KID	Major depression: 16% Suicidality (past month): 14%
Lwidiko et al. (2018)	Tanzania	7–17	Total = 900 HIV+ = 300 HIV– = 600	– Depressive symptoms	CDI-II	Depressive symptoms: HIV+ vs HIV–: 27% vs 5.8%, $p < 0.001$

(Continued)

Table 13.2 Continued

Study	Country	Age (range or mean) (years)	Sample size	Mental disorder(s)	Mental health measures used	Key finding (prevalence estimates unless otherwise stated)
Kinyanda et al. (2019)	Uganda	5–17	1339	– Generalised anxiety disorder – Separation anxiety disorder – Major depression – ADHD – ODD – Conduct disorder	CASI (CgR) YI-4R (self-report)	Generalised anxiety disorder: 5.4%[d] Separation anxiety disorder: 2.1%[d] Major depression: 0.2%[d] ADHD: 3.1%[d] ODD: 2.9%[d] Conduct disorder: 2.9%[d]
West et al. (2019)	South Africa	9–19	278	– Depressive symptoms – Anxiety symptoms – PTSD	CDI RCMAS Child PTSD Checklist	Depressive symptoms: 7.6% Anxiety symptoms: 6.7% PTSD: 27%
Durteste et al. (2019)	Ukraine	13–25	Total = 204 PHIV = 104 BHIV = 100	– Anxiety symptoms – Depressive symptoms	HADS	**Moderate/severe anxiety symptoms** Whole sample: 13% PHIV: 11% BHIV: 16% **Moderate/severe depressive symptoms** Whole sample: 5% PHIV: 3% BHIV: 7%

Aurpibul et al. (2021)	Cambodia, Thailand	13–17	195	– Depressive symptoms
				– Behavioural problems
					CDI (for young people <15 years)
					CES-D (for young people ≥15 years)
					CBCL
						Depressive symptoms: 20.7%
						CBCL (cutoff score ≥ 60):
						  Total: 14.6%
						  Externalising problems: 12.7%
						  Internalising problems: 18.2%

Table13.2 Continued

Study	Country	Age (range or mean) (years)	Sample size	Mental disorder(s)	Mental health measures used	Key finding (prevalence estimates unless otherwise stated)
Molinaro et al. (2021)	Zambia	8–17	Total = 416 PHIV = 208 PHEU = 208	– Depressive symptoms	PHQ-9 NIH Toolbox Sadness module	**PHQ-9 score, mean** PHIV vs PHEU: 2.0 vs 1.5, $p = 0.03$ **Sadness module t-score, mean** PHIV vs PHEU: 50 vs 44, $p < 0.01$ **Depression index Z-score, mean** PHIV vs PHEU: 0.23 vs 0.21, $p < 0.001$

Notes:

$*p = 0.02$ for HIV+ vs HIV−; all other $p > 0.12$ for psychiatric disorders between HIV+ and HIV− in that study.

[#]Odd ratios.

[‡]Includes obsessive compulsve disorder, psychosis, personality disorder, eating disorder, and substance use disorder; [a]reported prevalence based on caregiver report tool; [b]reported prevalence is at entry (baseline) and when symptom score for either tool equalled or exceeded the threshold necessary for a *DSM-IV* diagnosis; [c]prevalence estimates for current mental diagnoses based on the neuropsychological diagnoses interview tool, *p*-values for all comparisons were >0.05; [d]based on the self-report tool.

Abbreviations: ADHD: attention-deficit/hyperactivity disorder; BASC-2: Behavior Assessment System for Children, Second Edition; BDI: Beck Depression Inventory; BHIV: behaviourally infected with HIV; CASI: Child and Adolescent Symptom Inventory; CBCL: Child Behaviour Checklist; CDI: Child Depression Inventory; CES-DC: Centre for Epidemiologic Studies Depression Scale; CgR: caregiver report; DISC: Diagnostic Interview Schedule for Children (versions IV & 2.3); HADS: Hospital Anxiety and Depression Scale; MINI-KID: Mini-international Neuropsychiatric Interview for Children; NPD: Neuropsychological Diagnoses Interview; ODD: oppositional defiant disorder; PHEU: perinatally HIV exposed uninfected; PHIV: perinatally infected with HIV; PHQ-9: 9-item Patient Health Questionnaire; PTSD: post-traumatic stress disorder; RCMAS: Revised Children's Manifest Anxiety Scale; SDQ: Strengths and Difficulties Questionnaire; STAIC: State Trait Anxiety Inventory for Children; SUDs: substance use disorders; UCLA-PTSD: University of California Los Angeles Post-traumatic Stress Disorder; YI-4R: Revised Youth Inventory, Fourth Edition; YSR: Young person self-report.

The findings from the existing literature from select studies across contexts since 2010 suggest that psychiatric disorders among HIV-infected adolescents are still prevalent, depression and anxiety being the most common mental disorders. Suicidality and behavioural problems are also evident in these adolescents. Overall, studies including comparison groups of uninfected adolescents are limited, more so from LMICs. Some studies with comparison groups reported a significantly higher prevalence of psychiatric problems among HIV-infected adolescents compared to uninfected adolescents, while others observed insignificant between-group differences (Table 13.2). Additional epidemiological studies that compare the burden of psychiatric disorders between HIV-infected and uninfected adolescents are needed to inform intervention approaches appropriately.

Factors associated with mental disorders in HIV-infected adolescents are numerous and can be classified broadly as sociodemographic, psychosocial, and HIV-related. Studies in HICs have identified significant correlations for emotional and behavioural problems in HIV-infected adolescents. These include sociodemographic factors such as older age (Elkington et al. 2011; Mellins et al. 2011, 2012; Smith et al. 2019) and ethnicity, i.e. being black (Elkington et al. 2011); psychosocial factors like self-awareness of HIV infection (for younger age group) (Gadow et al. 2010), experience of stressful life events (Smith et al. 2019), caregiver HIV status (Elkington et al. 2011), caregiver depression (Elkington et al. 2011), birth mother as primary caregiver (Mellins et al. 2011), and poor adolescent–caregiver communication (Elkington et al. 2011); and HIV-related factors like undetectable viral load (Mellins et al. 2012).

Factors significantly associated with frequently occurring mental disorders in HIV-infected adolescents, i.e. depression and anxiety, have also been documented in HICs. For depression, these include sociodemographic factors such as sex (male sex) (Elkington et al. 2011), female sex (Le Prevost et al. 2018), older age (Mellins et al. 2012), ethnicity, i.e. being black (Elkington et al. 2011), and HIV-positive status (Elkington et al. 2011; Mellins et al. 2012); psychosocial factors like higher caregiver anxiety (Elkington et al. 2011), death of a parent (Le Prevost et al. 2018), exclusion from school activities (Le Prevost et al. 2018), low self-esteem (Le Prevost et al. 2018), and low social functioning (Le Prevost et al. 2018); and HIV-related factors like higher CD4+ count levels at entry into care (Gadow et al. 2012), higher viral load at study entry (Nachman et al. 2012), and poor antiretroviral adherence (Kacanek et al. 2015). For anxiety, identified sociodemographic correlates include sex (male sex) (Elkington et al. 2011), female sex (Mellins et al. 2012), and older age (Elkington et al. 2011; Mellins et al. 2012). Psychosocial factors such as higher caregiver depression (Elkington et al. 2011), having many caregivers (Le Prevost et al. 2018), history of suicidal ideation (Le Prevost et al. 2018), low self-esteem (Le Prevost et al. 2018), and low social functioning (Le Prevost et al. 2018) have been reported as significant correlates of anxiety. In their USA study, Kapetanovic et al. (2011) found that the presence of at least one of three risky health behaviours (pre-adult sexual activity, antiretroviral adherence problems, or substance abuse) was significantly associated with at least one psychiatric diagnosis (Table 13.2) among HIV-infected adolescents.

In LMICs, the literature on correlates of mental disorders among HIV-infected adolescents is largely based on SSA studies. These studies are primarily cross-sectional surveys, a large number of them focusing on common mental disorders – depression and anxiety. Findings must be interpreted with caution as inference on causality is limited with a cross-sectional study design. Some of the important correlates of common mental disorders in HIV-infected adolescents from SSA include sociodemographic factors like older age and female sex (Betancourt et al. 2014; Dow et al. 2016) and HIV-positive status (Lwidiko et al. 2018); psychosocial factors like being off-school for long periods (Dow et al. 2016), being bullied (Ashaba et al. 2018), a history of childhood deprivation (Lwidiko et al. 2018), experiencing negative life events (Molinaro et al. 2021), daily hardship, caregiver psychological distress, and harsh punishment

(Betancourt et al. 2014); and HIV-related factors like poor antiretroviral adherence (Dow et al. 2016) and HIV stigma (Betancourt et al. 2014; Dow et al. 2016). According to studies conducted in South Africa (Boyes et al. 2019; West et al. 2019), higher social support was protective against depressive and anxiety symptomatology. In Tanzania, rural residency was protective against depressive symptoms (Lwidiko et al. 2018). A study from Kenya (Abubakar et al. 2017) found that cumulative psychosocial risk among perinatally HIV-infected adolescents (orphanhood, caregiver depression, and family poverty) was significantly associated with higher depression scores.

Correlates of emotional and behavioural problems among HIV-infected adolescents from SSA have been reported by a few studies and include sociodemographic factors such as female sex (Betancourt et al. 2014; Kinyanda et al. 2019), older age (Kinyanda et al. 2019), and higher levels of education (Betancourt et al. 2014; Kinyanda et al. 2019); psychosocial factors like harsh punishments (Betancourt et al. 2014) and caregiver depression (Louw et al. 2016); and HIV-related factors like poor antiretroviral adherence (Dow et al. 2016) and HIV stigma (Betancourt et al. 2014; Dow et al. 2016).

Outside SSA, Zhou et al. (2021) investigated the correlates of depression in perinatally HIV-infected Chinese adolescents aged 8 to 18 years. In this study, greater social support was protective against depression. Conversely, social desirability and catastrophising (i.e. believing that one is in a worse situation than one actually is) were significantly correlated with higher levels of depression. In Thailand, Aurpibul et al. (2021) found low household income and caregiver mental disorders as independent risk factors for depressive symptoms. In Ukraine, Durteste et al. (2019) identified HIV-related stigma, drug use, low self-esteem, and non-disclosure of HIV status to family members as significant risk factors for depression and anxiety symptoms. In the same study, drug use and an unstable living situation, defined as changing homes more than twice in the past 3 years, were other major risk factors.

Little is known about interventions that address mental disorders among HIV-infected adolescents. Bhana et al. (2021), reviewing the state of the evidence on interventions to address the mental health of HIV-infected adolescents, identified only eight studies. Most intervention work has been carried out in SSA, understandably because this is the region where many HIV-infected adolescents live. Most of the interventions are targeted to treat depression in these adolescents. Even though few studies used evidence-based approaches such as cognitive behaviour therapy, Bhana et al. (2021) note that most applied approaches are promising, i.e. they show positive intervention effects on mental health.

In summary, mental disorders are prevalent among HIV-infected adolescents, depression and anxiety being the most frequent. These mental disorders are significantly associated with a range of sociodemographic, psychosocial, and HIV-related factors. More research on evidence-based intervention methods is needed to address the mental health of HIV-infected adolescents. A transdiagnostic model has been proposed to address co-occurring mental disorders (Remien et al. 2019). Factors that improve the mental health of HIV-infected adolescents, such as social capital, should also be incorporated into the treatment package (Too et al. 2021). Considering resource constraints in LMICs, integrating mental health treatment into primary health care services and digital health approaches can support scalable treatments (Bhana et al. 2021).

PSYCHOSOCIAL OR BEHAVIOURAL ADJUSTMENT

Adherence to Antiretroviral Therapy

The UNAIDS' Fast-Track target of 95-95-95 HIV treatment highlights the importance of adherence in preventing new HIV infections, reducing mortality, and ending the HIV epidemic by 2030. Under the Fast-Track approach, governments have been called upon to exercise effective leadership and to invest in research, improved clinical experience, and diagnostic procedures (UNAIDS 2016b). In 2020, 54% (about 940 000) of adolescents living with HIV globally received antiretroviral treatment (ART). The lowest ART coverage was in West and Central Africa (43%) and the highest in South Asia (61%). In general, access to ART globally was slightly higher for males than for females (55% vs 53%) (UNICEF 2021a). The level of access to ART improved from a figure of 9% for females and 13% for males to 53% for females and 55% for males by 2021. Maintaining adherence to ART presents significant challenges for optimising health outcomes in HIV-infected adolescents (WHO 2003, 2013). AIDS-related deaths (estimated at 32 000 in 2020 among adolescents) have reduced at the slowest rate among adolescents compared to any other age group (UNICEF 2021a). This is explained by delayed treatment initiation and poor treatment adherence in the adolescent group (UNAIDS 2016a). It is suspected that HIV-infected adolescents are worse ART adherents compared to their adult counterparts. One South African observational cohort study reported a two-fold or higher proportion of adults that achieved 100% adherence when compared to adolescent patients at 6 months (20.7% vs 40.5%), 12 months (14.3% vs 27.9%), and 24 months (6.6% vs 20.6%) follow-up periods (Nachega et al. 2009). A 2014 systematic review of 50 studies on ART adherence in adolescent and young adult populations (12–24 years) reported that 62.3% of this subpopulation was adherent to ART. It also indicated that adherence was higher in Africa and Asia compared to Europe and North America (Kim et al. 2014). Another systematic review on pediatric adherence to ART documents adherence rates of 49% to 100% (Vreeman et al. 2008) among children and adolescents from LMICs compared to 20% to 100% among high-income settings (Simoni et al. 2007). Of note is that single-time assessment of adherence may mask high rates of variability in adherence over time. Findings from a prospective cohort among South African adolescents showed that whereas 'past-week' ART adherence was high (66%, 65%, and 75% at baseline, wave 2, and wave 3 respectively), only 37% of the adolescents sustained 'past-week' ART adherence over the three waves (3 years) of the study. The majority of adolescents reported inconsistent adherence over the three waves (Zhou et al. 2021).

Other studies have reported poorer virological suppression among adolescents compared to the older HIV-positive patient population. These results reveal worse ART adherence in younger age groups (Nglazi et al. 2011; Evans et al. 2013; Hassan et al. 2014). One Kenyan study of 232 HIV-infected people aged 15 years and older reported three-fold odds of virological failure among patients with unsatisfactory adherence. Prevalence of virological failure (53.3%) and drug resistance (40%) was highest in the 15 to 24-year-old age group (Hassan et al. 2014). Self-reported non-adherence was 16.6%, and viral non-suppression was 17.4% among Ugandan adolescents (Brathwaite et al. 2021). Poor ART adherence, along with other treatment gaps like late ART initiation and poor treatment retention (WHO 2013), may underlie the elevated rate of HIV-related deaths among adolescents when compared to the decreasing trends in all other age categories (WHO 2013; UNAIDS 2016b). It is estimated that between 2005 and 2012 there was a 30% reduction in overall HIV-related deaths yet, among adolescents, the HIV-related deaths increased by 50% during the same period (WHO 2013). Poor adherence is also associated with drug resistance, which dramatically increases the per capita costs of maintaining patients on second-line treatments (Muya et al. 2015). Likewise, it causes unnecessary suffering to patients due to accelerated disease progression, psychosocial disease-related complications, comorbidities, and mortality (Chesney 2000; WHO 2003, 2013). Adolescents must be supported in overcoming and coping with the numerous challenges they face during long-term HIV treatment (WHO 2013). Adherence problems manifest in most situations that necessitate self-administration of treatment, regardless of disease severity and accessibility to health resources (WHO 2003). Poor adherence is attributed to numerous factors, including patient-related, therapy-related, health system-related, and social–economic factors (WHO 2003, 2013). Adolescents increasingly seek autonomy and independence from their parents and authorities, which is often a contributing factor to poor treatment adherence (Taddeo, Egedy, and Frappier 2008). Adolescents also transition from HIV-paediatric services, where parents and guardians make treatment and care decisions, to adult health care services, where patient autonomy and full responsibility are expected (WHO 2013). Additionally, HIV-positive adolescents need to withstand numerous challenges, including HIV-associated stigma, depression, fatigue, pill burden, complexity of regimens, medical side effects, lack of caregiver availability, lack of youth-friendly services, household poverty, mental ill health, inadequate planning, and poor organisation skills (Taddeo, Egedy, and Frappier 2008; Vreeman et al. 2008; Reisner et al. 2009; WHO 2013; Nabukeera-Barungi et al. 2015; Foster, Ayers, and Fidler 2020).

Community, group, and individual adherence support, e-Health, and youth-friendly services are promising interventions for improving ART adherence among HIV-infected adolescents (Foster, Ayers, and Fidler 2020). Engagement with community-based support workers or peer-to-peer treatment support networks has been shown to improve adherence to ART, adolescents' self-esteem, linkage to services and retention in HIV care in various settings, for example, in Zimbabwe (Willis et al. 2019) and South Africa (Fatti et al. 2018). A systematic review of 27 studies on the use of mobile health technologies to promote adherence and retention to ART in LMICs indicated that more than half (56%) the studies had statistically significant effects (Demena et al. 2020). Effective mobile health interventions included those using SMS health messages and appointment reminders and interactive voice responses. There is also growing evidence demonstrating that conditional economic incentive programmes, such as cash transfer programmes, can improve ART adherence, viral suppression, and retention in HIV care for HIV-positive adolescents (Cluver et al. 2016; El-Sadr et al. 2017; Galárraga et al. 2020). However, there is a need for more rigorously evaluated ART adherence intervention since many studies comprise small sample sizes without appropriate comparison groups, some have an inadequate length of follow-up, and there is a common tendency to utilise surrogate measures of adherence rather than plasma HIV viral load (Foster, Ayers, and Fidler 2020).

Health Risk Behaviour

Health risk behaviour (HRB) is a major public health concern for adolescents. By the age of 15 years, adolescents have fully developed their logical-reasoning abilities; however, their psychosocial capacities for decision-making and moderating risk-taking behaviours will not be fully mature until young adulthood (Steinberg 2008). Adolescents often struggle with emotional regulation, peer influence, delayed gratification, and impulse control, all of which make them prone to risk-taking behaviours (Kelley, Schochet, and Landry 2004; Steinberg 2008; Chein et al. 2011). HRBs like alcohol abuse, drug use, risky sexual behaviour, sedentary lifestyle, poor dietary habits, and behaviour resulting in injury are the leading causes of disabilities and death in adolescents. By 2019, globally one-third of all adolescent deaths were attributable to unintentional injuries or interpersonal violence and conflict. Self-harm also accounted for 8% globally of all adolescent deaths in the same period (Ward et al. 2021). Unsafe sexual behaviour also accounted for most of the 150 000 new HIV infections among adolescents in 2020 (UNICEF 2021a).

Most research on adolescents' HRB focuses on the general adolescent population. In regions with high HIV prevalence, such as SSA and South Asia, reports indicate that adolescent females become sexually active before age 15 years at higher rates than adolescent males (Doyle et al. 2012; Idele et al. 2014). Surveys from South Asia indicate that up to 8% of females and 3% of males age 15 through 19 years have had early sexual activity (Idele et al. 2014). Similarly, national survey data of young people from 24 SSA countries indicate that between 2% and 27% of adolescents have had early sexual activity. This is disproportionately higher in females in West Africa, but it is equal among males and females from Central, Eastern, and Southern Africa (Doyle et al. 2012). The occurrence of early sexual activity is often coupled with non-condom use, sexual violence, and multiple sexual partnerships, as well as child sexual exploitation in the form of early marriages, transactional sex, and sex in the context of power and age asymmetries (Doyle et al. 2012; Joint United Nations Programme on HIV/AIDS 2014; Idele et al. 2014; WHO 2014). High occurrence of multiple sexual partnerships among adolescents has been reported in both low and high HIV-prevalence countries, including Jamaica (39%), the Ivory Coast (32%), and Mozambique (18%) (Doyle et al. 2012; Idele et al. 2014).

Among HIV-infected adolescents, the occurrence of HRB (e.g. risky sexual behaviour, violence and injury, substance use, and unhealthy dietary habits) is of major concern because of its implications for retention in HIV care, ART adherence, and the prevention of HIV transmission (Toska et al. 2017; Ross et al. 2019). There is growing research on HRB among HIV-infected adolescents. Systematic reviews on HRB from SSA have found no significant differences in the burden of HRB among HIV-infected adolescents compared to their non-infected peers (Toska et al. 2017; Ssewanyana et al. 2018; Zgambo, Kalembo, and Mbakaya 2018). Notably, the HRB burden is unacceptably high. The burden of sexual related behaviour (e.g. not using a condom, transactional sex, early sexual debut) among HIV-infected adolescents in SSA, for example, ranges somewhere from 14% to 64% (Ssewanyana et al. 2018; Zgambo, Kalembo, and Mbakaya 2018). Some studies reveal that between 12% and 60% of HIV-infected adolescents have exchanged sex for goods or gifts, which increases the concern about their ability to negotiate for safe sex in such relationships (Gavin et al. 2006; Jaspan et al. 2006; Jewkes et al. 2006; Test et al. 2012). A study conducted in Ugandan HIV-treatment centres found that 53% of sexually active individuals were not using condoms (Birungi et al. 2009). Similar findings were reported in Rwanda, where 56% of adolescents attending an ART clinic reported inconsistent condom use (Test et al. 2012). Elsewhere, a prospective cohort study among HIV-infected adolescents conducted in Malaysia, Thailand, and Vietnam also found that there were no significant differences between the proportions of HIV-infected adolescents and controls who drank alcohol (58% vs 65%), had been sexually active (31% vs 21%), and consistently used condoms (42% vs 44%) (Ross et al. 2019). A study from the USA found that 57% of perinatally HIV-infected adolescents had engaged in vaginal/anal sex. Of those who reported sexual intercourse, 13% had condomless sex in the previous 3 months (Benson et al. 2018). Another longitudinal study from the USA found that the occurrence of unprotected sex among sexually active, HIV-infected young people was 52.6% at baseline and 48.8% at follow-up (Elkington et al. 2015). HIV-infected adolescents are also likely to experience coerced sexual intercourse. High prevalence of rape by coercion – for example, 30% (Gavin et al. 2006) and 27% (Birungi et al. 2009) – has been reported in this patient subpopulation. Substance use is increasingly documented among HIV-infected adolescents and has been shown to co-occur with other forms of HRB and with mental illness in this subpopulation (Gavin et al. 2006; Test et al. 2012; Elkington et al. 2015; Mutumba et al. 2016b; Ssewanyana et al. 2020). Prevalence of substance use symptoms rose from 35.7% at baseline to 75.5% during follow-up (Mutumba et al. 2016b), and another study (Alperen et al. 2014) reported a 60% prevalence of lifetime alcohol use, 27% marijuana use, and 25% tobacco use among HIV-infected adolescents in the USA. Another study found that substance use disorder increased from 1.8% when perinatally HIV-infected adolescents were, on average, 12 years old, to 4.2% when they were 14 years old (Mellins et al. 2012). Depression and anxiety are significantly associated with the onset of sexual behaviour and substance use during early to middle adolescence (9–16 years) among HIV-infected adolescents (Mellins et al. 2009; Benson et al. 2018; Ssewanyana et al. 2020).

Evidence suggests that HIV-infected adolescents experience conditions that predispose them to various forms of HRB. These include the psychosocial impact of negative life events, such as the loss of close family members, orphanhood, stigma, social exclusion, household poverty, the quality of the caregiver's relationship with the adolescent, personal sickness, and living with a sick caregiver (Swendeman et al. 2006; Birdthistle et al. 2008; Mellins et al. 2011; Nakigozi et al. 2012; Alperen et al. 2014; Mutumba et al. 2016b). Biological factors, such as mental illness, and neurocognitive deficits, such as executive function deficits, are predisposing factors for HRB in HIV-infected adolescents (Brown and Lourie 2000; Anand et al. 2010; Romer et al. 2011; Benson et al. 2018).

The Disclosure of HIV Status to Adolescents

Disclosing the disease status of an HIV-infected patient is a difficult but necessary part of HIV care (Wiener et al. 2007; Hazra, Siberry, and Mofenson 2010). Knowledge about HIV status positively impacts ART adherence, lifestyle choices, and health care decision-making participation (Lesch et al. 2007; Hazra, Siberry, and Mofenson 2010). HIV-infected adolescents from Zambia indicated that disclosure led to better ART access and improved psychosocial support from family and peers (Mburu et al. 2014). Many caregivers view disclosing disease status as a one-time event (Vreeman et al. 2013); however, disclosure is a dynamic, longitudinal process that should be tailored to a patient's age and cognitive level. Both the adolescent and their family should be seen as a treatment unit, with consideration for unique familial and contextual concerns (Lesch et al. 2007; Hazra, Siberry, and Mofenson 2010). Fortunately, research interest in disease-status disclosure among children and adolescents is growing. Available evidence suggests that disclosure to HIV-infected children and adolescents, especially from regions with high HIV prevalence, is still poor (Oberdorfer et al. 2006; Turissini et al. 2013; Vreeman et al. 2013). Only 10% of Western Kenyan caregivers of children aged 6 through 14 years enrolled in an HIV care programme had disclosed the child's HIV status to the child (Turissini et al. 2013). Another study from Thailand found an HIV disclosure rate of 30%, with a mean age of disclosure of 9 years. Most (84.3%) patients had only received partial disclosure about their disease status (Oberdorfer et al. 2006). Similarly, a systematic review on disclosure of HIV status to children from resource-limited settings – including SSA, parts of Europe, Asia, and South America – found that between 0% and 69% of children living with HIV had been told by their caregivers that they had HIV(Vreeman et al. 2013). Overall, disclosure of HIV status to HIV-infected children and adolescents in LMICs is lower and occurs later (approximately 20% at a median age of 10 years) compared to HICs (about 43% at a median age of 8 years) (Pinzón-Iregui, Beck-Sagué, and Malow 2013).

Children and adolescents living with HIV often have limited control over when and how they are informed of their HIV status (Lesch et al. 2007). While some caregivers understand the benefits of timely disclosure, many caregivers who disclose disease status do so secondary to concerns regarding accidental disclosure, adolescent sexual activity, questions regarding medication, a high number of clinic visits, and recurring sickness (Lesch et al. 2007; Turissini et al. 2013). Many caregivers often presume that the child or adolescent is too young to comprehend the consequences of an HIV diagnosis (Lesch et al. 2007; Mburu et al. 2014; Ubesie et al. 2016). Caregivers and health providers also often have different perceptions of what entails disclosure (Lesch et al. 2007). Disclosure of HIV status can be daunting for health care providers due to unclear guidelines and insufficient training in paediatric HIV disclosure (Sariah et al. 2016). Other factors that influence non-disclosure or late disclosure include caregiver related factors (sex, HIV status, disclosure experiences, guilt and anxiety about being asked about their own infection), adolescent patient characteristics (age, sex, cognitive abilities, child–caregiver relationship), and community-related factors (community norms surrounding sexuality communication, family related dynamics, fear of stigma, level of support from health care providers fear for stigma) (Oberdorfer et al. 2006; Lesch et al. 2007; Turissini et al. 2013; Kidia et al. 2014; Mburu et al. 2014).

The State of Adolescent HIV Care During the COVID-19 Pandemic

The coronavirus outbreak that began in 2019 (COVID-19) has led to massive disruptions to economies, health systems, and social life across the globe. This threatens to reverse the gains in preventing and treating HIV (UNICEF 2021b). By early 2020, about 2.8 million children and adolescents (age 0–19 years) and 1.3 million pregnant females living with HIV were estimated to face a significant risk of experiencing adverse effects due to COVID-19 control measures (UNICEF 2020). The mitigation strategies being undertaken in response to COVID-19 have led to a scaling back of certain activities and care-seeking; reduced capabilities of the health system as a result of high demand for the care of patients with COVID-19; and disruptions to domestic and international supply chains of various commodities (Hogan et al. 2020).

For adolescents, the most significant concerns were that the complex adolescent-specific challenges to adhering to ART and remaining in HIV care, in addition to the mental health challenges related to HIV stigma, isolation, and trauma, might be compounded during the COVID-19 pandemic (Banati and Idele 2021; Enane et al. 2021; Waterfield et al. 2021). COVID-19 related restrictions and health consequences have led to isolation and trauma, besides heightening disruptions to adolescents' schooling, work, and social activities. A Kenyan study on the effects of the pandemic on the well-being of HIV-infected adolescents identified numerous challenges, including an increase in school disengagement (46% during COVID-19 compared to 36% pre-COVID); a third of adolescents reporting lost income for someone they relied on; 40% experiencing food insecurity; and several adolescents described challenges in taking ART. In the same study, a large proportion (15%) of HIV-infected adolescents reported at least one mental health symptom from depression or anxiety screening tools (Enane et al. 2021). Research indicates that although ART provision was generally maintained during the COVID-19 lockdown, HIV testing and ART initiations were heavily impacted. A South African study from 65 primary care clinics estimated a 48% decline in HIV testing and a 46% decrease in ART initiations during the COVID-19 lockdown periods; however, these gradually improved when restrictions eased (Dorward et al. 2021). In many countries, orphans and vulnerable children have been severely affected as a result of HIV care and treatment clinic hours being reduced, medical personnel being re-deployed from HIV services to COVID-19 services, and the movement of community health workers being restricted such that they are unable to do mobile outreach or home visits (Waterfield et al. 2021). Furthermore, during the COVID-19 lockdown, females disproportionately experienced increased abuse, maltreatment, and violence in their households (Banati and Idele 2021; Waterfield et al. 2021).

While a path to ending the COVID-19 pandemic appears closer with the introduction of vaccines, evidence-informed policies and strategies among countries are needed to support engagement in care and positive mental health among HIV-infected adolescents across settings. On a practical level, this includes developing strategies for clinics to identify and respond to the emerging needs of HIV-infected adolescents, facilitation of in-person care whenever needed, and a need to adapt clinic services to virtual/phone modalities. It is imperative to expand the reach of helplines to address those issues that are sensitive to adolescents, to expand virtual safe spaces to combat violence or abuse, and to provide online counselling. It is important to adapt programmes to the COVID-19 situation and expand the reach of programmes that mitigate economic impacts, including child grants, income-generating activities for caregivers, food distribution, health care vouchers, and other economic empowerment interventions (Banati and Idele 2021; UNICEF 2021b). Working across sectors to address multiple vulnerabilities, utilising evidence-driven programming, building on the strengthening of community systems, and providing people-centred service and support are crucial for improved HIV care and prevention during (and after) the COVID-19 era (UNICEF 2021b).

CONCLUSION

The population of HIV-infected adolescents is expected to continue increasing, especially in LMICs, where HIV has had its greatest impact over the past three decades. This chapter has illustrated the existing regional disparities in research on HIV and the implications for adolescence. This lack of research is even more evident in specific populations, including adolescents residing in SSA, which accounts for the greatest share of HIV-infected adolescents. There is a major dearth of research and tailored interventions for key adolescent populations: for example, adolescent sex workers, adolescents who inject drugs, and adolescents who are LGBTQIA+. More research is required to better understand the implications of HIV exposure and infection on adolescents and throughout the life course. There is also a need for a more pragmatic and human-rights centred approach to research and service delivery, which will enable the inclusion of marginalised and under-represented segments of the HIV-infected adolescent community. Research oriented toward improving the quality of life in HIV-infected adolescents is a reasonable 'next step', especially considering improved access to ART. Although monitoring medical and treatment outcomes, including viral suppression and ART adherence, is essential, other issues for HIV-infected adolescents, including mental health, neurocognitive outcomes, stigma, psychosocial well-being, and HIV disclosure status should also be prioritised. Of note, the burden, mechanisms, relatedness, implications, risk factors, and protective factors underlying neurocognitive impairment, mental illness, and HRB among HIV-positive adolescents are still poorly understood, especially in high-prevalence settings like SSA. These determinant factors for self-regulation, quality of life, independence, and productivity during adolescence and adulthood require more research. Such research requires that utilised models extensively explore risk and protective factors across various ecological domains (e.g. individuals, peers, family, community, school environment, and public policy) and that testing of age- and context-appropriate interventions to address neurocognitive impairment, mental illness, and HRB in HIV-infected adolescents is conducted. Implementation research is critical for understanding scalability and for guiding future policy and interventions. It is imperative that interventions utilise existing resources within communities and that caregivers and family members are engaged in intervention methods. Future epidemiological and implementation research on the health and well-being of HIV-infected adolescents and on implementation strategies and their impact on policy is the next logical step in establishing both increased survival and increased quality of life in this population, especially in low-resource settings with a high HIV prevalence.

REFERENCES

Abas M, Ali GC, Nakimuli-Mpungu E et al. (2014) Depression in people living with HIV in sub-Saharan Africa: Time to act. *Tropical Medicine & International Health*, 19: 1392–1396.

Abubakar A, Van de Vijver FJ, Hassan AS et al. (2017) Cumulative psychosocial risk is a salient predictor of depressive symptoms among vertically HIV-infected and HIV-affected adolescents at the Kenyan Coast. *Annals of Global Health*, 83. 743–752.

Ali G-C, Ryan G, De Silva MJ (2016) Validated screening tools for common mental disorders in low and middle income countries: A systematic review. *PLoS One*, 11: e0156939.

Alperen J, Brummel S, Tassiopoulos K et al. (2014) Prevalence of and risk factors for substance use among perinatally human immunodeficiency virus–infected and perinatally exposed but uninfected youth. *Journal of Adolescent Health*, 54: 341–349.

Anand P, Springer SA, Copenhaver MM et al. (2010) Neurocognitive impairment and HIV risk factors: A reciprocal relationship. *AIDS and Behavior*, 14: 1213–1226.

Ashaba S, Cooper-Vince C, Maling S et al. (2018) Internalized HIV stigma, bullying, major depressive disorder, and high-risk suicidality among HIV-positive adolescents in rural Uganda. *Global Mental Health*, 5: e22–e22.

Atkinson J, McCurdy S, Williams M et al. (2011) HIV risk behaviours, perceived severity of drug use problems, and prior treatment experience in a sample of young heroin injectors in Dar es Salaam, Tanzania. *African Journal of Drug and Alcohol Studies*, 10: 1–9.

Aurpibul L, Sophonphan J, Malee K et al. (2021) HIV-related enacted stigma and increased frequency of depressive symptoms among Thai and Cambodian adolescents and young adults with perinatal HIV. *International Journal of STD & AIDS*, 32: 246–256.

Baggaley R, Armstrong A, Dodd Z et al. (2015) Young key populations and HIV: A special emphasis and consideration in the new WHO Consolidated Guidelines on HIV Prevention, Diagnosis, Treatment and Care for Key Populations. *Journal of the International AIDS Society*, 18(2 Suppl 1): 19438.

Banati P, Idele P (2021) Addressing the mental and emotional health impacts of COVID-19 on children and adolescents: Lessons from HIV/AIDS. *Frontiers in Psychiatry*, 12: 589827.

Bankole KO, Bakare MO, Edet BE et al. (2017) Psychological complications associated with HIV/AIDS infection among children in South-South Nigeria, sub-Saharan Africa. *Cogent Medicine*, 4: 1372869.

Becker ML, Bhattacharjee P, Blanchard JF et al. (2018) Vulnerabilities at first sex and their association with lifetime gender-based violence and HIV prevalence among adolescent girls and young women engaged in sex work, transactional sex, and casual sex in Kenya. *Journal of Acquired Immune Deficiency Syndromes (1999)*, 79: 296.

Bekker L-G, Johnson L, Wallace M et al. (2015) Building our youth for the future. *Journal of the International AIDS Society*, 18: 20027.

Benson S, Elkington KS, Leu C-S et al. (2018) Association between psychiatric disorders, substance use, and sexual risk behaviors in perinatally HIV-exposed youth. *Journal of the Association of Nurses in AIDS Care*, 29: 538–549.

Betancourt T, Scorza P, Kanyanganzi F et al. (2014) HIV and child mental health: A case-control study in Rwanda. *Pediatrics*, 134: e464–e472.

Bhana A, Kreniske P, Pather A et al. (2021) Interventions to address the mental health of adolescents and young adults living with or affected by HIV: State of the evidence. *Journal of the International AIDS Society*, 24: e25713.

Bhatia A, Fabbri C, Cerna-Turoff I et al. (2021) Violence against children during the COVID-19 pandemic. *Bulletin of the World Health Organization*, 99: 730.

Birdthistle IJ, Floyd S, Machingura A et al. (2008) From affected to infected? Orphanhood and HIV risk among female adolescents in urban Zimbabwe. *Aids*, 22: 759–766.

Birungi H, Obare F, Mugisha JF et al. (2009) Preventive service needs of young people perinatally infected with HIV in Uganda. *AIDS Care*, 21: 725–731.

Boyes ME, Cluver LD, Meinck F et al. (2019) Mental health in South African adolescents living with HIV: Correlates of internalising and externalising symptoms. *AIDS Care*, 31: 95–104.

Brackis-Cott E, Kang E, Dolezal C et al. (2009) The impact of perinatal HIV infection on older school-aged children's and adolescents' receptive language and word recognition skills. *AIDS Patient Care and STDs*, 23: 415–421.

Brathwaite R, Ssewamala FM, Neilands TB et al. (2021) Predicting the individualized risk of poor adherence to ART medication among adolescents living with HIV in Uganda: The Suubi+ Adherence study. *Journal of the International AIDS Society*, 24: e25756.

Brown LK, Lourie KJ (2000) Children and adolescents living with HIV and AIDS: A review. *Journal of Child Psychology and Psychiatry*, 41: 81–96.

CDC (2015) *HIV Among Youth*. Available at: https://www.cdc.gov/hiv/group/age/youth/.

Chein J, Albert D, O'Brien L et al. (2011) Peers increase adolescent risk taking by enhancing activity in the brain's reward circuitry. *Developmental Science* 14: F1–F10.

Chesney MA (2000) Factors affecting adherence to antiretroviral therapy. *Clinical Infectious Diseases*, 30: S171–S176.

Clark H, Babu AS, Wiewel EW et al. (2017) Diagnosed HIV infection in transgender adults and adolescents: Results from the National HIV Surveillance System, 2009–2014. *AIDS and Behavior*, 21: 2774–2783.

Cluver L, Toska E, Orkin F et al. (2016) Achieving equity in HIV-treatment outcomes: Can social protection improve adolescent ART-adherence in South Africa? *AIDS Care*, 28: 73–82.

Couture M-C, Sansothy N, Sapphon V et al. (2011) Young women engaged in sex work in Phnom Penh, Cambodia, have high incidence of HIV and sexually transmitted infections, and amphetamine-type stimulant use: New challenges to HIV prevention and risk. *Sexually Transmitted Diseases*, 38: 33.

Day S, Kapogiannis BG, Shah SK et al. (2020) Adolescent participation in HIV research: Consortium experience in low- and middle-income countries and scoping review. *The Lancet HIV*, 7: e844–e852.

de Andrade ME, Santos IHF, de Souza AAM et al. (2017) Experimentation with psychoactive substances by public school students. *Revista de Saúde Pública*, 51: 82.

Demena BA, Artavia-Mora L, Ouedraogo D et al. (2020) A systematic review of mobile phone interventions (SMS/IVR/calls) to improve adherence and retention to antiretroviral treatment in low-and middle-income countries. *AIDS Patient Care and STDs*, 34: 59–71.

Dorward J, Khubone T, Gate K et al. (2021) The impact of the COVID-19 lockdown on HIV care in 65 South African primary care clinics: An interrupted time series analysis. *The Lancet HIV*, 8: e158–e165.

Dow DE, Turner EL, Shayo AM et al. (2016) Evaluating mental health difficulties and associated outcomes among HIV-positive adolescents in Tanzania. *AIDS Care*, 28: 825–833.

Doyle AM, Mavedzenge SN, Plummer ML et al. (2012) The sexual behaviour of adolescents in sub-Saharan Africa: Patterns and trends from national surveys. *Tropical Medicine & International Health*, 17: 796–807.

Durteste M, Kyselyova G, Volokha A et al. (2019) Anxiety symptoms and felt stigma among young people living with perinatally or behaviourally-acquired HIV in Ukraine: A cross-sectional survey. *PloS One*, 14: e0210412.

El-Sadr WM, Donnell D, Beauchamp G et al. (2017) Financial incentives for linkage to care and viral suppression among HIV-positive patients: A randomized clinical trial (HPTN 065). *JAMA Internal Medicine*, 177: 1083–1092.

Elkington KS, Robbins RN, Bauermeister JA et al. (2011) Mental health in youth infected with and affected by HIV: The role of caregiver HIV. *Journal of Pediatric Psychology*, 36: 360–373.

Elkington KS, Bauermeister JA, Santamaria EK et al. (2015) Substance use and the development of sexual risk behaviors in youth perinatally exposed to HIV. *Journal of Pediatric Psychology*, 40: 442–454.

Enane LA, Apondi E, Aluoch J et al. (2021) Social, economic, and health effects of the COVID-19 pandemic on adolescents retained in or recently disengaged from HIV care in Kenya. *PloS One*, 16: e0257210.

Evans D, Menezes C, Mahomed K et al. (2013) Treatment outcomes of HIV-infected adolescents attending public-sector HIV clinics across Gauteng and Mpumalanga, South Africa. *AIDS Research and Human Retroviruses*, 29: 892–900.

Ezeamama AE, Kizza FN, Zalwango SK et al. (2016) Perinatal HIV status and executive function during school-age and adolescence: A comparative study of long-term cognitive capacity among children from a high HIV prevalence setting. *Medicine*, 95: 17.

Fatti G, Jackson D, Goga AE et al. (2018) The effectiveness and cost-effectiveness of community-based support for adolescents receiving antiretroviral treatment: An operational research study in South Africa. *Journal of the International AIDS Society*, 21: e25041.

Foster C, Ayers S, Fidler S (2020) Antiretroviral adherence for adolescents growing up with HIV: Understanding real life, drug delivery and forgiveness. *Therapeutic Advances in Infectious Disease*, 7: 2049936120920177.

Gadow KD, Chernoff M, Williams PL et al. (2010) Co-occuring psychiatric symptoms in children perinatally infected with HIV and peer comparison sample. *Journal of Developmental and Behavioral Pediatrics*, 31: 116.

Gadow KD, Angelidou K, Chernoff M et al. (2012) Longitudinal study of emerging mental health concerns in youth perinatally infected with HIV and peer comparisons. *Journal of Developmental and Behavioral Pediatrics*, 33: 456.

Galárraga O, Enimil A, Bosomtwe D et al. (2020) Group-based economic incentives to improve adherence to antiretroviral therapy among youth living with HIV: Safety and preliminary efficacy from a pilot trial. *Vulnerable Children and Youth Studies*, 15: 257–268.

Garvie PA, Zeldow B, Malee K et al. (2014) Discordance of cognitive and academic achievement outcomes in youth with perinatal HIV exposure. *The Pediatric Infectious Disease Journal*, 33: e232.

Gavin L, Galavotti C, Dube H et al. (2006) Factors associated with HIV infection in adolescent females in Zimbabwe. *Journal of Adolescent Health*, 39: 596. e511–e596. e518.

Guessoum SB, Lachal J, Radjack R et al. (2020) Adolescent psychiatric disorders during the COVID-19 pandemic and lockdown. *Psychiatry Research*, 291: 113264.

Hassan AS, Nabwera HM, Mwaringa SM et al. (2014) HIV-1 virologic failure and acquired drug resistance among first-line antiretroviral experienced adults at a rural HIV clinic in coastal Kenya: A cross-sectional study. *AIDS Research and Therapy*, 11: 1.

Hazra R, Siberry GK, Mofenson LM (2010) Growing up with HIV: Children, adolescents, and young adults with perinatally acquired HIV infection. *Annual Review of Medicine*, 61: 169–185.

Hermetet-Lindsay KD, Correia KF, Williams PL et al. (2017) Contributions of disease severity, psychosocial factors, and cognition to behavioral functioning in US youth perinatally exposed to HIV. *AIDS and Behavior*, 21: 2703–2715.

Hogan AB, Jewell BL, Sherrard-Smith E et al. (2020) Potential impact of the COVID-19 pandemic on HIV, tuberculosis, and malaria in low-income and middle-income countries: A modelling study. *The Lancet Global Health*, 8: e1132–e1141.

Idele P, Gillespie A, Porth T et al. (2014) Epidemiology of HIV and AIDS among adolescents: Current status, inequities, and data gaps. *Journal of Acquired Immune Deficiency Syndromes*, 66: S144–S153.

Jaspan HB, Berwick JR, Myer L et al. (2006) Adolescent HIV prevalence, sexual risk, and willingness to participate in HIV vaccine trials. *Journal of Adolescent Health*, 39: 642–648.

Jewkes R, Dunkle K, Nduna M et al. (2006) Factors associated with HIV sero-status in young rural South African women: Connections between intimate partner violence and HIV. *International Journal of Epidemiology*, 35: 1461–1468.

Jewkes RK, Dunkle K, Nduna M et al. (2010) Intimate partner violence, relationship power inequity, and incidence of HIV infection in young women in South Africa: A cohort study. *The Lancet*, 376: 41–48.

Joffres C, Mills E, Joffres M et al. (2008) Sexual slavery without borders: Trafficking for commercial sexual exploitation in India. *International Journal for Equity in Health*, 7: 1.

Joint United Nations Programme on HIV/AIDS (UNAIDS) (2014) *The Gap Report*. Geneva: UNAIDS.

Kacanek D, Angelidou K, Williams PL et al. (2015) Psychiatric symptoms and antiretroviral non-adherence in US youth with perinatal HIV: A longitudinal study. *AIDS (London, England)*, 29: 1227.

Kamau JW, Kuria W, Mathai M et al. (2012) Psychiatric morbidity among HIV-infected children and adolescents in a resource-poor Kenyan urban community. *AIDS Care*, 24: 836–842.

Kapetanovic S, Wiegand RE, Dominguez K et al. (2011) Associations of medically documented psychiatric diagnoses and risky health behaviors in highly active antiretroviral therapy-experienced perinatally HIV-infected youth. *AIDS Patient Care and STDs*, 25: 493–501.

Kelley AE, Schochet T, Landry CF (2004) Risk taking and novelty seeking in adolescence: Introduction to part I. *Annals of the New York Academy of Sciences*, 1021: 27–32.

Kerr SJ, Puthanakit T, Malee KM et al. (2019) Increased risk of executive function and emotional behavioral problems among virologically well-controlled perinatally HIV-infected adolescents in Thailand and Cambodia. *Journal of Acquired Immune Deficiency Syndromes*, 82: 297–304.

Kidia KK, Mupambireyi Z, Cluver L et al. (2014) HIV status disclosure to perinatally-infected adolescents in Zimbabwe: A qualitative study of adolescent and healthcare worker perspectives. *PloS One*, 9: e87322.

Kim S-H, Gerver SM, Fidler S et al. (2014) Adherence to antiretroviral therapy in adolescents living with HIV: Systematic review and meta-analysis. *AIDS (London, England)*, 28: 1945.

Kinyanda E, Salisbury TT, Levin J et al. (2019) Rates, types and co-occurrence of emotional and behavioural disorders among perinatally HIV-infected youth in Uganda: The CHAKA study. *Social Psychiatry and Psychiatric Epidemiology*, 54: 415–425.

Koekkoek S, de Sonneville LM, Wolfs TF et al. (2008) Neurocognitive function profile in HIV-infected school-age children. *European Journal of Paediatric Neurology*, 12: 290–297.

Kreniske P, Mellins CA, Dolezal C et al. (2021) Predictors of attempted suicide among youth living with perinatal HIV infection and perinatal HIV-exposed uninfected counterparts. *JAIDS Journal of Acquired Immune Deficiency Syndromes*, 88: 348–355.

Lau C (2008) Child prostitution in Thailand. *Journal of Child Health Care*, 12: 144–155.

Le Prevost M, Arenas-Pinto A, Melvin D et al. (2018) Anxiety and depression symptoms in young people with perinatally acquired HIV and HIV affected young people in England. *AIDS Care*, 30: 1040–1049.

Lesch A, Swartz L, Kagee A et al. (2007) Paediatric HIV/AIDS disclosure: Towards a developmental and process-oriented approach. *AIDS Care*, 19: 811–816.

Lewis-de Los Angeles CP, Alpert KI, Williams PL et al. (2016) Deformed subcortical structures are related to past HIV disease severity in youth with perinatally acquired HIV infection. *Journal of the Pediatric Infectious Diseases Society*, 5: S6–S14.

Lewis-de Los Angeles CP, Williams PL, Huo Y et al. (2017) Lower total and regional grey matter brain volumes in youth with perinatally-acquired HIV infection: Associations with HIV disease severity, substance use, and cognition. *Brain, Behavior, and Immunity*, 62: 100–109.

Lewis-de Los Angeles CP, Williams PL, Jenkins LM et al. (2020) Brain morphometric differences in youth with and without perinatally-acquired HIV: A cross-sectional study. *NeuroImage: Clinical*, 26: 102246.

Louthrenoo O, Oberdorfer P, Sirisanthana V (2014) Psychosocial functioning in adolescents with perinatal HIV infection receiving highly active antiretroviral therapy. *Journal of the International Association of Providers of AIDS Care*, 13: 178–183.

Louw K-A, Ipser J, Phillips N et al. (2016) Correlates of emotional and behavioural problems in children with perinatally acquired HIV in Cape Town, South Africa. *AIDS Care*, 28: 842–850.

Lwidiko A, Kibusi SM, Nyundo A et al. (2018) Association between HIV status and depressive symptoms among children and adolescents in the Southern Highlands Zone, Tanzania: A case-control study. *PloS One*, 13: e0193145.

Martin SC, Wolters PL, Toledo-Tamula MA et al. (2006) Cognitive functioning in school-aged children with vertically acquired HIV infection being treated with highly active antiretroviral therapy (HAART). *Developmental Neuropsychology*, 30: 633–657.

Mbewe EG, Kabundula PP, Mwanza-Kabaghe S et al. (2022) Socioeconomic status and cognitive function in children with HIV: Evidence from the HIV-associated neurocognitive disorders in Zambia (HANDZ) Study. *JAIDS Journal of Acquired Immune Deficiency Syndromes*, 89: 56–63.

Mburu G, Hodgson I, Kalibala S et al. (2014) Adolescent HIV disclosure in Zambia: Barriers, facilitators and outcomes. *Journal of the International AIDS Society*, 17: 18866.

Mellins CA, Elkington KS, Bauermeister JA et al. (2009) Sexual and drug use behavior in perinatally HIV-infected youth: Mental health and family influences. *Journal of the American Academy of Child & Adolescent Psychiatry*, 48: 810–819.

Mellins CA, Tassiopoulos K, Malee K et al. (2011) Behavioral health risks in perinatally HIV-exposed youth: Co-occurrence of sexual and drug use behavior, mental health problems, and nonadherence to antiretroviral treatment. *AIDS Patient Care and STDs*, 25: 413–422.

Mellins CA, Elkington KS, Leu C-S et al. (2012) Prevalence and change in psychiatric disorders among perinatally HIV-infected and HIV-exposed youth. *AIDS Care*, 24: 953–962.

Mellins CA, Malee KM (2013) Understanding the mental health of youth living with perinatal HIV infection: Lessons learned and current challenges. *Journal of the International AIDS Society*, 16: 18593.

Molinaro M, Adams HR, Mwanza-Kabaghe S et al. (2021) Evaluating the relationship between depression and cognitive function among children and adolescents with HIV in Zambia. *AIDS and Behavior*, 25: 2669–2679.

Moore AM, Awusabo-Asare K, Madise N et al. (2007) Coerced first sex among adolescent girls in sub-Saharan Africa: Prevalence and context. *African Journal of Reproductive Health*, 11: 62.

Mughal AY, Devadas J, Ardman E et al. (2020) A systematic review of validated screening tools for anxiety disorders and PTSD in low to middle income countries. *BMC Psychiatry*, 20: 1–18.

Mustanski B, Fisher CB (2016) HIV rates are increasing in gay/bisexual teens: IRB barriers to research must be resolved to bend the curve. *American Journal of Preventive Medicine*, 51: 249–252.

Mutumba M, Bauermeister JA, Elkington KS et al. (2016a) A prospective longitudinal study of mental health symptoms among perinatally HIV-infected and HIV-exposed but uninfected urban youths. *Journal of Adolescent Health*, 58: 460–466.

Mutumba M, Elkington K, Bauermeister J et al. (2016b) Changes in substance use symptoms across adolescence in youth perinatally infected with HIV. *AIDS and Behavior*, 21: 1117–1128.

Muya AN, Geldsetzer P, Hertzmark E et al. (2015) Predictors of nonadherence to antiretroviral therapy among HIV-infected adults in Dar es Salaam, Tanzania. *Journal of the International Association of Providers of AIDS Care (JIAPAC)*, 14: 163–171.

Nabukeera-Barungi N, Elyanu P, Asire B et al. (2015) Adherence to antiretroviral therapy and retention in care for adolescents living with HIV from 10 districts in Uganda. *BMC Infectious Diseases*, 15: 520.

Nachega JB, Hislop M, Nguyen H et al. (2009) Antiretroviral therapy adherence, virologic and immunologic outcomes in adolescents compared with adults in southern Africa. *Journal of Acquired Immune Deficiency Syndromes (1999)*, 51: 65.

Nachman S, Chernoff M, Williams P et al. (2012) Human immunodeficiency virus disease severity, psychiatric symptoms, and functional outcomes in perinatally infected youth. *Archives of Pediatrics & Adolescent Medicine*, 166: 528–535.

Nakigozi G, Atuyambe L, Kamya M et al. (2012) A qualitative study of barriers to enrollment into free HIV care: Perspectives of never-in-care HIV-positive patients and providers in Rakai, Uganda. *BioMed Research International*, 2013: 470245–470245.

Napierala S, Chabata ST, Fearon E et al. (2018) Engagement in HIV care among young female sex workers in Zimbabwe. *JAIDS Journal of Acquired Immune Deficiency Syndromes*, 79: 358–366.

Nglazi MD, Lawn SD, Kaplan R et al. (2011) Changes in programmatic outcomes during 7 years of scale-up at a community-based antiretroviral treatment service in South Africa. *Journal of Acquired Immune Deficiency Syndromes (1999)*, 56: e1.

Nichols SL, Brummel SS, Smith RA et al. (2015) Executive functioning in children and adolescents with perinatal HIV infection. *The Pediatric Infectious Disease Journal*, 34: 969.

Nichols SL, Chernoff MC, Malee K et al. (2016) Learning and memory in children and adolescents with perinatal HIV infection and perinatal HIV exposure. *The Pediatric Infectious Disease Journal*, 35: 649.

Oberdorfer P, Puthanakit T, Louthrenoo O et al. (2006) Disclosure of HIV/AIDS diagnosis to HIV-infected children in Thailand. *Journal of Paediatrics and Child Health*, 42: 283–288.

Paramesparan Y, Garvey LJ, Ashby J et al. (2010) High rates of asymptomatic neurocognitive impairment in vertically acquired HIV-1–infected adolescents surviving to adulthood. *JAIDS Journal of Acquired Immune Deficiency Syndromes*, 55: 134–136.

Patel PB, Belden A, Handoko R et al. (2021) Behavioral impairment and cognition in Thai adolescents affected by HIV. *Global Mental Health*, 8: e3.

Phillips N, Thomas KG, Mtukushe B et al. (2021) Youth perinatal HIV-associated neurocognitive disorders: Association with functional impairment. *AIDS Care*: 1–5.

Pinzón-Iregui MC, Beck-Sagué CM, Malow RM (2013) Disclosure of their HIV status to infected children: A review of the literature. *Journal of Tropical Pediatrics*, 59: 84–89.

Puthanakit T, Aurpibul L, Louthrenoo O et al. (2010) Poor cognitive functioning of school-aged children in Thailand with perinatally acquired HIV infection taking antiretroviral therapy. *AIDS Patient Care and STDs*, 24: 141–146.

Redmond SM, Yao T-J, Russell JS et al. (2016) Longitudinal evaluation of language impairment in youth with perinatally acquired human immunodeficiency virus (HIV) and youth with perinatal HIV exposure. *Journal of the Pediatric Infectious Diseases Society*, 5: S33–S40.

Reisner MSL, Mimiaga MJ, Skeer MM et al. (2009) A review of HIV antiretroviral adherence and intervention studies among HIV-infected youth. *Topics in HIV Medicine: A Publication of the International AIDS Society, USA*, 17: 14.

Remien RH, Stirratt MJ, Nguyen N et al. (2019) Mental health and HIV/AIDS: the need for an integrated response. *AIDS (London, England)* 33: 1411.

Rice ML, Buchanan AL, Siberry GK et al. (2012) Language impairment in children perinatally infected with HIV compared to children who were HIV-exposed and uninfected. *Journal of Developmental and Behavioral Pediatrics*, 33: 112.

Robbins RN, Zimmerman R, Korich R et al. (2020) Longitudinal trajectories of neurocognitive test performance among individuals with perinatal HIV-infection and-exposure: Adolescence through young adulthood. *AIDS Care*, 32: 21–29.

Romer D, Betancourt LM, Brodsky NL et al. (2011) Does adolescent risk-taking imply weak executive function? A prospective study of relations between working memory performance, impulsivity, and risk-taking in early adolescence. *Developmental Science*, 14: 1119–1133.

Ross JL, Teeraananchai S, Lumbiganon P et al. (2019) A longitudinal study of behavioral risk, adherence and virologic control in adolescents living with HIV in Asia. *Journal of Acquired Immune Deficiency Syndromes (1999)*, 81: e28.

Santoro AF, Ferraris C, Phillips N et al. (2021) Childhood adversity's impact on neurocognitive functioning: Findings from South African adolescents living with HIV. *Archives of Clinical Neuropsychology*, 36: 1027–1028.

Sariah A, Rugemalila J, Somba M et al. (2016) 'Experiences with disclosure of HIV-positive status to the infected child': Perspectives of healthcare providers in Dar es Salaam, Tanzania. *BMC Public Health*, 16: 1083.

Scharko A (2006) DSM psychiatric disorders in the context of pediatric HIV/AIDS. *AIDS Care* 18: 441–445.

Shiau S, Yu W, Jacobson DL et al. (2021) Components of metabolic syndrome associated with lower neurocognitive performance in youth with perinatally acquired HIV and youth who are HIV-exposed uninfected. *Journal of NeuroVirology*, 27: 702–715.

Simoni JM, Montgomery A, Martin E et al. (2007) Adherence to antiretroviral therapy for pediatric HIV infection: A qualitative systematic review with recommendations for research and clinical management. *Pediatrics*, 119: e1371–e1383.

Smith R, Chernoff M, Williams PL et al. (2012) Impact of human immunodeficiency virus severity on cognitive and adaptive functioning during childhood and adolescence. *The Pediatric Infectious Disease Journal*, 31: 592–598.

Smith R, Huo Y, Tassiopoulos K et al. (2019) Mental health diagnoses, symptoms, and service utilization in US youth with perinatal HIV infection or HIV exposure. *AIDS Patient Care and STDs*, 33: 1–13.

Ssewanyana D, Mwangala PN, Van Baar A et al. (2018) Health risk behaviour among adolescents living with HIV in sub-Saharan Africa: A systematic review and meta-analysis. *BioMed Research International*, 2018: 1–18.

Ssewanyana D, Newton CR, Van Baar A et al. (2020) Beyond their HIV status: The occurrence of multiple health risk behavior among adolescents from a rural setting of sub-Saharan Africa. *International Journal of Behavioral Medicine*, 27: 426–443.

Steinberg L (2008) A social neuroscience perspective on adolescent risk-taking. *Developmental Review*, 28: 78–106.

Swendeman D, Rotheram-Borus MJ, Comulada S et al. (2006) Predictors of HIV-related stigma among young people living with HIV. *Health Psychology*, 25: 501.

Taddeo D, Egedy M, Frappier J (2008) Adherence to treatment in adolescents. *Paediatrics & Child Health*, 13: 19–24.

Test F, Mehta S, Handler A et al. (2012) Gender inequities in sexual risks among youth with HIV in Kigali, Rwanda. *International Journal of STD & AIDS*, 23: 394–399.

Too EK, Abubakar A, Nasambu C et al. (2021) Prevalence and factors associated with common mental disorders in young people living with HIV in sub-Saharan Africa: A systematic review. *Journal of the International AIDS Society*, 24: e25705.

Toska E, Pantelic M, Meinck F et al. (2017) Sex in the shadow of HIV: A systematic review of prevalence, risk factors, and interventions to reduce sexual risk-taking among HIV-positive adolescents and youth in sub-Saharan Africa. *PloS One*, 12: e0178106.

Turissini ML, Nyandiko WM, Ayaya SO et al. (2013) The prevalence of disclosure of HIV status to HIV-infected children in Western Kenya. *Journal of the Pediatric Infectious Diseases Society*, 2: 136–143.

Ubesie A, Iloh K, Emodi I et al. (2016) HIV status disclosure rate and reasons for non-disclosure among infected children and adolescents in Enugu, southeast Nigeria. *SAHARA-J: Journal of Social Aspects of HIV/AIDS*, 13: 136–141.

UNAIDS (2013) *Global Report: UNAIDS Report on the Global AIDS Epidemic 2013*. Geneva: UNAIDS.

UNAIDS (2014) *Joint United Nations Programme on HIV/AIDS. The Gap Report*. Geneva: UNAIDS. Available at: https://files.unaids.org/en/media/unaids/contentassets/documents/unaidspublication/2014/UNAIDS_Gap_report_en.pdf

UNAIDS (2016a) *Ending the AIDS Epidemic for Adolescents, with Adolescents. A Practical Guide to Meaningfully Engage Adolescents in the AIDS Response*. Geneva: UNAIDS.

UNAIDS (2016b) *Global AIDS Update 2016*. Geneva: UNAIDS.

UNAIDS (2016c) *Prevention Gap Report*. Geneva: UNAIDS.

UNAIDS (2020) *UNAIDS Data 2020*. Geneva: UNAIDS.

UNAIDS (2021) *Global AIDS Monitoring 2021 and UNAIDS 2021 Estimates*. Available at: https://www.unaids.org/en/global-aids-monitoring.

UNICEF (2016) *For Every Child, End AIDS: Seventh Stocktaking Report 2016*. New York: UNICEF.

UNICEF (2020) *Children, HIV and AIDS. How will progress be impacted by COVID-19?* Available at: https://data.unicef.org/resources/children-hiv-and-aids-how-will-progress-be-impacted-by-covid-19/.

UNICEF (2021a) *HIV and AIDS in Adolescents. Turning the Tide Against AIDS Will Require More Concetrated Focus on Adolescents and Young People*. Available at: https://data.unicef.org/topic/adolescents/hiv-aids/.

UNICEF (2021b) *UNICEF's HIV Programming in the Context of COVID-19: Building Back Better for Children, Adolescents and Women. Compendium of Innovative Approaches in Eastern and Southern Africa. Volume II*. Nairobi: UNICEF.

Van den Hof M, ter Haar AM, Scherpbier HJ et al. (2020) Neurocognitive development in perinatally human immunodeficiency virus–infected adolescents on long-term treatment, compared to healthy matched controls: A longitudinal study. *Clinical Infectious Diseases*, 70: 1364–1371.

Vreeman RC, Wiehe SE, Pearce EC et al. (2008) A systematic review of pediatric adherence to antiretroviral therapy in low- and middle-income countries. *The Pediatric Infectious Disease Journal*, 27: 686–691.

Vreeman RC, Gramelspacher AM, Gisore PO et al. (2013) Disclosure of HIV status to children in resource-limited settings: A systematic review. *Journal of the International AIDS Society*, 16: 18466.

Vreeman RC, McCoy BM, Lee S (2017) Mental health challenges among adolescents living with HIV. *Journal of the International AIDS Society*, 20: 21497.

Ward JL, Azzopardi PS, Francis KL et al. (2021) Global, regional, and national mortality among young people aged 10–24 years, 1950–2019: A systematic analysis for the Global Burden of Disease Study 2019. *The Lancet*, 398: 1593–1618.

Waterfield KC, Shah GH, Etheredge GD et al. (2021) Consequences of COVID-19 crisis for persons with HIV: The impact of social determinants of health. *BMC Public Health*, 21: 1–7.

West N, Schwartz S, Mudavanhu M et al. (2019) Mental health in South African adolescents living with HIV. *AIDS Care*, 31: 117–124.

WHO (2003) *Adherence to Long-term Therapies. Evidence for Action*. Geneva: World Health Organization.

WHO (2013) *HIV and Adolescents: Guidance for HIV testing and Counselling and Care for Adolescents Living with HIV: Recommendations for a Public Health Approach and Considerations for Policy-makers and Managers*. Geneva: World Health Organization. Available at https://apps.who.int/iris/handle/10665/94334.

WHO (2014) *Health for the World's Adolescents. A Second Chance in the Second Decade*. Geneva: World Health Organization.

Wiener L, Mellins C, Marhefka S et al. (2007) Disclosure of an HIV diagnosis to children: History, current research, and future directions. *Journal of Developmental & Behavioral Pediatrics*, 28: 155–166.

Willis N, Milanzi A, Mawodzeke M et al. (2019) Effectiveness of community adolescent treatment supporters (CATS) interventions in improving linkage and retention in care, adherence to ART and psychosocial well-being: A randomised trial among adolescents living with HIV in rural Zimbabwe. *BMC Public Health*, 19: 1–9.

Woods SP, Rippeth JD, Frol AB et al. (2004) Interrater reliability of clinical ratings and neurocognitive diagnoses in HIV. *Journal of Clinical and Experimental Neuropsychology*, 26: 759–778.

Zielińska-Wieniawska A, Bielecki M, Wolańczyk T et al. (2022) Cognitive impairments in Polish children and adolescents with perinatal HIV infection. *Psychiatria Polska*, 56(5): 1061–1077.

Zgambo M, Kalembo FW, Mbakaya BC (2018) Risky behaviours and their correlates among adolescents living with HIV in sub-Saharan Africa: A systematic review. *Reproductive Health*, 15: 1–12.

Zhang X-D, Temmerman M, Li Y et al. (2013) Vulnerabilities, health needs and predictors of high-risk sexual behaviour among female adolescent sex workers in Kunming, China. *Sexually Transmitted Infections*, 89: 237–244.

Zhou S, Cluver L, Shenderovich Y et al. (2021) Uncovering ART adherence inconsistencies: An assessment of sustained adherence among adolescents in South Africa. *Journal of the International AIDS Society*, 24: e25832.

Long-term Outcomes in Adults Living with HIV

Patrick N Mwangala, Derrick Ssewanyana, Moses K Nyongesa,
Felix Hosea, and Amina Abubakar

INTRODUCTION

Before the groundbreaking discovery of antiretroviral therapy (ART), a human immunodeficiency virus (HIV) diagnosis was considered a death sentence, with many people living with HIV (PLWH) dying from AIDs-related illnesses (Borrell et al. 2006). Nonetheless, two decades later, the life expectancy of adults living with HIV is approaching that of the general population (Marcus et al. 2020). In a collaborative analysis of 18 European and North American HIV cohort studies, adults who initiated combination antiretroviral therapy (cART) at age 20 years between 2003 and 2005 were expected to live an additional 49 years (Trickey et al. 2017). A similar retrospective observational cohort study in Rwanda registered an overall life expectancy of an additional 25 years 7 months among adults who initiated cART at 20 years of age (Nsanzimana et al. 2015). A recent policy recommendation by the World Health Organization (WHO) to initiate cART for all people regardless of their disease staging and cluster of differentiation–4 (CD4) cell count, has led to a tremendous reduction in HIV transmissions and AIDS-related mortality (WHO 2021). Unfortunately, the ongoing progress is being threatened by the extended time lag in adopting and implementing such guidelines, especially in HIV-endemic countries, partly because of inadequate resources (Gupta and Granich 2016; Songo et al. 2021). For instance, by the end of 2020, about 10 million eligible adults were still not accessing ART (Joint United Nations Programme on HIV/AIDS 2020) worldwide. By extension, this delays the realisation of the Sustainable Development Goal target 3.3, which aims to eliminate HIV/AIDS as a public health threat by 2030 through treatment as prevention (Rosa 2017).

Despite the ongoing global efforts in tackling the HIV epidemic thus far, a variety of new challenges with an adverse effect on the quality of life of adults living with HIV still exists. Of particular concern is the array of neuropsychiatric comorbidities associated with HIV, including common mental disorders, drug and substance use and abuse, and HIV-associated neurocognitive disorders HAND (Watkins and Treisman 2012; Remien et al. 2019). The persistent incidence of these complications in the cART period has been associated with direct effects of HIV on the brain, emergence of virologic failure, direct and indirect effects of some antiretroviral drugs, decreased effectiveness of cART in the central nervous system, and concurrent illnesses (Harezlak et al. 2011; Singer and Thames 2016).

Understanding the nature and burden of HIV-associated comorbidities is an important first step in addressing these problems and ensuring that we fast track the UNAIDS target of eradicating the HIV epidemic by 2030. If left unmanaged, these conditions have far-reaching effects, including poor quality of life, reduced functional ability, poor medication adherence, and increased mortality (Watkins and Treisman 2012), thus complicating the care of adults living with HIV and their families at large. Also important is the occurrence of such comorbidities even in well-controlled viremia (Van Lelyveld et al. 2012; Ingle et al. 2014), and the significant contributions of these comorbidities to the global burden of disease (Whiteford et al. 2015). There is an important need to design, evaluate, and subsequently scale up appropriate interventions to address these problems (Hoeft et al. 2018), which would ultimately improve the quality of life of adults living with HIV.

To better understand some of these comorbidities in adults living with HIV, this chapter consolidates existing evidence of some of the long-term outcomes in adults living with HIV globally. Specifically, the chapter is divided into six sections. First, a discussion on HIV-associated neurocognitive impairment is provided. Related to this is a discussion on HIV and age-associated dementias. Subsequently, we describe the neuropsychiatric outcomes among these adults. The health-related quality of life (HRQoL) of adults living with HIV is then discussed. The following section highlights cART adherence among these adults. Thereafter, we highlight the risk of HIV infection among key population groups and their vulnerability to poor health outcomes. Finally, we provide an overall summary of the issues discussed in this chapter. For clarity, in this chapter an 'adult' refers to anyone more than 19 years of age, unless national law delimits an earlier age as stipulated by WHO (2013).

NEUROCOGNITIVE IMPAIRMENT

Three decades have elapsed since the earliest account of HIV-associated neurological complications by Grant et al. (1987). Despite the significant advances in the management of HIV in the cART era, these complications are still a major challenge in PLWH. These complications are commonly referred to as HAND according to the Frascati criteria (widely recognised as the 'criterion standard diagnostic schema') (Antinori et al. 2007). Frascati criteria classify HAND into three categories based on increasing severity of cognitive impairment: asymptomatic neurocognitive impairment (ANI), mild neurocognitive disorder (MND), and HIV-associated dementia (HAD). Classification considers clinical features, particularly those associated with daily functioning, exclusion of alternative causes, and comprehensive neuropsychological measurement. The mechanisms underlying the development of these complications incorporate an intricate mix of viral factors, antiretroviral factors, chronic HIV inflammation, and individual factors (Alford and Vera 2018).

Before the widespread use of ART, the cognitive and functional impacts of HIV were devastating (Holland and Tross 1985). Before widespread cART, more than half of PLWH experienced severe cognitive impairments, particularly dementia and HIV-associated encephalopathy, before succumbing to an HIV-related death (Navia, Jordan, and Price 1986). Nonetheless, in the era of potent cART, there is a growing consensus that the severity profile of HAND is milder (Wei et al. 2020). Though less severe, the mild impairments have a clinical and functional impact on the individual, including a heightened risk of mortality (Vivithanaporn et al. 2010), poor treatment adherence (Hinkin et al. 2002; Becker et al. 2011), poor quality of life (Alford et al. 2021), increased risk-taking behaviours (Doyle et al. 2016), and disruptions to everyday functioning (Weber, Blackstone, and Woods 2013).

Clinical Presentation/Profile

The onset of neurological signs is believed to occur as early as during the acute HIV infection phase. Hellmuth and colleagues demonstrated that the acute phase of HIV infection is associated with a high prevalence of mild neurological symptoms, including cognitive symptoms (33%), motor problems (34%), and neuropathy (11%), which mainly remit while on cART (Hellmuth et al. 2016). This evidence supports the recent WHO recommendations of initiating cART as early as possible regardless of the CD4 count and HIV viral load (WHO 2021). Overall, the profile of HAND in the present era of widespread cART differs considerably from what was witnessed in the pre-cART era. Noticeably, there has been a sharp reduction in the severe forms of HAND, i.e. HAD, and an increase in the milder forms (Wei et al. 2020). Moreover, the current manifestations of HAND show a subtle subcortical involvement and more cortical involvement. This contrasts with the progressive subcortical dementia with marked deterioration of cognitive and motor functions observed in the pre-cART era (Guha et al. 2016). Furthermore, a majority of adults living with HIV in the pre-cART era exhibited their greatest cognitive impairments in the speed of information processing, verbal fluency, and motor skills compared to the concentration, attention, and memory domains in the present era of effective cART (Eggers et al. 2017). Nonetheless, geographical discrepancies may still be observed in the patterning of HAND, owing to differences in cART access especially when comparing high-income countries (HICs) and low- and middle-income countries (LMICs). Evidence on the temporal sequence of HAND over time is mixed. In one longitudinal study, the Multicenter AIDS Cohort Study, a diagnosis of MND and HAD was not progressive in about 70% of virally suppressed individuals over a 4-year period (Sacktor et al. 2016). In a different cohort study, the CHARTER Study, patients diagnosed with ANI at baseline were 2 to 6 times more likely to manifest HAND symptoms during the follow-up period (3 years) than those who had no cognitive impairments at baseline (Heaton et al. 2010). Similarly, O'Connor and colleagues reported grey and white matter atrophy as well as subcortical atrophy in people with well-controlled viremia in a recent meta-analysis of brain structural changes following HIV infection (O'Connor, Zeffiro, and Zeffiro 2018). This potentially highlights the issue of neuropsychological measures lacking sensitivity compared to biological markers.

DIAGNOSIS AND SCREENING

HAND typically manifests with clinically important deteriorations in several domains of cognitive functioning, for example, motor skills, speed of information processing, learning and memory, attention and working memory, speech and language, and visuoperception (Eggers et al. 2017). Some of the important procedures that may aid the diagnosis of HAND include neuropsychological testing, radiological studies, biochemical analyses (such as cerebrospinal fluid), and electrophysiological studies (such as electroencephalogram) (Eggers et al. 2017). Quantitative cognitive testing is the most appropriate method and the criterion standard in ascertaining HAND. The Frascati criteria are the most commonly utilised nosology of HAND in the cART era (Antinori et al. 2007). Nonetheless, the accuracy of this method has been criticised in recent years (Gisslén, Price, and Nilsson 2011) with some of the researchers suggesting it overestimates the actual prevalence of HAND. Such criticisms have given rise to other HAND diagnostic criteria such as the Gisslén criteria (Gisslén, Price, and Nilsson 2011). Recently, other researchers have recommended the use of multivariate normative comparison (MNC) criteria, a statistical method specifically designed to control false-positive rates while retaining sensitivity (Agelink van Rentergem, Murre, and Huizenga 2017). In one study, Su and colleagues assessed whether the MNC improves HAND detection compared with Frascati and Gisslén criteria (Su et al. 2015). The authors found that the prevalence of HAND estimated by MNC was much higher than that estimated by the Gisslén criteria, while the false-positive rate was significantly reduced compared with the Frascati criteria. In contexts where comprehensive neuropsychological testing is not feasible, brief screening tests, for example, the International HIV Dementia Scale, may be applied. Nonetheless, a recent scoping review identified a lack of adequately standardised and contextually relevant HAND screening tools in sub-Saharan Africa (SSA) (Mwangala et al. 2019). Most studies in the scoping review only reported the diagnostic accuracy of the tools identified, with specificity ranging from 37% to 81% and sensitivity ranging from 45% to 100% (Mwangala et al. 2019). Current screening tools performed well in screening for severe forms of HAND but rarely so for moderate forms of HAND. Of critical concern is the lack of evidence on the clinical application of these tools. Feasibility studies on the clinical utility of these tools will generate vital information needed to address the next steps in the clinical pathway.

PREVALENCE AND CORRELATES

The prevalence estimates of HAND vary extensively depending on the populations studied and the methods utilised (such as tools of assessment). The varying sensitivity and specificity of the neurobehavioural tests is an important determinant of the prevalence of HAND. Gisslén and colleagues argue that the Frascati criteria are less stringent diagnostic criteria resulting in 16% to 21% of the population being classified as false positive (Gisslén, Price, and Nilsson 2011). The POPPY Study, conducted in the UK and Ireland, has provided the most stringent estimate of HAND, by comparing the agreement of different diagnostic criteria (De Francesco et al. 2016). The authors registered a prevalence range of 14% to 28% (De Francesco et al. 2016). In a recent meta-analysis, the global prevalence of Frascati-criteria based HAND in adults living with HIV was 44.9% (26.2% ANI, 8.5% MND, and 2.1% HAD) (Wei et al. 2020). A similar review assessing the global prevalence and burden of HAND, recorded a prevalence of 42.6%, which did not differ with diagnostic criteria (Wang et al. 2020). The prevalence of ANI, MND, and HAD was 23.5%, 13.3%, and 5% respectively. The varying prevalence of HAND may also be explained by the different presentations of the health-related chronic ailments commonly associated with long-term HIV, including cardiovascular conditions, diabetes, cerebrovascular injuries, and cancers across regions (Milic et al. 2019). This could also be related to the variation in treatment characteristics among participants (e.g. duration on ART, adherence). Some of the factors associated with an increased risk for HAND include comorbidities such as cardiovascular disease and diabetes (Fabbiani et al. 2013), coinfections such as hepatitis C (Vance et al. 2014), lifestyle factors such as drug and substance use, psychiatric problems (e.g. depression, anxiety), ageing, potential neurotoxicity from HIV medication, and previous infections of the central nervous system (Alford and Vera 2018).

MANAGEMENT

Considering HIV infection of the central nervous system as the underlying mechanism for the development of HAND, the fundamental principle of a causal treatment is the suppression of viral replication in the brain. Indeed different studies have demonstrated that cART leads to a reduced viral load in the brain and the degree of clinical improvement is higher in more severely affected patients (Eggers et al. 2017). Nonetheless, this is not to mean that cART can completely reverse HAND. It is not yet clear which substances and combinations of antiretroviral drugs are most appropriate for the treatment and prevention of HAND. While it is widely accepted that all HIV-untreated patients with HAND should be started on cART, the question of how to manage HAND is less clear with patients already on cART. Ongoing or worsening cognitive decline warrants a review of the ART regimen. The Mind Exchange working group has suggested a useful algorithm on this matter (Mind Exchange Working Group 2012). For instance, good practice suggests that all PLWH should be screened for HAND early in the disease using standardised tools and that the follow-up frequency is dependent on whether HAND is already present or whether clinical data suggest elevated risk. Deteriorating cognitive impairment may necessitate cART review when other causes have been excluded.

A few clinical guidelines from HICs recommend the screening of HAND in clinical settings (Eggers et al. 2017). In the event of a confirmed diagnosis, central nervous system antiretroviral drugs should be considered (Eggers et al. 2017). During the differential diagnosis of HAND, the toxic effect of cART ought to be considered (Mind Exchange Working Group 2012). In low-income settings, however, such guidelines are non-existent and hardly any clinic screens for such impairments. This may be attributed partly to a lack of contextually relevant screening tools, lack of clinical expertise to adequately identify and manage cases of HAND, poorly resourced health facilities, and many competing health care needs that make HAND a lesser priority. It is also possible that many stakeholders in these settings are not aware of the clinical and public health importance of this condition. It is not surprising, therefore, that there are hardly any recommendations on how to adequately follow up and manage PLWH and having symptoms of HAND. In addition, there are no recommendations on how to address the clinical, social, and psychological needs of adults living with HIV with worsening cognitive symptoms, especially in the context of LMICs.

A recent scoping review of putative rehabilitative interventions for HAND identified two intervention options, namely cognitive training (psycho-cognitive training) and physical activity interventions (Nweke et al. 2021). All articles reporting on cognitive training for HAND showed improved post-treatment interventions, while two of the six interventional physical activity studies recorded improved post-treatment cognitive performance, highlighting the need for further research. In another systematic review of studies investigating cognitive training in PLWH, it was found that cognitive ability can be moderately improved in the domain that was targeted (i.e. working memory, attention, and speed of processing); however, most of the studies had small sample sizes, limiting their reliability and generalisability (Vance et al. 2019). Although computerised cognitive training has been a massive initiative in HICs, it is now making its way to LMICs as one of the options in the management of HAND. The potential utility of computerised cognitive rehabilitation therapy has also been demonstrated in SSA, for example, in Ugandan seniors living with HIV (Ezeamama et al. 2020), as well as among Ugandan children living with HIV (Boivin et al. 2010, 2016). Although more evidence is needed to establish treatment guidelines, current evidence suggests that cognitive training is beneficial to cognitive function, as it can improve everyday functioning, mood, and quality of life among PLWH with HAND.

Several non-ART substances (adjuvant therapies), including memantine, selegiline, minocycline, lithium, valproate, lexipafant, psychostimulants, nimodipine, and rivastigmine have also been tested for the management of HAND. However, results on their clinical benefit are mixed and inconclusive (Bougea et al. 2019; Omeragic et al. 2020). Other management approaches include preventative and treatment strategies supporting biopsychosocial aspects of cognition, such as reducing alcohol and substance use, improving nutrition, treating comorbidities (e.g. depression), and promoting social contact (Waldrop et al. 2021).

HIV and Age-associated Dementias

Effective use of cART has led to phenomenal health improvements among PLWH, including significant reductions in the incidence of the most severe form of HAND (HAD) from around 30% in the early years of the epidemic to 2% to 4% currently among people infected with advanced chronic HIV, and less in PLWH treated early. However, given that many PLWH are now over 50 years of age and have a near-normal life expectancy (Autenrieth et al. 2018), a growing concern is that they will experience a disproportionate burden of age-associated dementia, such as Alzheimer disease. Indeed, neuroimaging studies have exhibited persistent microstructural brain abnormalities and progressive brain atrophy in PLWH despite viral suppression (Clifford et al. 2017; Kallianpur et al. 2020), contributing to an expanding body of literature suggesting that adults ageing with HIV may experience premature or accelerated cognitive impairment, and greater neurocognitive morbidity and dementia than their HIV-uninfected peers. A recent systematic review identified an increase in risk factors for dementia in the global HIV population entering the dementia-risk age range, that is ≥60 years, in relation to both traditional and HIV-specific risk factors. These included age, HIV-related and non-HIV-related cardiovascular diseases, HAND, high mental health burden, low education/socioeconomic status, historical immune compromise, and persistent immune activation (Aung et al. 2019).

Much of the published research to date exploring the risk of dementia in PLWH has focused on the risks of HAD. The evidence on other types of dementia, including Alzheimer's disease in PLWH, is minimal, especially in SSA (Aung et al. 2019). The minimal evidence of PLWH with diagnosed age-associated dementias may potentially be because most cohort studies, including the Women's Interagency HIV Study (Adimora et al. 2018), Multicenter AIDS Cohort Study (Becker et al. 2015), the Ugandan Non-Communicable Diseases and Aging Cohort (US Clinical Trials Registry 2021), and Health and Aging in Africa: A Longitudinal Study of an INDEPTH Community in South Africa (Gómez-Olivé et al. 2018), have focused on mid-life participants (around 40 years of age). Most likely, large-scale data will continue to emerge over the next decade with continued follow up of these studies. Also, multiple prospective cohort studies with a focus on ageing among PLWH have been set up, including the Veterans Aging Cohort Study (Justice et al. 2006), the Pharmacokinetic and Clinical Observations in People Over Fifty (Bagkeris et al. 2018), and a 12-year follow-up study of individuals enrolled in the CNS HIV Anti-Retroviral Therapy Effects Research Study (Blackstone et al. 2012). So far, the emerging data appear mixed. In a cohort of 2228 mostly male veterans (1114 PLWH of whom 61% were ART treated), HIV infection increased the risk of incident dementia by 50%, while exposure to cART did not offset this risk (Bobro et al. 2020). In another large observational study in the USA (involving 5381 ART-treated PLWH and 119 022 HIV-uninfected peers) PLWH were at a 58% higher risk for incident dementia despite HIV treatment with ART (Lam et al. 2021). These results contrast with a nationwide cohort study conducted in Taiwan (Yang et al. 2019), which evaluated whether HIV infection was associated with the risk of developing dementia in 1261 PLWH and 3783 age- and sex-matched controls. The authors of the Taiwanese study concluded that PLWH were not at increased risk for dementia. Results from a cross-sectional study screening older adults in South Africa for dementia registered higher but not significantly different dementia point-prevalence estimates in PLWH compared to those without (Joska et al. 2019). Notably, the sample for the South African study only included 55 PLWH and registered only 10 screen-positive dementia cases.

Clearly, more research is needed to unravel the mechanisms by which dementia risk is increased (particularly dementia subtypes) in PLWH, whether biological or socially patterned. As the population of PLWH rapidly ages globally, an understanding of the general and unique dementia risk factors for this group is needed to develop appropriate mitigation strategies. Clinicians and researchers should also aim to distinguish between HAND and age-associated dementia, including Alzheimer disease. Clinically, the more degenerative profile of age-associated dementias requires different life planning and treatment options compared to the HAND profile, where cognitive impairment is typically more stable. Besides, a delayed dementia diagnosis in PLWH would limit the opportunity to intervene early when interventions – for example, cognitive interventions – are most effective and can help in better life planning.

Although there are no known effective treatments to mitigate ageing or HIV-associated cognitive decline, it has been shown that cognitive training programmes can buffer against age-associated dementias in adults living with HIV (Waldrop et al. 2021). In several studies, participants engaged in 10 to 20 hours of exercises to improve specific cognitive ability or overall cognitive functioning (Vance et al. 2019). Generally, these exercises become increasingly complex, thereby challenging the brain to strengthen the efficiency of cognitive processing via a process called neuroplasticity (Vance et al. 2019).

MENTAL HEALTH PROBLEMS

Mental health problems remain the most prevalent comorbidities in the HIV population (Jallow et al. 2017; Remien et al. 2019). Depression, anxiety disorders, adjustment disorders, sexual dysfunction, drug and substance use disorders, mania, and schizophreniform and personality disorders are some of the principal psychiatric diagnoses in HIV (Adams et al. 2016). The global burden of these disorders rises in late adolescence and peaks in young adulthood, which emulates the global HIV burden. Adults living with HIV could develop these neuropsychiatric problems indirectly as a psychosocial consequence of the disease (e.g. gross caregiving burden, lack of social support, HIV-related stigma, interpersonal conflicts) or as a direct impact of HIV infection on the brain (Owe-Larsson et al. 2009). These problems often complicate health-seeking behaviour, treatment and its outcomes, and the general quality of life of these adults. Together, these conditions contribute significantly to the global burden of mental disorders (Rehm and Shield 2019). Regrettably, these illnesses are often under-diagnosed and inadequately managed, especially in LMICs (Cohen et al. 2017; Ruffieux et al. 2021).

Depression

Depression is a common psychiatric disorder in adults living with HIV (Remien et al. 2019). It is an important but widely ignored disorder of public health concern, especially in LMICs. Screening and subsequent management of depression have been recommended as a key priority for comprehensive HIV care services, especially in SSA (Abas et al. 2014). This is informed by the prevailing evidence of high rates of depression in adults living with HIV, the severity of disabilities associated with depression, as well as the adverse impact of depression on HIV progression (Abas et al. 2014).

In a recent systematic review and meta-analysis, the global prevalence of depression in PLWH was estimated to be 31% (Rezaei et al. 2019). Meanwhile, the highest prevalence rate of depression measured by continent was South America at 44%, and the lowest was Europe at 22%. In SSA, 9% to 32% of adults living with HIV are estimated to be depressed (Bernard, Dabis, and de Rekeneire 2017). Moreover, higher estimates are shown in specific contexts and population groups such as postnatal mothers living with HIV (Chibanda et al. 2010) and key populations (WHO 2017; see also 'Key Populations' section, of this chapter). This is against a backdrop of the 2016 Global Burden of Disease Study, which showed that major depressive disorder is still a leading cause of years lived with disability across the world (Vos et al. 2017). Some of the excess depression rates witnessed in adults living with HIV can be attributed to factors such as the challenges of coping with diagnosis, HIV prognosis, grief and bereavement, HIV-related stigma and discrimination, loneliness and relationship crises, financial difficulties, and the potential side effects of certain antiretroviral drugs (Slavich and Irwin 2014). Inflammation processes brought about by chronic stress, HIV infection itself, or other coexisting conditions could also elevate the risk of depression in these adults. Depression could also precede and even heighten the risk of HIV infection (Sherr et al. 2011).

The co-occurrence of depressive disorders and HIV has been associated with reduced economic productivity, decreased quality of life, impaired functional abilities, difficulties in solving problems, and a decline in physical health (Abas et al. 2014). Depression has also been shown to be an important predictor of ART non-adherence. In one study, non-adherent individuals had a threefold heightened risk of having depressive symptoms compared to those adhering to their medication (Nel and Kagee 2013). In SSA, depression has also been correlated with poorer health status generally, including low weight gain, low CD4 count (Kingori, Haile, and Ngatia 2015), suicide (Kinyanda et al. 2012), poor quality of life (Nyongesa et al. 2018), faster advancement to AIDS, and elevated mortality rates (Abas et al. 2014). Such impacts could potentially compromise the achievement of the 95-95-95

UNAIDS targets. This is especially so given that optimal ART adherence is crucial to attaining sustained virologic suppression, achieving better management outcomes, and preventing issues of drug resistance; all of which are core UNAIDS targets in the prevention and eradication of HIV by 2030 (UNAIDS 2014).

Several studies have indicated that both pharmacological and psychological treatments are effective in addressing depression comorbid with HIV in both HICs and LMICs (Sherr et al. 2011; Sikkema et al. 2015; van Luenen et al. 2018). Various studies have tested pharmacological interventions (e.g. various antidepressants) and psychological and psychosocial interventions (e.g. cognitive behavioural therapy, interpersonal therapy, group therapy, motivational interviewing, stress management, meditation, and psycho-educational family interventions) (Nakimuli-Mpungu et al. 2021). Reviews of the literature report small to moderate positive effects of these interventions on mental health among PLWH, with demonstrated reductions in depression and anxiety and improved quality of life and psychological well-being (van Luenen et al. 2018; Nakimuli-Mpungu et al. 2021). In Cameroon and Zimbabwe, studies have reported initial effectiveness of counselling and antidepressants in reducing depressive symptoms in adults living with HIV (Chibanda et al. 2011; Gaynes et al. 2015). Counselling interventions have also been shown to promote ART adherence (Sin and DiMatteo 2013), improve CD4 cell count, and to improve viral load suppression (Gaynes et al. 2015). While this evidence is encouraging, the progress made thus far in addressing depression comorbid with HIV is alarmingly low, particularly in LMICs. Overall, there is a need for large and well-designed implementation studies (Lofgren, Nakasujja, and Boulware 2018). Many national strategic plans on HIV in various LMICs recognise the need to address mental health services for adults living with HIV, such as the screening for depression with the PHQ-9 in Kenya (Ministry of Health 2018). Nonetheless, the nationwide implementation of existing guidelines remains a challenge. Screening should be supported with a clear continuum of care. However, this is not the case in most LMICs, which rely on antidepressants with no alternative treatment options. Fortunately, South Africa is currently evaluating the effectiveness and cost-effectiveness of scalable interventions in a bid to reduce the mental health treatment gap posed by the increasing burden of depression among adults on ART (Petersen et al. 2018). In the context of an overburdened primary health care system and limited mental health expertise in LMICs, there is a critical need to consider task shifting, which is promoted by the WHO and the global mental health movement as an efficient and effective way of improving access to mental health services (Patel and Prince 2010). Managing depression using simple psychological therapy and/or antidepressants (for severe cases) has been recommended by the World Federation for Mental Health as a 'best buy' intervention providing good value for money spent (Ganju 2011). This strategy has been shown to be cost effective, affordable, and feasible for delivery through primary care, and hence easily scalable to benefit a greater number of individuals. It is therefore crucial for HIV prevention and treatment services to implement screening and diagnosis of depression, at least for adults with poor viral and immunological indicators, as well as those with suboptimal ART adherence. With the effective use of cART, there is also a need for a smooth transition of children and adolescents from paediatric to adult HIV care services.

Mania

Adults with HIV-associated mania are described as being agitated, disruptive, sleepless, having high energy levels, and being excessively talkative (Puri, Hall, and Ho 2014). Reports of HIV mania have reduced considerably due to the widespread use of cART but it remains a problem, especially among individuals with untreated or under-treated HIV or among those with advancing HIV infection (Singer and Thames 2016). Generally, the occurrence of mania in the context of HIV is uncommon. Hypomanic or manic behaviour presents problems for optimising HIV care and treatment: for example, an increased tendency to sexual activity and substance use by those affected with mania heightens the risk for contracting new HIV strains and/or transmitting HIV (Hinkin et al. 2001). Mania in HIV infection may occur as a result of a coexisting bipolar disorder (Schmidt and Miller 1988), HIV treatment effects, or secondary effects of HIV infection on the central nervous system (Nakimuli-Mpungu et al. 2006). Its prevalence ranges from 1.2% (Ellen et al. 1999) among individuals with early HIV infection to 8% among individuals with AIDS symptoms (Lyketsos et al. 1993). This amplified occurrence of mania around the time of onset of AIDS has been closely linked with neurocognitive changes or dementia and is characterised as a secondary manic syndrome due to the effect of HIV on the central nervous system (Lyketsos et al. 1993). Occasionally referred to as 'AIDS mania', this disorder is phenomenologically different from the characteristic manic syndrome of bipolar disorder in its symptom profile and severity (Lyketsos et al. 1993). It is frequently characterised by irritability rather than the normal euphoria (Lyketsos et al. 1997). It is important to note is that the prevalence of AIDS mania has greatly reduced over the years following the introduction of effective cART. A common manifestation of AIDS mania, either early or late, is the delusional belief that the individual has either been cured of HIV or has discovered the cure (Venugopal et al. 2001). This delusion frequently results in resumption of high-risk sexual behaviour and medication non-adherence. With the interruption of medication, this disorder usually becomes worse (Mijch et al. 1999). Unfortunately, these patients usually have cognitive deficits that render them less able to pursue treatment independently or consistently. Descriptive and clinical studies of HIV-related mania are not well described in either LMICs or HICs. More so, there is a dearth of population-based studies documenting the prevalence of HIV-related mania in HIV-endemic regions.

Anxiety Disorders

Anxiety is a usual reaction to distress. Its symptoms can vary from a mild feeling of unease to critical and debilitating symptoms that meet the criteria for an anxiety disorder such as generalised anxiety disorder, panic disorder, or post-traumatic stress disorder (Brandt et al. 2017). It is one of the most common psychiatric conditions across the globe (Bandelow and Michaelis 2015). These disorders can precede HIV infection or be triggered by an HIV diagnosis. It is associated with a myriad of psychosocial or clinical challenges encountered by individuals living with HIV over the course of the infection, from diagnosis, treatment effects, illness episodes, and lifelong adjustments to living with HIV (Clucas et al. 2011). Often, anxiety coexists with other common mental disorders, particularly depression (Pence et al. 2006). Sometimes, when anxiety becomes more severe, individuals may be at increased risk of suicidality when experiencing a stressful life event, even in the absence of depression (Gizachew et al. 2021). Although a lot of scientific and clinical attention has been given to depression and psychopathology among adults living with HIV globally, less attention has been given to anxiety disorders. In a recently published systematic review of the mental health and well-being of older adults living with HIV in SSA, only two studies examined anxiety in this population (Mwangala et al. 2021). The dearth of research in this area is of great concern from a public health perspective, given that anxiety disorders are one of the most common mental problems with a huge negative impact on functional abilities (Bandelow and Michaelis 2015; Brandt et al. 2017).

For anxiety disorders, prevalence rates as high as 82% (Morrison et al. 2011) have been reported in some parts of the world among adults living with HIV, compared to 33.7% for the general population (Bandelow and Michaelis 2015). The high prevalence has been associated with several factors, including clinical and psychosocial factors, opportunistic infections, the demise of a significant other, deterioration in CD4 cell count, the progression of HIV disease, and HIV-stigma (Tucker et al. 2003). The increasing life expectancy of adults living with HIV is also hypothesised to be an important factor in the increasing prevalence of anxiety disorders (Nüesch et al. 2009).

While not as well studied as depression, anxiety disorders may interrupt the cascade of HIV care by making people less likely to present for HIV testing, remain engaged in HIV care, adhere to ART, and more likely to engage in risky sexual behaviour (Brandt et al. 2017; Beer et al. 2019). In a recent meta-analysis, PLWH who reported anxiety in LMICs had 59% higher odds of poor adherence to ART compared to those who did not report an anxiety disorder (Wykowski et al. 2019). Evidence also suggests that elevated anxiety symptoms are predictive of higher viral load (Lampe et al. 2010). This evidence highlights the critical need to screen for these conditions in primary care and to intervene accordingly to ensure healthy ageing among adults living with HIV. Unfortunately, there are few well-designed studies seeking to develop novel treatments to address this condition. A comprehensive global review by Clucas and colleagues evaluated interventions for anxiety in adults living with HIV (Clucas et al. 2011). The authors identified that psychological interventions (particularly cognitive behavioural stress management interventions and cognitive behavioural therapy-based interventions) were more effective than pharmacological interventions. However, additional research is needed to tailor and thus enhance the effectiveness of these interventions. There is also a need to extend this research to LMICs given that most of the available studies originate from HICs. Additionally, given the increased co-occurrence of depression and anxiety, there is a need for transdiagnostic interventions for an integrated response (Remien et al. 2019).

Psychotic Disorders

The most common psychotic diagnoses in this population include schizophrenia, schizoaffective disorder, and bipolar disorders (Chandra et al. 1999). Prevalence rates range from 0.5% to nearly 15%, depending upon the method of surveillance globally (Grant and Atkinson 1999). The pathogenesis of HIV-related psychosis is unclear. There is suggestive evidence that subcortical neurodegeneration due to HIV itself or to opportunistic infections of the brain may be partly responsible (Perry and Jacobsen 1986). These disorders may have several aetiologies in HIV infection (Cournos et al. 1991). The psychotic symptomatology may also precede HIV infection because adults living with schizophrenia have an increased risk for HIV infection due to their elevated likelihood of poor impulse control, impaired judgment, substance abuse, and high sexual risk behaviour. Psychosis could also be a consequence of ART side effects (Hinsch, Reichelt, and Husstedt 2014). Overall, a significant proportion of the available evidence on psychosis originates from HICs. Moreover, the volume of studies examining HIV-associated psychotic disorders has stagnated in the post-cART era. Evidence of the appropriate management of these conditions in adults living with HIV is scantily addressed. More studies are still needed on this subject in the cART era, especially in HIV-endemic settings, to better understand and to find improved ways of managing these outcomes.

Drug and Substance Use Disorders

Alcohol, tobacco and illicit drug consumption are major risk factors for disability and premature deaths globally (Degenhardt et al. 2018). In the context of HIV, the commonly abused substances include alcohol, tobacco, heroin, marijuana, and cocaine (Durvasula and Miller 2014; Edelman, Tetrault, and Fiellin 2014). Taken together, these disorders have far-reaching consequences on the health, economy, productivity, as well as social aspects of an individual and the society at large. Moreover, it is well documented that tobacco and alcohol abuse are important risk factors for cancer and cardiovascular diseases, which are the leading causes of death (O'Keefe et al. 2014). In the 2016 estimates of the Global Burden of Disease Study, alcohol use disorders (AUDs) were the most prevalent of all substance use disorders (Degenhardt et al. 2018). The most common drug use disorders were cannabis and opioid dependence. Importantly, much of this burden was because of the effect of substance use on other health outcomes globally. Among adults living with HIV, alcohol, tobacco, and illicit drug use have been shown to occur at a higher rate than in the general population (Shokoohi et al. 2018). In a recent systematic review and meta-analysis, the pooled prevalence of AUDs among PLWH was 29.3% globally (Duko, Ayalew, and Ayano 2019). In a subgroup analysis of LMICs and HICs, the authors found a significantly higher prevalence of AUDs in HICs (42.1%) compared to LMICs (24.5%). Similar findings were reported in a different review in SSA (Necho, Belete, and Getachew 2020).

There is an extensive body of literature showing that alcohol, tobacco, and illicit drug use can have deleterious effects on HIV care and general health outcomes by interacting with access and adherence to ART medication (Deren et al. 2019). This, in turn, affects HIV pathogenesis and disrupts important sources of social and financial support. Adults who use substances of abuse are likely to have suboptimal engagement in the HIV continuum of care, including delayed diagnosis/entry into HIV care services, reduced likelihood of initiating ART, reduced rates of retention in HIV care, as well as viral non-suppression (Golin et al. 2002; Kuchinad et al. 2016). The potential negative effects include drug resistance/treatment failure, cognitive decline, and premature mortality. Suboptimal adherence increases the risk of treatment failure, which presents a huge setback in the fight against the HIV epidemic.

The substantial morbidity brought about by substance use disorders among adults living with HIV and the various complications resulting from AIDS warrants management strategies to improve the quality of life of these adults. Fortunately, evidence on the effectiveness of a range of cost-effective interventions addressing these problems is growing (Durvasula and Miller 2014). What is concerning, however, is the slow rate of scaling up of such interventions to improve outcomes and increase the number of individuals reached in each step of the continuum of care (Parcesepe et al. 2020). Intervention efforts on drug and substance use disorders are particularly hampered by the complex health and social needs of affected individuals. There is evidence suggesting that adults using substances are more likely to be homeless, experience unemployment, live in poverty, and experience several forms of violence, which could negatively affect the management of their disease conditions (CDC 2018). This highlights the need for multisectoral and integrated approaches to address their needs. Screening for drug and substance use disorders in primary health care will facilitate early detection, treatment, and referral for these comorbidities. Some of the brief screening tools for these disorders include CRAFFT (Gamarel et al. 2017), AUDIT (Surah et al. 2013), CAGE (Ewing 1984), and ASSIST (Humeniuk et al. 2010). It is encouraging that some countries have integrated the screening of these disorders into their national HIV care guidelines (Ministry of Health 2018).

HEALTH-RELATED QUALITY OF LIFE

HRQoL refers to how health influences an individual's perceived and actual level of functioning and well-being in important aspects of life (Degroote, Vogelaers, and Vandijck 2014). Key among these aspects of life are feelings of well-being, control and autonomy, a positive self-perception, a sense of belonging, participation in enjoyable and meaningful life activities, and a positive view of the future. The concept of HRQoL has become a salient measure of the impact of HIV in the cART era considering that many adults living with HIV are increasingly achieving near-normal life expectancy, albeit with a myriad of HIV-associated comorbidities. In the wake of the changing dynamics of HIV infection, it is imperative to assess HRQoL because it reflects the patients' experiences of living with HIV, thereby serving as a proxy for understanding HIV treatment and care outcomes. It is vital to monitor HIV outcomes beyond clinical endpoints such as viral suppression or improvement in CD4 cell count. This need stems from accumulating research evidence showing that adults living with HIV manifest with significantly lower HRQoL than the general population (Miners et al. 2014). It is with this understanding that Lazarus and colleagues proposed a 'fourth 90' to the WHO's '90-90-90' testing and treatment target: ensure that 90% of people with viral suppression have a good HRQoL with special attention on two domains – comorbidities and self-perceived quality of life (Lazarus et al. 2016). The authors argue that the original WHO target fails to consider the needs of PLWH who have attained viral suppression but must still cope with several other health challenges, including non-communicable diseases, psychosocial problems, and mental health comorbidities.

The vast majority of the empirical evidence on HRQoL is cross-sectional and conducted over relatively shorter periods. There are also a few longitudinal and interventional studies (Degroote, Vogelaers, and Vandijck 2014). The overall consensus on the subject is that adults living with HIV present with lower HRQoL compared to the general population (Degroote, Vogelaers, and Vandijck 2014). Some recent studies, however, show that the HRQoL of PLWH is comparable to that of adults in the general population (Popping et al. 2021). Some of the predictors of poor HRQoL include lower ART adherence rates, depressive symptoms, impaired social support, low socioeconomic status, virological and immunological status, and comorbidity (Degroote, Vogelaers, and Vandijck 2014). Reports about the association of age, sex, ethnicity, and ART with HRQoL are mixed (Degroote, Vogelaers, and Vandijck 2014). One study showed improvement in HRQoL and attributed this to lifestyle modification following HIV diagnosis (Tsevat et al. 2009). Other studies have shown that ART initiation improves the quality of life of adults living with HIV within the first year (Booysen et al. 2007). However, little research has been conducted looking beyond this period, especially in Africa. A longitudinal study of adult outpatients living with HIV, of whom most were consistently on ART, recorded moderate stability overall in HRQoL ratings over 4 years (Burgoyne et al. 2004), a finding that contrasts with pre-cART longitudinal research, which showed progressive HRQoL decline over time (Lenderking et al. 1994; Revicki, Wu, and Murray 1995). It is clear from the literature that good mental health and pain relief remain among the important factors in improving the HRQoL of adults living with HIV (Degroote, Vogelaers, and Vandijck 2014). Patient-centred management approaches should be adopted in the care of adults living with HIV to improve the quality of life of these adults.

MEDICAL ADHERENCE

High levels of cART adherence (≥90%) are needed to attain viral suppression, to avoid potential drug resistance, and to minimise HIV-associated morbidity and mortality (Mathes et al. 2013). Unfortunately, a published meta-analysis of adherence to cART revealed that the average rate of reporting ≥90% cART adherence was 62% (Ortego et al. 2011). The UNAIDS flagship project – the 95-95-95 treatment goals – aims to eradicate the AIDS scourge by 2030 (UNAIDS 2014). The 'third 95' seeks to achieve viral suppression for all individuals living with HIV and is based on the principle of universal testing and treatment, which ultimately aims to reduce HIV incidence at the level of the general population. However, these targets have been criticised as unrealistic and almost unattainable (Bain, Nkoke, and Noubiap 2017). By the end of 2017, for instance, the world had attained 75-79-81 of the 95-95-95 targets. Only six countries (Cambodia, Denmark, Botswana, Eswatini [previously known as Swaziland], Namibia, and the Netherlands) had achieved these targets, while seven others were on track (UNAIDS 2018).

A vital step to achieving these targets is improving ART adherence. The WHO defines this concept as 'the degree to which the person's behaviour (taking medications, following a diet and/or executing lifestyle changes) corresponds with the agreed recommendations from a health care provider' (WHO 2016). Several barriers to achieving optimal ART adherence have been identified in the published literature. These include forgetting to take medication, household food insecurity, HIV-related stigma and discrimination, adverse effects of ART drugs, travelling/movements (Croome et al. 2017), male sex, alcohol use, use of traditional/herbal medicine, dissatisfaction with health care providers, depression (Heestermans et al. 2016), and inadequate training and compensation for lay health workers (Ma et al. 2016). On the other hand, some of the facilitators of optimal ART adherence include social support, reminders/memory aids, improvements after taking ART, disclosure of one's HIV status, having a good relationship with a health care provider, ART adherence counselling, and education interventions (Heestermans et al. 2016; Croome et al. 2017). Clearly, adults living with HIV face multiple barriers to ART adherence, and no one-size-fits-all intervention is adequate to promote optimal adherence.

Evidence of the effectiveness of interventions for enhancing adherence to ART is mixed. In a recent systematic review of high-quality studies, only 10 out of the 49 eligible studies reported improvement in ART adherence and other clinical outcomes (Mbuagbaw et al. 2015). Some of the effective interventions reported were routine counselling, text messages, counselling plus alarm device, life-steps programme (computer-delivered stress, mood, and ART adherence management), integrated intervention enhancing patients' decision-making skills, and contingency management to promote ART adherence. In another review, of 21 clinical trials, only one trial showed statistically significant results for adherence rates and viral load in favour of the interventions (Mathes et al. 2013). Evidence for technology-based interventions to promote ART adherence in adult populations is promising (Amico 2015). Given the quantitative nature of the prevailing reviews on the assessment of interventions for ART adherence, Ma and colleagues sought to provide global qualitative evidence on the barriers to and facilitators of interventions for improving ART adherence (Ma et al. 2016). Qualitative studies are particularly important in summarising data on participant and stakeholder experiences of various interventions. The evidence suggests that strengthening the social relationships of adults living with HIV, as well as empowering and developing culturally appropriate interventions, could promote fidelity to interventions (Ma et al. 2016).

KEY POPULATIONS

Key populations refer to specific groups at high risk of HIV infection irrespective of the epidemic type or local context, stigmatised by the society due to their identities or behaviours, and less likely than other groups to be reached by interventions (WHO 2017). The UNAIDS and the WHO include males who have sex with males (MSM), transgender persons, sex workers, people who inject drugs (PWIDs) and incarcerated persons (those in prisons and closed settings) as key populations (WHO 2017; Joint United Nations Programme on HIV/AIDS 2020). In contrast, vulnerable populations are people particularly vulnerable to HIV infection in certain situations or contexts. They include adolescents (particularly adolescent females in SSA), orphans, homeless/street families, people with disabilities, people in conflict areas, and migrants and mobile workers who are not affected by HIV uniformly across all countries.

Worldwide, approximately 65% of new HIV infections occur within key populations. In East and Southern Africa (where the majority of all incident HIV infections are), 17% of new HIV infections occur in key populations, whereas in West and Central Africa 42% of new HIV infections occur in key populations (Joint United Nations Programme on HIV/AIDS 2020). Nonetheless, these are likely underestimations given the limited data. The percentages for new HIV infections in key populations in SSA are expected to continue rising in the future. Compared with the general population, the average risk for HIV infection is 26 times higher for sex workers, 25 times higher for MSM, 35 times higher for PWIDs and 34 times higher for transgender females (Joint United Nations Programme on HIV/AIDS 2020). A range of complex individual factors explains the disproportionate HIV risks, including biological (e.g. unprotected anal sex) and behavioural (e.g. lack of condom use and the use of psychoactive substances), together with structural factors such as HIV-related stigma and discrimination (Joint United Nations Programme on HIV/AIDS 2020; Jin, Restar, and Beyrer 2021; Kloek et al. 2022). In SSA, the estimated HIV prevalence for MSM is about 20% and 30% for transgender females (Kloek et al. 2022). However, data remain largely scarce in the region (Jin, Restar, and Beyrer 2021; Kloek et al. 2022). Although the highest burden of HIV is in SSA, where heterosexual sex has been the primary mode of transmission, HIV epidemics in Eastern Europe and Central Asia continue to be driven by drug injecting (Larney et al. 2020). Key-populations programmes, particularly in SSA, struggle to meet the same ART treatment, retention, and viral suppression rates. In South and Southeast Asia, complex epidemics involving sex workers, MSM, transgender persons and PWIDs challenge service provision. There is an urgent need for scaling up tailored HIV prevention and the treatment interventions for these populations.

Accumulating evidence highlights that the implications and consequences of challenging health care systems, internal and public HIV-related stigma, homophobia, and health comorbidities among key populations can lead to suicide attempts, poor quality of life, poor retention in HIV care, virological failure, isolation, risky behaviour, substance use and abuse, non-adherence to ART, and mortality (Christopoulos, Das, and Colfax 2011; Lyons, Heywood, and Rozbroj 2016; Sandfort et al. 2017). For instance, transgender populations and MSM have been shown to experience a high burden of depression, anxiety, substance use, suicidality, HIV infection and unmet health care needs (Rich et al. 2020; Kirwan et al. 2021). Until recently, these health inequities were rendered largely invisible by the systematic exclusion of key populations in health research and information systems. However, there has been a remarkable increase in health research on key populations across the globe. Nonetheless, research remains concentrated in HICs, and hence the existing research is limited in its ability to inform interventions in LMICs.

SUMMARY AND CONCLUDING REMARKS

Over the past few decades, improved access to cART has effectively transformed HIV into a chronic and manageable condition. A growing number of adults living with HIV are attaining viral suppression thanks to the scale-up of the lifesaving cART. Although the incidence of AIDS-defining illnesses has dramatically reduced in the cART era, adults living with HIV still have an increased risk of chronic complications and comorbidities, such as mental, neurological, and substance use disorders, and noncommunicable diseases. These complications and comorbidities have been described as a 'double-edged sword' threatening the global vision of containing the epidemic by 2030, given that they are associated with increased mortality, poor treatment adherence, poor HRQoL, increased risk-taking behaviours, and disruptions to everyday functioning, especially among key populations. Despite their negative impact, the treatment gap for many of these conditions is appalling, especially in LMICs. For instance, the treatment gap for mental disorders in adults enrolled in HIV treatment programmes in SSA is about 40% for PLWH in private health care, 97% for PLWH in public primary care, and 65% for PLWH in public tertiary care ART programmes (Ruffieux et al. 2021). Furthermore, many frontline health care workers are not conversant with certain conditions, for example, HAND, according to recent surveys (Gouse et al. 2021; Munsami et al. 2021). Health care workers seldom suspect HAND among PLWH and screening practices are uncommon, and referrals for cognitive impairment are never requested. Addressing these complications and comorbidities will improve the quality of life of PLWH and prevent HIV disease progression, the development of drug-resistant strains, and HIV transmission.

The next important challenge for HIV neuropsychiatric researchers is to translate the wealth of observational knowledge regarding neurobehavioural outcomes into effective, theory-driven, and evidence-based treatments that can improve the health and well-being of adults living with HIV. The evidence on the effectiveness of interventions for the treatment and prevention of HIV- associated complications and comorbidities is promising. Common mental disorders can be treated effectively across the globe with low-cost medications or psychological intervention. Stepped care and collaborative models provide a good framework for integrating a range of interventions for better health outcomes (Goodrich et al. 2013). Brief interventions delivered by primary health care providers are effective for managing hazardous alcohol use, for instance. Overall, most of the research on mental health interventions has been conducted in HICs (especially in the USA) rather than LMICs, which is a mismatch of the global burden of HIV. Moreover, mental health interventions have generally focused on short-term over long-term outcomes, and the research could benefit from improved quality and rigour. There is also a paucity of studies that examine neuropsychiatric interventions related to HIV care outcomes. Furthermore, few evidence-based interventions have been tested among older adults living with HIV, despite their growing population across regions. The literature on HAND is increasing in both LMICs and HICs and, while this is promising, a significant proportion of the existing literature documents the general epidemiology of HAND but has little focus on how to identify and manage it in primary health care settings. More work needs to be done on improving current screening tools for this condition in clinical settings and on addressing the next step in their management. There is also a need for clinicians and researchers to distinguish between HAND and age-associated dementia, including Alzheimer's disease. Clinically, the more degenerative profile of age-associated dementias requires different life planning and treatment options compared to the HAND profile, in which cognitive impairment is typically more stable. Besides, a delayed dementia diagnosis in PLWH would limit the opportunity to intervene early when interventions – for example, cognitive interventions – are most effective.

Overall, it is imperative for policymakers to act on available evidence to scale-up cost-effective forms of treatment and care to improve the quality of life and the well-being of adults living with HIV. Clearly, there is a need for collaboration between health systems and individual communities to deliver the required services to the many people who need them the most. Task-shifting is a promising approach, especially in such settings where there are inadequate human resources.

REFERENCES

Abas M, Ali GC, Nakimuli-Mpungu E, Chibanda D (2014) Depression in people living with HIV in sub-Saharan Africa: Time to act. *Tropical Medicine & International Health,* 19(12): 1392–1396.

Adams, C, Zacharia S, Masters L, Coffey C, Catalan P (2016) Mental health problems in people living with HIV. Changes in the last two decades: The London experience 1990–2014. *AIDS Care,* 28(Suppl 1): 56–59.

Adimora AA, Ramirez C, Benning L et al. (2018) Cohort profile: The women's interagency HIV study (WIHS). *International Journal of Epidemiology,* 47(2): 393–394i.

Agelink van Rentergem JA, Murre JM, Huizenga HM (2017) Multivariate normative comparisons using an aggregated database. *PloS One,* 12(3): e0173218.

Alford K, Vera J (2018) Cognitive impairment in people living with HIV in the ART era: A review. *British Medical Bulletin,* 127(1): 55–68.

Alford K, Daley S, Banerjee S, Vera JH (2021) Quality of life in people living with HIV-associated neurocognitive disorder: A scoping review study. *PloS One,* 16(5): e0251944.

Amico KR (2015) Evidence for technology interventions to promote ART adherence in adult populations: A review of the literature 2012–2015. *Current HIV/AIDS Reports*, 12(4): 441–450.

Antinori A, Arendt G, Becker J et al. (2007) Updated research nosology for HIV-associated neurocognitive disorders. *Neurology*, 69(18): 1789–1799.

Aung HL, Kootar S, Gates TM, Brew BJ, Cysique LA (2019) How all-type dementia risk factors and modifiable risk interventions may be relevant to the first-generation aging with HIV infection? *European Geriatric Medicine*, 10(2): 227–238.

Autenrieth CS, Beck EJ, Stelzle D, Mallouris C, Mahy M, Ghys P (2018) Global and regional trends of people living with HIV aged 50 and over: Estimates and projections for 2000–2020. *PloS One*, 13(11): e0207005.

Bagkeris E, Burgess L, Mallon PW et al. (2018) Cohort profile: The pharmacokinetic and clinical observations in PeoPle over fiftY (POPPY) study. *International Journal of Epidemiology*, 47(5): 1391–1392e.

Bain LE, Nkoke C, Noubiap JJN (2017) UNAIDS 90–90–90 targets to end the AIDS epidemic by 2020 are not realistic: Comment on 'Can the UNAIDS 90–90–90 target be achieved? A systematic analysis of national HIV treatment cascades'. *BMJ Global Health*, 2(2): e000227.

Bandelow B, Michaelis S (2015) Epidemiology of anxiety disorders in the 21st century. *Dialogues in Clinical Neuroscience*, 17(3): 327.

Becker BW, Thames AD, Woo E, Castellon SA, Hinkin CH (2011) Longitudinal change in cognitive function and medication adherence in HIV-infected adults. *AIDS and Behavior*, 15(8): 1888–1894.

Becker JT, Kingsley LA, Molsberry S et al. (2015) Cohort profile: Recruitment cohorts in the neuropsychological substudy of the Multicenter AIDS Cohort Study. *International Journal of Epidemiology*, 44(5): 1506–1516.

Beer L, Tie Y, Padilla M, Shouse RL (2019) Generalized anxiety disorder symptoms among persons with diagnosed HIV in the United States. *Aids*, 33(11): 1781–1787.

Bernard C, Dabis F, de Rekeneire N (2017) Prevalence and factors associated with depression in people living with HIV in sub-Saharan Africa: A systematic review and meta-analysis. *PloS One*, 12(8): e0181960.

Blackstone K, Moore D, Heaton R et al. (2012) CNS HIV Antiretroviral Therapy Effects Research (CHARTER) group diagnosing symptomatic HIV-associated neurocognitive disorders: Self-report versus performance-based assessment of everyday functioning. *J Int Neuropsychol Soc*, 18(1): 79–88.

Bobrow K, Xia F, Hoang T, Valcour V, Yaffe K (2020) HIV and risk of dementia in older veterans. *Aids*, 34(11): 1673–1679.

Boivin MJ, Busman RA, Parikh SM et al. (2010) A pilot study of the neuropsychological benefits of computerized cognitive rehabilitation in Ugandan children with HIV. *Neuropsychology*, 24(5): 667.

Boivin MJ, Nakasujja N, Sikorskii A, Opoka RO, Giordani B (2016) A randomized controlled trial to evaluate if computerized cognitive rehabilitation improves neurocognition in Ugandan children with HIV. *AIDS Research and Human Retroviruses*, 32(8): 743–755.

Booysen FlR, Van Rensburg H, Bachmann M, Louwagie G, Fairall L (2007) The heart in HAART: Quality of life of patients enrolled in the public sector antiretroviral treatment programme in the Free State Province of South Africa. *Social Indicators Research*, 81(2): 283–329.

Borrell C, Rodríguez-Sanz M, Pasarín MI et al. (2006) AIDS mortality before and after the introduction of highly active antiretroviral therapy: Does it vary with socioeconomic group in a country with a National Health System? *The European Journal of Public Health*, 16(6): 601–608.

Bougea A, Spantideas N, Galanis P, Gkekas G, Thomaides T (2019) Optimal treatment of HIV-associated neurocognitive disorders: Myths and reality. A critical review. *Therapeutic Advances in Infectious Disease*, 6: 2049936119838228.

Brandt C, Zvolensky MJ, Woods SP, Gonzalez A, Safren SA, O'Cleirigh CM (2017) Anxiety symptoms and disorders among adults living with HIV and AIDS: A critical review and integrative synthesis of the empirical literature. *Clinical Psychology Review*, 51: 164–184.

Burgoyne RW, Rourke SB, Behrens DM, Salit IE (2004) Long-term quality-of-life outcomes among adults living with HIV in the HAART era: The interplay of changes in clinical factors and symptom profile. *AIDS and Behavior*, 8(2): 151–163.

CDC (2018) HIV and substance use in the United States. Available at https://www.cdc.gov/hiv/risk/substanceuse.html.

Chandra P, Krishna V, Ravi V, Desai A, Puttaram S (1999) HIV related admissions in a psychiatric hospital: A five year profile. *Indian Journal of Psychiatry*, 41(4): 320.

Chibanda D, Mangezi W, Tshimanga M et al. (2010) Postnatal depression by HIV status among women in Zimbabwe. *Journal of Women's Health,* 19(11): 2071–2077.

Chibanda D, Mesu P, Kajawu L, Cowan F, Araya R, Abas MA (2011) Problem-solving therapy for depression and common mental disorders in Zimbabwe: Piloting a task-shifting primary mental health care intervention in a population with a high prevalence of people living with HIV. *BMC Public Health*, 11(1): 1–10.

Christopoulos KA, Das M, Colfax GN (2011) Linkage and retention in HIV care among men who have sex with men in the United States. *Clinical Infectious Diseases*, 52(Suppl 2): S214–S222.

Clifford KM, Samboju V, Cobigo Y et al. (2017) Progressive brain atrophy despite persistent viral suppression in HIV over age 60. *Journal of Acquired Immune Deficiency Syndromes (1999)*, 76(3): 289.

Clucas C, Sibley E, Harding R, Liu L, Catalan J, Sherr L (2011) A systematic review of interventions for anxiety in people with HIV. *Psychology, Health & Medicine*, 16(5): 528–547.

Cohen MA, Gorman JM, Volberding P, Letendre SL (2017) *Comprehensive Textbook of AIDS Psychiatry: A Paradigm for Integrated Care.* Oxford: Oxford University Press.

Cournos F, Empfield M, Horwath E et al. (1991) HIV seroprevalence among patients admitted to two psychiatric hospitals. *Am J Psychiatry*, 148(9): 1225–1230.

Croome N, Ahluwalia M, Hughes LD, Abas M (2017) Patient-reported barriers and facilitators to antiretroviral adherence in sub-Saharan Africa. *AIDS (London, England)*, 31(7): 995.

De Francesco D, Underwood J, Post FA et al. (2016) Defining cognitive impairment in people-living-with-HIV: The POPPY study. *BMC Infectious Diseases*, 16(1): 617.

Degenhardt L, Charlson F, Ferrari A et al. (2018) The global burden of disease attributable to alcohol and drug use in 195 countries and territories, 1990–2016: A systematic analysis for the Global Burden of Disease Study 2016. *The Lancet Psychiatry*, 5(12): 987–1012.

Degroote S, Vogelaers D, Vandijck DM (2014) What determines health-related quality of life among people living with HIV: An updated review of the literature. *Archives of Public Health*, 72(1): 40.

Deren S, Cortes T, Dickson VV et al. (2019) Substance use among older people living with HIV: Challenges for health care providers. *Frontiers in Public Health*, 7: 94.

Doyle KL, Woods SP, Morgan EE et al. (2016) Health-related decision-making in HIV disease. *Journal of Clinical Psychology in Medical Settings*, 23(2): 135–146.

Duko B, Ayalew M, Ayano G (2019) The prevalence of alcohol use disorders among people living with HIV/AIDS: A systematic review and meta-analysis. *Substance Abuse Treatment, Prevention, and Policy*, 14(1): 1–9.

Durvasula R, Miller TR (2014) Substance abuse treatment in persons with HIV/AIDS: Challenges in managing triple diagnosis. *Behavioral Medicine*, 40(2): 43–52.

Edelman EJ, Tetrault JM, Fiellin DA (2014) Substance use in older HIV-infected patients. *Current Opinion in HIV and AIDS*, 9(4): 317.

Eggers C, Arendt G, Hahn K et al. (2017) HIV-1-associated neurocognitive disorder: Epidemiology, pathogenesis, diagnosis, and treatment. *Journal of Neurology*, 264(8): 1715–1727.

Ellen SR, Judd FK, Mijch AM, Cockram A (1999) Secondary mania in patients with HIV infection. *Australian and New Zealand Journal of Psychiatry*, 33(3): 353–360.

Ewing JA (1984) Detecting alcoholism: The CAGE questionnaire. *Jama*, 252(14): 1905–1907.

Ezeamama AE, Sikorskii A, Sankar PR et al. (2020) Computerized cognitive rehabilitation training for Ugandan seniors living with HIV: A validation study. *Journal of Clinical Medicine*, 9(7): 2137.

Fabbiani M, Ciccarelli N, Tana M et al. (2013) Cardiovascular risk factors and carotid intima-media thickness are associated with lower cognitive performance in HIV-infected patients. *HIV Medicine*, 14(3): 136–144.

Gamarel KE, Nelson KM, Brown L, Fernandez MI, Nichols S, The Adolescent Medicine Trials Network for HIV/AIDS Intervention (2017) The usefulness of the CRAFFT in screening for problematic drug and alcohol use among youth living with HIV. *AIDS and Behavior*, 21(7): 1868–1877.

Ganju V (2011) *The Great Push: Investing in Mental Health.* World Federation for Mental Health.

Gaynes BN, Pence BW, Atashili J et al. (2015) Changes in HIV outcomes following depression care in a resource-limited setting: Results from a pilot study in Bamenda, Cameroon. *PloS One*, 10(10): e0140001.

Gisslén M, Price RW, Nilsson S (2011) The definition of HIV-associated neurocognitive disorders: Are we overestimating the real prevalence? *BMC Infectious Diseases*, 11(1): 356.

Gizachew KD, Chekol YA, Basha EA, Mamuye SA, Wubetu AD (2021) Suicidal ideation and attempt among people living with HIV/AIDS in selected public hospitals: Central Ethiopia. *Annals of General Psychiatry*, 20(1): 1–18.

Golin CE, Liu H, Hays RD et al. (2002) A prospective study of predictors of adherence to combination antiretroviral medication. *Journal of Ggeneral Internal Medicine*, 17(10): 756–765.

Gómez-Olivé FX, Montana L, Wagner RG et al. (2018) Cohort profile: Health and ageing in Africa: A longitudinal study of an INDEPTH community in South Africa (HAALSI). *International Journal of Epidemiology*, 47(3): 689–690j.

Goodrich DE, Kilbourne AM, Nord KM, Bauer MS (2013) Mental health collaborative care and its role in primary care settings. *Current Psychiatry Reports*, 15(8): 383.

Gouse H, Masson CJ, Henry M et al. (2021) Assessing HIV provider knowledge, screening practices, and training needs for HIV-associated neurocognitive disorders. A short report. *AIDS Care*, 33(4): 468–472.

Grant I, Atkinson JH, Hesselink JR et al. (1987) Evidence for early central nervous system involvement in the acquired immunodeficiency syndrome (AIDS) and other human immunodeficiency virus (HIV) infections: Studies with neuropsychologic testing and magnetic resonance imaging. *Annals of Internal Medicine*, 107(6): 828–836.

Grant I, Atkinson J (1999) Neuropsychiatric aspects of HIV infection and AIDS. In: Sadock B, Sadock J, editors, *Kaplan and Sadock's Comprehensive Textbook of Psychiatry. 7th Edition*. Philadelphia, PA: Lippincott Williams and Wilkins, pp. 308–335.

Group MEW, Antinori A, Arendt G et al. (2012) Assessment, diagnosis, and treatment of HIV-associated neurocognitive disorder: A consensus report of the mind exchange program. *Clinical Infectious Diseases*, 56(7): 1004–1017.

Guha A, Brier MR, Ortega M, Westerhaus E, Nelson B, Ances BM (2016) Topographies of cortical and subcortical volume loss in HIV and aging in the cART era. *Journal of Acquired Immune Deficiency Syndromes (1999)*, 73(4): 374.

Gupta S, Granich R (2016) When will sub-Saharan Africa adopt HIV treatment for all? *Southern African Journal of HIV Medicine,* 17(1): 1–6.

Harezlak J, Buchthal S, Taylor M et al. (2011) Persistence of HIV-associated cognitive impairment, inflammation and neuronal injury in era of highly active antiretroviral treatment. *AIDS (London, England)*, 25(5): 625.

Heaton R, Clifford D, Franklin D et al. (2010) HIV-associated neurocognitive disorders persist in the era of potent antiretroviral therapy: CHARTER Study. *Neurology*, 75(23): 2087–2096.

Heestermans T, Browne JL, Aitken SC, Vervoort SC, Klipstein-Grobusch K (2016) Determinants of adherence to antiretroviral therapy among HIV-positive adults in sub-Saharan Africa: A systematic review. *BMJ Global Health*, 1(4): e000125.

Hellmuth J, Fletcher JL, Valcour V et al. (2016) Neurologic signs and symptoms frequently manifest in acute HIV infection. *Neurology*, 87(2): 148–154.

Hinkin C, Castellon S, Atkinson J, Goodkin K (2001) Neuropsychiatric aspects of HIV infection among older adults. *Journal of Clinical Epidemiology*, 54(12): S44–S52.

Hinkin C, Castellon S, Durvasula R et al. (2002) Medication adherence among HIV+ adults: Effects of cognitive dysfunction and regimen complexity. *Neurology*, 59(12): 1944–1950.

Hinsch M, Reichelt D, Husstedt I (2014) Acute psychosis as a side effect of efavirenz therapy with metabolic anomalies: An important differential diagnosis of HIV-associated psychoses. *Der Nervenarzt*, 85(10): 1304–1308.

Hoeft TJ, Fortney JC, Patel V, Unützer J (2018) Task-sharing approaches to improve mental health care in rural and other low-resource settings: A systematic review. *The Journal of Rural Health*, 34(1): 48–62.

Holland JC, Tross S (1985) The psychosocial and neuropsychiatric sequelae of the acquired immunodeficiency syndrome and related disorders. *Annals of Internal Medicine*, 103(5): 760–764.

Humeniuk R, Henry-Edwards S, Ali R, Poznyak V, Monteiro MG (2010) *The Alcohol, Smoking and Substance Involvement Screening Test (ASSIST): Manual for Use in Primary Care*. Geneva: World Health Organization.

Ingle SM, May MT, Gill MJ et al. (2014) Impact of risk factors for specific causes of death in the first and subsequent years of antiretroviral therapy among HIV-infected patients. *Clinical Infectious Diseases*, 59(2): 287–297.

Jallow A, Ljunggren G, Wändell P, Wahlström L, Carlsson AC (2017) HIV-infection and psychiatric illnesse: A double-edged sword that threatens the vision of a contained epidemic: The Greater Stockholm HIV Cohort Study. *Journal of Infection*, 74(1): 22–28.

Jin H, Restar A, Beyrer C (2021) Overview of the epidemiological conditions of HIV among key populations in Africa. *Journal of the International AIDS Society*, 24: e25716.

Joint United Nations Programme on HIV/AIDS (2014) *90-90-90: An Ambitious Treatment Target to Help End the AIDS Epidemic*. Geneva: UNAIDS.

Joint United Nations Programme on HIV/AIDS (2020). *Global AIDS Update 2020. Seizing the Moment: Tackling Entrenched Inequalities to End Epidemics*. [online] Available at https://www.unaids.org/en/resources/documents/2020/global-aids-report.

Joska JA, Dreyer AJ, Nightingale S, Combrinck MI, De Jager CA (2019) Prevalence of HIV-1 infection in an elderly rural population and associations with neurocognitive impairment. *Aids*, 33(11): 1765–1771.

Justice AC, Dombrowski E, Conigliaro J et al. (2006) Veterans aging cohort study (VACS): Ooverview and description. *Medical Care*, 44(8 Suppl 2): S13.

Kallianpur KJ, Jahanshad N, Sailasuta N et al. (2020) Regional brain volumetric changes despite two years of treatment initiated during acute HIV infection. *AIDS (London, England)*, 34(3): 415.

Kingori C, Haile ZT, Ngatia P (2015) Depression symptoms, social support and overall health among HIV-positive individuals in Kenya. *International Journal of STD & AIDS*, 26(3): 165–172.

Kinyanda E, Hoskins S, Nakku J, Nawaz S, Patel V (2012) The prevalence and characteristics of suicidality in HIV/AIDS as seen in an African population in Entebbe district, Uganda. *BMC Psychiatry*, 12(1): 63.

Kirwan P, Hibbert M, Kall M et al. (2021) HIV prevalence and HIV clinical outcomes of transgender and gender-diverse people in England. *HIV Medicine*, 22(2): 131–139.

Kloek M, Bulstra CA, van Noord L, Al-Hassany L, Cowan FM, Hontelez J (2022) HIV prevalence among men who have sex with men, transgender women and cisgender male sex workers in sub-Saharan Africa: A systematic review and meta-analysis. *Journal of the International AIDS Society*, 25: e26022.

Kuchinad KE, Hutton HE, Monroe AK, Anderson G, Moore RD, Chander G (2016) A qualitative study of barriers to and facilitators of optimal engagement in care among PLWH and substance use/misuse. *BMC Research Notes*, 9(1): 229.

Lam JO, Hou CE, Hojilla JC et al. (2021) Comparison of dementia risk after age 50 between individuals with and without HIV infection. *Aids*, 35(5): 821–828.

Lampe FC, Harding R, Smith CJ, Phillips AN, Johnson M, Sherr L (2010) Physical and psychological symptoms and risk of virologic rebound among patients with virologic suppression on antiretroviral therapy. *JAIDS Journal of Acquired Immune Deficiency Syndromes*, 54(5): 500–505.

Larney S, Leung J, Grebely J et al. (2020) Global systematic review and ecological analysis of HIV in people who inject drugs: National population sizes and factors associated with HIV prevalence. *International Journal of Drug Policy*, 77: 102656.

Lazarus JV, Safreed-Harmon K, Barton SE et al. (2016) Beyond viral suppression of HIV: The new quality of life frontier. *BMC Medicine*, 14(1): 94.

Lenderking WR, Gelber RD, Cotton DJ et al. (1994) Evaluation of the quality of life associated with zidovudine treatment in asymptomatic human immunodeficiency virus infection. *New England Journal of Medicine*, 330(11): 738–743.

Lofgren SM, Nakasujja N, Boulware DR (2018) Systematic review of interventions for depression for People Living with HIV in Africa. *AIDS and Behavior*, 22(1): 1–8.

Lyketsos CG, Hanson AL, Fishman M, Rosenblatt A, McHugh PR, Treisman GJ (1993) Manic syndrome early and late in the course of HIV. *The American Journal of Psychiatry*, 150(2): 326–327.

Lyketsos CG, Schwartz J, Fishman M, Treisman G (1997) AIDS mania. *J Neuropsychiatry Clin Neurosci*, 9(2): 277–279. doi: 10.1176/jnp.9.2.277.

Lyons A, Heywood W, Rozbroj T (2016) Psychosocial factors associated with flourishing among Australian HIV-positive gay men. *BMC Psychology*, 4(1): 1–10.

Ma Q, Tso LS, Rich ZC et al. (2016) Barriers and facilitators of interventions for improving antiretroviral therapy adherence: A systematic review of global qualitative evidence. *Journal of the International AIDS Society*, 19(1): 21166.

Marcus JL, Leyden WA, Alexeeff SE et al. (2020) Comparison of overall and comorbidity-free life expectancy between insured adults with and without HIV infection, 2000–2016. *JAMA Network Open*, 3(6): e207954–e207954.

Mathes T, Pieper D, Antoine SL, Eikermann M (2013) Adherence-enhancing interventions for highly active antiretroviral therapy in HIV-infected patients – A systematic review. *HIV Medicine*, 14(10): 583–595.

Mbuagbaw L, Sivaramalingam B, Navarro T et al. (2015) Interventions for enhancing adherence to antiretroviral therapy (ART): A systematic review of high quality studies. *AIDS Patient Care and STDs*, 29(5): 248–266.

Mijch AM, Judd FK, Lyketsos CG, Ellen S, Cockram A (1999) Secondary mania in patients with HIV infection: Are antiretrovirals protective? *The Journal of Neuropsychiatry and Clinical Neurosciences*, 11(4): 475–480.

Milic J, Russwurm M, Calvino AC, Brañas F, Sánchez-Conde M, Guaraldi G (2019) European cohorts of older HIV adults: POPPY, AGE h IV, GEPPO, COBRA and FUNCFRAIL. *European Geriatric Medicine,* 10(2): 247–257.

Mind Exchange Working Group, Antinori A, Arendt G et al. (2012) Assessment, diagnosis, and treatment of HIV-associated neurocognitive disorder: A consensus report of the mind exchange program. *Clinical Infectious Diseases*, 56(7): 1004–1017.

Miners A, Phillips A, Kreif N et al. (2014) Health-related quality-of-life of people with HIV in the era of combination antiretroviral treatment: A cross-sectional comparison with the general population. *The Lancet HIV*, 1(1): e32–e40.

Ministry of Health (2018) *Guidelines on Use of Antiretroviral Drugs for Treating and Preventing HIV Infection in Kenya.* Nairobi, Kenya: National AIDS and STI Control Program (NASCOP).

Morrison SD, Banushi VH, Sarnquist C et al. (2011) Levels of self-reported depression and anxiety among HIV-positive patients in Albania: A cross-sectional study. *Croatian Medical Journal*, 52(5): 622–628.

Munsami A, Gouse H, Nightingale S, Joska JA (2021) HIV-associated neurocognitive impairment knowledge and current practices: A survey of frontline healthcare workers in South Africa. *Journal of Community Health*, 46(3): 538–544.

Mwangala PN, Newton CR, Abas M, Abubakar A (2019) Screening tools for HIV-associated neurocognitive disorders among adults living with HIV in sub-Saharan Africa: A scoping review. *AAS Open Research*, 1: 28.

Mwangala PN, Mabrouk A, Wagner R, Newton CR, Abubakar AA (2021) Mental health and well-being of older adults living with HIV in sub-Saharan Africa: A systematic review. *BMJ Open*, 11(9): e052810.

Nakimuli-Mpungu E, Musisi S, Mpungu SK, Katabira E (2006) Primary mania versus HIV-related secondary mania in Uganda. *American Journal of Psychiatry*, 163(8): 1349–1354.

Nakimuli-Mpungu E, Musisi S, Smith CM et al. (2021) Mental health interventions for persons living with HIV in low- and middle-income countries: A systematic review. *Journal of the International AIDS Society*, 24: e25722.

Navia BA, Jordan BD, Price RW (1986) The AIDS dementia complex: I. Clinical features. *Annals of Neurology: Official Journal of the American Neurological Association and the Child Neurology Society*, 19(6): 517–524.

Necho M, Belete A, Getachew Y (2020) The prevalence and factors associated with alcohol use disorder among people living with HIV/AIDS in Africa: A systematic review and meta-analysis. *Substance Abuse Treatment, Prevention, and Policy*, 15(1): 1–15.

Nel A, Kagee A (2013) The relationship between depression, anxiety and medication adherence among patients receiving antiretroviral treatment in South Africa. *AIDS Care*, 25(8): 948–955.

Nsanzimana S, Remera E, Kanters S et al. (2015) Life expectancy among HIV-positive patients in Rwanda: A retrospective observational cohort study. *The Lancet Global Health*, 3(3): e169–e177.

Nüesch R, Gayet-Ageron A, Chetchotisakd P et al. (2009) The impact of combination antiretroviral therapy and its interruption on anxiety, stress, depression and quality of life in Thai patients. *The Open AIDS Journal*, 3: 38.

Nweke M, Nombeko M, Govender N, Akineplu AO (2021) Rehabilitation of HIV-associated neurocognitive disorder: A systematic scoping review of available interventions. *Advances in Mental Health*, 20: 200–217.

Nyongesa MK, Mwangala PN, Mwangi P, Kombe M, Newton CR, Abubakar AA (2018) Neurocognitive and mental health outcomes and association with quality of life among adults living with HIV: A cross-sectional focus on a low-literacy population from coastal Kenya. *BMJ Open,* 8(9): e023914.

O'Connor E, Zeffiro TA, Zeffiro TA (2018) Brain structural changes following HIV Infection: Meta-analysis. *American Journal of Neuroradiology*, 39(1): 54–62.

O'Keefe JH, Bhatti SK, Bajwa A, DiNicolantonio JJ, Lavie CJ (2014) Alcohol and cardiovascular health: The dose makes the poison… or the remedy. *Mayo Clinic Proceedings*, 89(3): 382–393.

Omeragic A, Kayode O, Hoque MT, Bendayan R (2020) Potential pharmacological approaches for the treatment of HIV-1 associated neurocognitive disorders. *Fluids and Barriers of the CNS*, 17(1): 1–30.

Ortego C, Huedo-Medina TB, Llorca J et al. (2011) Adherence to highly active antiretroviral therapy (HAART): A meta-analysis. *AIDS and Behavior*, 15(7): 1381–1396.

Owe-Larsson M, Säll L, Salamon E, Allgulander C (2009) HIV infection and psychiatric illness. *African Journal of Psychiatry*, 12(2): 115–128.

Parcesepe AM, Lancaster K, Edelman EJ et al. (2020) Substance use service availability in HIV treatment programs: Data from the global IeDEA consortium, 2014-2015 and 2017. *PloS One*, 15(8): e0237772.

Patel V, Prince M (2010) Global mental health: A new global health field comes of age. *Jama,* 303(19): 1976–1977.

Pence BW, Miller WC, Whetten K, Eron JJ, Gaynes BN (2006) Prevalence of DSM-IV-defined mood, anxiety, and substance use disorders in an HIV clinic in the Southeastern United States. *JAIDS Journal of Acquired Immune Deficiency Syndromes*, 42(3): 298–306.

Perry S, Jacobsen P (1986) Neuropsychiatric manifestations of AIDS-spectrum disorders. *Psychiatric Services*, 37(2): 135–142.

Petersen I, Bhana A, Folb N et al. (2018) Collaborative care for the detection and management of depression among adults with hypertension in South Africa: Study protocol for the PRIME-SA randomised controlled trial. *Trials*, 19(1): 192.

Popping S, Kall M, Nichols BE et al. (2021) Quality of life among people living with HIV in England and the Netherlands: A population-based study. *The Lancet Regional Health-Europe*, 8: 100177.

Puri BK, Hall AD, Ho R (2014) *Revision Notes in Psychiatry:* CRC Press.

Rehm J, Shield KD (2019) Global burden of disease and the impact of mental and addictive disorders. *Current Psychiatry Reports*, 21(2): 1–7.

Remien RH, Stirratt MJ, Nguyen N, Robbins RN, Pala AN, Mellins CA (2019) Mental health and HIV/AIDS: The need for an integrated response. *AIDS (London, England)*, 33(9): 1411.

Revicki DA, Wu AW, Murray MI (1995) Change in clinical status, health status, and health utility outcomes in HIV-infected patients. *Medical Care*, 33(4 Suppl): AS173–AS182.

Rezaei S, Ahmadi S, Rahmati J et al. (2019) Global prevalence of depression in HIV/AIDS: A systematic review and meta-analysis. *BMJ Supportive & Palliative Care*, 9(4): 404–412.

Rich AJ, Scheim AI, Koehoorn M, Poteat T (2020) Non-HIV chronic disease burden among transgender populations globally: A systematic review and narrative synthesis. *Preventive Medicine Reports*, 20: 101259.

Rosa W (ed.) (2017) *A New Era in Global Health: Nursing and the United Nations 2030 Agenda for Sustainable Development:* New York: Springer Publishing Company.

Ruffieux Y, Efthimiou O, Van den Heuvel LL et al. (2021) The treatment gap for mental disorders in adults enrolled in HIV treatment programmes in South Africa: A cohort study using linked electronic health records. *Epidemiology and Psychiatric Sciences*, 30: e37.

Sacktor N, Skolasky RL, Seaberg E et al. (2016) Prevalence of HIV-associated neurocognitive disorders in the Multicenter AIDS Cohort Study. *Neurology*, 86(4): 334–340.

Sandfort TG, Knox JR, Alcala C, El-Bassel N, Kuo I, Smith LR (2017) Substance use and HIV risk among men who have sex with men in Africa: A systematic review. *Journal of Acquired Immune Deficiency Syndromes (1999)*, 76(2): e34.

Schmidt U, Miller D (1988) Two cases of hypomania in AIDS. *The British Journal of Psychiatry*, 152(6): 839–842.

Sherr L, Clucas C, Harding R, Sibley E, Catalan J (2011) HIV and depression – A systematic review of interventions. *Psychology, Health & Medicine*, 16(5): 493–527.

Shokoohi M, Bauer GR, Kaida A et al. (2018) Substance use patterns among women living with HIV compared with the general female population of Canada. *Drug and Alcohol Dependence*, 191: 70–77.

Sikkema KJ, Dennis AC, Watt MH, Choi KW, Yemeke TT, Joska JA (2015) Improving mental health among people living with HIV: A review of intervention trials in low-and middle-income countries. *Global Mental Health*, 2: e19.

Sin NL, DiMatteo MR (2013) Depression treatment enhances adherence to antiretroviral therapy: A meta-analysis. *Annals of Behavioral Medicine*, 47(3): 259–269.

Singer EJ, Thames AD (2016) Neurobehavioral manifestations of human immunodeficiency virus/AIDS: Diagnosis and treatment. *Neurologic Clinics*, 34(1): 33–53. doi: 10.1016/j.ncl.2015.08.003.

Slavich GM, Irwin MR (2014) From stress to inflammation and major depressive disorder: A social signal transduction theory of depression. *Psychological Bulletin*, 140(3): 774.

Songo J, Wringe A, Hassan F et al. (2021) Implications of HIV treatment policies on the health workforce in rural Malawi and Tanzania between 2013 and 2017: Evidence from the SHAPE-UTT study. *Global Public Health*, 16(2): 256–273.

Su T, Schouten J, Geurtsen GJ et al. (2015) Multivariate normative comparison, a novel method for more reliably detecting cognitive impairment in HIV infection. *Aids*, 29(5): 547–557.

Surah S, Kieran J, O'Dea S (2013) Use of the Alcohol Use Disorders Identification Test (AUDIT) to determine the prevalence of alcohol misuse among HIV-infected individuals. *International Journal of STD & AIDS*, 24(7): 517–521.

Trickey A, May MT, Vehreschild J-J et al. (2017) Survival of HIV-positive patients starting antiretroviral therapy between 1996 and 2013: A collaborative analysis of cohort studies. *The Lancet HIV*, 4(8): e349–e356.

Tsevat J, Leonard AC, Szaflarski M et al. (2009) Change in quality of life after being diagnosed with HIV: A multicenter longitudinal study. *AIDS Patient Care and STDs*, 23(11): 931–937.

Tucker JS, Burnam MA, Sherbourne CD, Kung FY, Gifford AL (2003) Substance use and mental health correlates of nonadherence to antiretroviral medications in a sample of patients with human immunodeficiency virus infection. *The American Journal of Medicine*, 114(7): 573–580.

UNAIDS (2014) *Fast Track: Ending the AIDS Epidemic by 2030.* Geneva: UNAIDS.

UNAIDS (2018) 90-90-90 Treatment target. Retrieved from: http://www.unaids.org/en/90-90-90.

US Clinical Trials Registry (2021) Ugandan non-communicable diseases and aging cohort. Retrieved from https://ichgcp.net/clinical-trials-registry/NCT02445079.

Van Lelyveld SF, Gras L, Kesselring A et al. (2012) Long-term complications in patients with poor immunological recovery despite virological successful HAART in Dutch ATHENA cohort. *Aids*, 26(4): 465–474.

van Luenen S, Garnefski N, Spinhoven P, Spaan P, Dusseldorp E, Kraaij V (2018) The benefits of psychosocial interventions for mental health in people living with HIV: A systematic review and meta-analysis. *AIDS and Behavior*, 22(1): 9–42.

Vance DE, Randazza J, Fogger S, Slater LZ, Humphrey SC, Keltner NL (2014) An overview of the biological and psychosocial context surrounding neurocognition in HIV. *Journal of the American Psychiatric Nurses Association*, 20(2): 117–124.

Vance DE, Fazeli PL, Cheatwood J, Nicholson WC, Morrison SA, Moneyham LD (2019) Computerized cognitive training for the neurocognitive complications of HIV infection: A systematic review. *Journal of the Association of Nurses in AIDS Care*, 30(1): 51–72.

Venugopal D, Patil P, Gupta D, Murali N, Kar N, Sharma P (2001) Mania in HIV infection. *Indian Journal of Psychiatry*, 43(3): 242.

Vivithanaporn P, Heo G, Gamble J et al. (2010) Neurologic disease burden in treated HIV/AIDS predicts survival: A population-based study. *Neurology*, 75(13): 1150–1158.

Vos T, Abajobir AA, Abate KH et al. (2017) Global, regional, and national incidence, prevalence, and years lived with disability for 328 diseases and injuries for 195 countries, 1990–2016: A systematic analysis for the Global Burden of Disease Study 2016. *The Lancet*, 390(10100): 1211–1259.

Waldrop D, Irwin C, Nicholson WC et al. (2021) The intersection of cognitive ability and HIV: A review of the state of the nursing science. *The Journal of the Association of Nurses in AIDS Care: JANAC*, 32(3): 306.

Wang Y, Liu M, Lu Q et al. (2020) Global prevalence and burden of HIV-associated neurocognitive disorder: A meta-analysis. *Neurology*, 95(19): e2610–e2621.

Watkins CC, Treisman GJ (2012) Neuropsychiatric complications of aging with HIV. *Journal of Neurovirology*, 18(4): 277–290.

Weber E, Blackstone K, Woods SP (2013) Cognitive neurorehabilitation of HIV-associated neurocognitive disorders: A qualitative review and call to action. *Neuropsychology Review*, 23(1): 81–98.

Wei J, Hou J, Su B et al. (2020) The prevalence of Frascati-criteria-based HIV-associated neurocognitive disorder (HAND) in HIV-infected adults: A systematic review and meta-Analysis. *Frontiers in Neurology*, 11: 1613.

Whiteford HA, Ferrari AJ, Degenhardt L, Feigin V, Vos T (2015) The global burden of mental, neurological and substance use disorders: An analysis from the Global Burden of Disease Study 2010. *PloS One*, 10(2): e0116820.

WHO (2013) Definition of key terms. In: *Consolidated Guidelines on the Use of Antiretroviral Drugs for Treating and Preventing HIV Infection (2013)*. Geneva: World Health Organization, pp. 13–16. Retrieved from http://www.who.int/hiv/pub/guidelines/arv2013/intro/keyterms/en/.

WHO (2016) *Consolidated Guidelines on HIV Prevention, Diagnosis, Treatment and Care for Key Populations – 2016 Update*. Geneva: World Health Organization.

WHO (2017) *Policy Brief: Consolidated Guidelines on HIV Prevention, Diagnosis, Treatment and Care for Key Populations*. Retrieved from https://apps.who.int/iris/handle/10665/258967

WHO (2021) *Consolidated Guidelines on HIV Prevention, Testing, Treatment, Service Delivery and Monitoring: Recommendations for a Public Health Approach*. Geneva: World Health Organization.

Wykowski J, Kemp CG, Velloza J, Rao D, Drain PK (2019) Associations between anxiety and adherence to antiretroviral medications in low-and middle-income countries: A systematic review and meta-analysis. *AIDS and Behavior*, 23(8): 2059–2071.

Yang C-C, Chien W-C, Chung C-H et al. (2019) No association between human immunodeficiency virus infections and dementia: A nationwide cohort study in Taiwan. *Neuropsychiatric Disease and Treatment*, 15: 3155.

Neurodevelopment of Children who are HIV-exposed and Uninfected

Catherine J Wedderburn, Shunmay Yeung, and Kirsten A Donald

INTRODUCTION

The successful scale-up of antiretroviral therapy (ART) during pregnancy has resulted in a substantial decline in infant human immunodeficiency virus (HIV) infections, therefore, most children born to women living with HIV will remain uninfected. However, the health outcomes of children exposed to HIV and ART during pregnancy who remain uninfected are only recently becoming apparent. Worldwide, there are more than 15 million children who are HIV-exposed and uninfected (HEU), the majority living in sub-Saharan Africa (SSA). It is important for health care workers in areas with a high HIV prevalence to address this growing vulnerable population. This chapter presents the evidence to date on the neurodevelopment of children who are HEU, and discusses recommendations for assessment, management, and future research.

DEFINITIONS

Children who are HEU are defined as HIV-uninfected children born to mothers living with HIV. Children born to mothers with HIV may be exposed to HIV in utero, during the birth process, and through breastfeeding in the postnatal period. In areas where ART has been scaled up, many HIV-exposed children have also been exposed to antiretroviral drugs during pregnancy across the placenta, after birth through breast milk, and from receiving postnatal antiretroviral prophylaxis directly. ART refers to the combination of antiretroviral drugs given to treat HIV. In the post-ART era, the term HEU generally refers to the combination of HIV and ART exposure. Some literature separately refers to this group as HIV-affected children. Children who are HIV-unexposed and uninfected (HUU) are defined as children born to mothers without HIV infection.

CLASSIFICATION OF HIV EXPOSURE

The accurate classification of HIV status in children born to mothers living with HIV is critical to ensuring that either HIV infection is diagnosed and treated early or that uninfected children are correctly monitored (Evans, Jones, and Prendergast 2016; Slogrove, Archary, and Cotton 2016). Delayed diagnosis of HIV may have serious consequences for children's health outcomes, and misclassification of children as HIV-infected can impact the rest of their lives. HIV transmission may occur antenatally, perinatally, or postnatally. The risk of vertical transmission of HIV remains throughout the postnatal period until breastfeeding has stopped, and it is therefore important to perform repeat HIV testing on children born to mothers living with HIV until the period of risk is over. The World Health Organization (WHO) has published guidelines on HIV testing for children born to mothers living with HIV, which have informed country guidelines (WHO 2021).

There have been some concerns raised about HIV tests available for young infants. This has resulted in the need for careful interpretation of infant test results, recommendations around timing, and confirmatory testing (Evans, Jones, and Prendergast 2016; Slogrove, Archary, and Cotton 2016; WHO 2016). Given that maternal HIV antibodies cross the placenta, serological tests may not be used to diagnose HIV infection early in life and virological testing using nucleic acid technologies is needed. In some settings, birth testing using virological (nucleic acid) tests is becoming more common, which will detect infections acquired in utero. However, further testing is needed at 6 weeks of life or later, even if the baby is negative at birth, to detect intrapartum and postnatal infections. There are several additional challenges to testing. First, it has been found that infant antiretroviral drug prophylaxis may reduce HIV viral load enough to cause false negative test results. Infant prophylaxis is typically given for 6 weeks after birth and may be given for longer, depending on the risk status of the mother. Therefore, a child may only be confirmed as HIV-uninfected if tested over 4 to 6 weeks after the last dose of prophylaxis. Second, the decreasing vertical transmission rates have led to a reduction in the positive predictive value of diagnostic tests; therefore, positive HIV test results should be confirmed on a second specimen before a diagnosis of HIV is made. Third, given the possibility of transmission during breastfeeding and reports of declining maternal ART adherence in the postpartum period, children should receive a final HIV test 6 weeks or more following cessation of breastfeeding. Finally, females who seroconvert during pregnancy or breastfeeding are at extremely high risk of transmitting the virus to their child due to the high viral load experienced during acute infection. Thus, repeat testing for HIV in HIV-negative females should take place during the antenatal and postnatal periods. Any mother diagnosed postnatally with HIV infection should be referred for immediate testing of the child and for discussions concerning management. Children may be classified as HEU if their mother is diagnosed as HIV-infected and if the child has tested negative in a recent appropriate test or, depending on their age, a final test following cessation of breastfeeding and infant prophylaxis.

EPIDEMIOLOGY

Worldwide, an estimated 1.3 million pregnant women are living with HIV, and the vast majority of their children will remain uninfected due to the success of ART programmes (UNICEF 2016; Slogrove et al. 2020; UNAIDS 2021). In 2010, the WHO recommended that pregnant women living with HIV were started on ART if required for their own health or on short-term antiretroviral drug prophylaxis if they were not eligible for ART. In 2013, the guidelines changed so that initiation of ART was no longer determined by a women's health status; instead, ART was recommended for all pregnant women for the duration of breastfeeding or for life, depending on country guidance. Since 2015, the WHO advice has recommended lifelong ART, regardless of CD4 cell count, for all people living with HIV starting at the point of diagnosis (WHO 2015). ART continues to be scaled up across the world and, in 2020, it was estimated that 85% of pregnant women with HIV received antiretroviral drugs for prevention of mother-to-child transmission (PMTCT) of HIV (UNAIDS 2021).

In the pre-ART era, a substantial proportion of children born to HIV-infected mothers acquired HIV (between 15% and 45% depending on the duration of breastfeeding) (WHO 2017). However, the

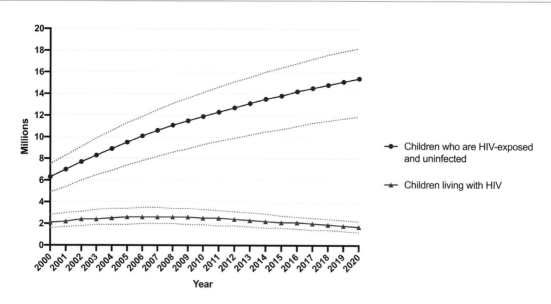

Figure 15.1   Children (aged 0–14 years) who are HIV-exposed and uninfected and children living with HIV: global numbers, 2000–2020. Data from UNAIDS (2021).

transition from the pre-ART to the post-ART era and the adoption of strategies to prevent vertical HIV transmission has led to a massive reduction in children acquiring HIV and a corresponding increase in children who are HEU (Figure 15.1). Due to the potent preventive effects of ART, the vertical transmission rate may decrease to less than 5%, and there were approximately 150 000 new HIV infections in children in 2020 (UNAIDS 2021). This leaves more than 1 million children born each year who are exposed to HIV but who remain uninfected.

Globally, there are more than 15 million children who are HEU and, in some countries, children who are HEU represent more than 20% of annual births (UNAIDS 2021). Any sequential neurodevelopmental problems will thus have a substantial impact at both the individual and national level (Filteau 2009). More than 90% of children who are HEU are living in SSA (UNICEF 2016). Many factors play a role in determining health outcomes in this population, which vary between countries, and children born to mothers living with HIV in high-income countries have different psychosocial, economic, and environmental influences compared to those in low- and middle-income countries (LMICs).

There is now substantial evidence to suggest that in utero exposure to HIV and/or ART can have potentially serious consequences for uninfected children despite avoiding HIV infection. Current research indicates that children who are HEU differ from children who are HUU in terms of mortality, morbidity, and growth (Filteau 2009; Evans, Jones, and Prendergast 2016). Although many of these studies are from the pre-ART era, recent studies support these same conclusions (Gonzalez et al. 2017; Ruperez et al. 2017). Studies from across the world have indicated that children who are HEU have higher mortality (Newell et al. 2004; Taron-Brocard et al. 2014), notably in the first 12 months, with varying reports across countries, although it is estimated to be around double that of HUU children (Arikawa et al. 2016; Brennan et al. 2016). This increased mortality appears to be primarily due to infectious causes, and in 2015 a report from South Africa showed that infants who are HEU have an increased risk of contracting invasive pneumococcal disease (von Mollendorf et al. 2015). Other studies have found that infants who are HEU have increased rates of hospitalisation and that they appear to suffer from more severe and unusual infectious diseases early in life (Slogrove et al. 2012). This is likely a result of alterations in their immune systems when compared to HUU infants (Abu-Raya et al. 2016). Differences in growth have also been observed, including shorter length at birth and reduced head circumference in the first year of life when compared to HUU children, suggesting that HIV-related changes occur early in the developmental process (Evans, Jones, and Prendergast 2016). Head circumference has been correlated with brain growth, which occurs most rapidly in the first few years of life. Given that brain growth is closely linked to neurodevelopment (Cheong et al. 2008), this raises concerns over the neurodevelopmental outcomes of children who are HEU.

THE NEURODEVELOPMENT OF CHILDREN WHO ARE HIV-EXPOSED AND UNINFECTED

Approximately 250 million (43%) children under the age of 5 years old in LMICs are at risk of not reaching their developmental potential because of stunting and extreme poverty (Black et al. 2017). SSA, where the majority of people living with HIV reside, has the highest prevalence of at-risk children (66% of children under 5 years of age) (Black et al. 2017). Poverty and stunting (of growth) encompass many risk factors; other specific factors that have been found to contribute to developmental outcomes include nutrition, parental physical and psychosocial health, environmental exposures, and infectious diseases, especially in resource-limited contexts. While the effects of child HIV infection have been described (see Chapters 11, 12, and 13), the impact of HIV and ART exposure without infection on neurodevelopment remains uncertain, although there is rising concern that the neurodevelopment of children who are HEU may be adversely affected when compared to their unexposed peers.

This chapter presents a summary of the major systematic reviews and meta-analyses to date on the topic of neurodevelopment in children who are HEU. Relevant publications were identified through a literature search carried out in SCOPUS and PubMed databases. Table 15.1 summarises the included systematic reviews and meta-analyses and their main outcomes by publication date.

Recent meta-analyses suggest that, in the first few years of life, children who are HEU may be at risk for impaired neurodevelopment in specific domains compared to HUU children. A meta-analysis of eight large studies found subtle deficits in expressive language and gross motor function in children who are HEU aged 12 to 24 months of age compared to children who are HUU (Wedderburn et al. 2022b). Similarly, a smaller meta-analysis of studies using the Bayley Scales of Infant and Toddler Development, Third Edition, reported poorer expressive language in children who are HEU (White and Connor 2020). An earlier network meta-analysis found worse cognitive and motor function in HEU children compared to HUU children, although they assessed using the Bayley Scales of Infant Development, First and Second Editions, where cognitive and language function are considered together (McHenry et al. 2018). These results build upon a prior systematic review that reported lower performance of children who are HEU compared to HUU across psychological measures in 7 out of 11 studies (Sherr et al. 2014). Similarly, other literature reviews have reported a modest but significant effect on the neurodevelopment of children exposed to HIV and ART (Desmonde et al. 2016), and delays in cognition, motor skills, and language expression in children who are HEU compared to HUU in resource-poor settings (Le Doare, Bland, and Newell 2012). Although another systematic review of studies in SSA found no difference in the preschool years between HEU and HUU children (le Roux et al. 2016), the review concluded that more evidence is needed to understand this population as most studies up to that time had substantial limitations.

Individual studies included in reviews differ in their results across age ranges and settings, although generally worse outcomes for children who are HEU compared to HUU children were reported in LMICs.

Table 15.1   Summary of systematic reviews and meta-analyses examining the neurodevelopment of children who are HIV-exposed and uninfected.

Study	Studies included	Region (number of studies included)	Findings
Wedderburn et al. (2022b)	31 studies (45 articles): 21 studies compared neurodevelopment of HEU and HUU children; 10 studies examined ART regimens; further, 13 studies reported on head circumference or neuroimaging. Meta-analysis included eight studies (seven Africa; one North America) and a total of 1856 HEU and 3067 HUU children.	Africa (22) South America (3) North America (4) Asia (2)	• Systematic review: 57% of studies found worse neurodevelopment among HEU children in at least one domain compared to HUU. • Meta-analysis: at 12–24 months of age, on average HEU children had poorer expressive language and gross motor development than HUU children. • Few studies examined ART. Limited evidence suggests little, if any, impact of specific maternal ART regimens on neurodevelopment, although concerns were raised regarding atazanavir and efavirenz. • Larger studies suggested HEU children may have smaller head circumferences in early life compared to HUU. There was only one neuroimaging study of children under 5 years.
White and Connor (2020)	24 studies: 15 studies assessed neurodevelopmental outcomes from birth to 36 months in infants born to mothers living with HIV; nine studies reported on early life nutrition-related variables and infant neurodevelopment. Meta-analysis included three studies (four articles) examining Bayley-III subscales for infants who are HEU compared to HUU (two Africa, one South America).	Africa (17) Asia (2) Europe (2) South America (2) North America (1)	• Review: HIV exposure was associated with lower scores in some studies, and child HIV infection with lower scores in many studies. • Meta-analysis: expressive language function was worse in HEU children compared to HUU in the first 3 years; other domain estimates were lower in HEU children but did not show significant differences. • Male infants were found to be more vulnerable to HIV exposure, although few studies specifically examined sex-dependent effects. • Maternal perinatal micronutrient supplementation improved motor outcomes at 6 months in HEU children. Infant supplementation alone did not affect neurodevelopment. Nutrient supplementation and education combined with a water, sanitation, and hygiene intervention improved neurodevelopment at 24 months in HEU children.
McHenry et al. (2019a)	Five studies of children (0–15 years) examining brain structure and function. A further 20 studies focused on behavioural assessments in animal models.	Africa (2) Asia (1) Europe (1) South America (1)	• Overall few clinical studies. • Four studies used MRI: two reported differences on diffusion tensor imaging between HEU and HUU children aged 2–6 weeks and 7 years; one found no group differences at mean age of 10 years; a final study examined individual qualitative outcomes of structural MRI of HEU children at 10–44 months presenting with neurological symptoms and found that 50% of children had MRI abnormalities. Another study found exposure to zidovudine +/- lamivudine may affect brainstem auditory evoked potentials in HEU infants.

Table 15.1 Continued

Study	Studies included	Region (number of studies included)	Findings
McHenry et al. (2018)	45 studies (containing 46 cohorts) were included in the review examining children with HIV, HEU, and HUU. Meta-analysis included four studies that compared HEU and HUU children from Africa ($n = 2$), South America ($n = 1$), North America ($n = 1$).	Africa (18) Asia (1) Europe (4) North America (20) South America (3)	• Systematic review: HEU children were described as having worse developmental outcomes compared with HUU children in a few studies; HIV-infected children had worse outcomes than comparison groups in many studies. • Meta-analysis: HEU children had lower mental developmental index (cognitive) and psychomotor developmental index (motor) scores compared to HUU peers up to age 8 years, although to a lesser extent than children living with HIV. • Studies outside the USA received a low-quality rating. In studies limited to high-quality assessments, HEU children had similar scores to HUU. • HEU children with ARV exposure had lower cognitive and motor scores than those without ARV exposure.
le Roux et al. (2016)	Eight studies contributed nine reports assessing early child development outcomes. Of these, four studies (five reports) had a low/moderate risk of bias with varying maternal ART use ($n = 1$ mothers received triple ART regardless of disease staging; $n = 2$ mothers received ARVs for PMTCT; $n = 1$ mothers received no ARVs).	All sub-Saharan Africa	• Limited studies from the current PMTCT era. • No difference was reported in preschool development in HEU children compared to HUU, or in 6–12-year-old children in the Democratic Republic of the Congo. • Lower educational achievement among school-age HEU children in Zambia compared to HUU children, as measured by lower mathematics grades.
Sherr et al. (2014)	11 studies	Africa (6) Asia (1) Europe (1) North America (3)	• Seven out of the 11 studies reported that HEU children performed lower in at least one psychological measure when compared to HUU children, spanning cognitive, developmental and behavioural parameters. However, findings differed across studies. • Cognitive: Overall, IQ scores were lower in preschool children who are HEU compared to HUU. However, mixed results were reported across countries. Lower scores for reading ability and language expression were reported in HEU children from studies in Africa, but not the USA. • Motor development: Some studies found that HEU children had poorer motor development, while others did not. • Behaviour: Varying reports of worse externalising and internalising behaviour in pre-adolescents who are HEU across countries.

Abbreviations: ART: antiretroviral therapy; ARV: antiretroviral; Bayley-III: Bayley Scales of Infant and Toddler Development, Third Edition; HEU: HIV-exposed and uninfected; HUU: HIV-unexposed and uninfected; MRI: magnetic resonance imaging; PMTCT: prevention of mother-to-child transmission.

Key domains of neurodevelopment that were first reported to be at risk include: language (Boivin et al. 1995), motor function (Le Doare, Bland, and Newell 2012), behaviour (Le Doare, Bland, and Newell 2012; Sherr et al. 2014), and cognition (Boivin et al. 1995; Van Rie, Mupuala, and Dow 2008; Kerr et al. 2014). Language delay was reported in the Democratic Republic of Congo in children aged 18 months to 6 years (Boivin et al. 1995; Van Rie, Mupuala, and Dow 2008), and this has been replicated more recently in large studies across Botswana (Chaudhury et al. 2017), South Africa (Wedderburn et al. 2019b), and Zimbabwe (Ntozini et al. 2020). The Sanitation, Hygiene, Infant Nutrition Efficacy (SHINE) trial in Zimbabwe also reported worse motor development in children who are HEU compared to HUU peers at 24 months (Ntozini et al. 2020). Further, a large South African study where all infants were born to mothers taking triple ART found increased risk of delayed motor development at 12 months, as well as increased risk of delayed cognitive development (le Roux et al. 2018). However, not all the results are consistent and other studies have found similar development between HEU children exposed to ART and HUU children, including a recent large study from Uganda and Malawi (Boivin et al. 2019).

Of note, the epidemiology of HIV infection differs across settings. In high-resource settings, adult infections are often found in groups with higher substance use, compared to the more generalised population-level epidemic seen in SSA. One study from Canada showed that any differences in neuro-development were not sustained after controlling for substance use (Alimenti et al. 2006). Reports from the Surveillance Monitoring for ART Toxicities in children who are HEU (SMARTT) study in the USA have given an insight into the effects of exposure to different antiretroviral drugs. This study revealed a few differences in language outcomes in HEU children who are less than 2 years of age, particularly associated with specific antiretroviral drugs (Rice et al. 2013; Caniglia et al. 2016). Further, some reports of negative cognitive and behavioural outcomes at older ages in high-income settings have emerged (Le Doare, Bland, and Newell 2012; Sherr et al. 2014), and one study found that cognitive scores in school-age HEU children fell below the population mean (Nozyce et al. 2014), a finding which requires further investigation. Persistent language impairment has also been documented in young people with perinatal HIV exposure in the USA, with similar performance deficits to those with HIV infection (Redmond et al. 2016).

Fewer studies have examined the neurodevelopment of older children and adolescents in LMICs to date and, as a result, these are often lacking from reviews (Sherr et al. 2014). One of the most common tools used to assess cognitive function in older children is the Kaufman Assessment Battery for Children (KABC) which has been used in children with HIV infection (van Wyhe et al. 2017). Studies embedded as neurodevelopmental follow-up of multi-site African randomised controlled trials of ART regimens in women and children living with HIV have compared longitudinal outcomes in HIV, HEU, HUU cohorts, including the PROMISE and P1060/P1104s trials (Boivin et al. 2018, 2019, 2020b). Similar cognitive development, attention, motor skills, and behaviour have been found comparing groups of HEU and HUU children aged 4 to 11 years using the KABC inventory and other assessments when controlling for other proximal (comorbidities) and distal (caregiving, socioeconomic status, nutrition) factors known to impact neuropsychological outcomes. The CHER plus study in South Africa also reported similar findings (Laughton et al. 2018; van Wyhe et al. 2021), although poorer auditory memory in HEU children was described (van Wyhe et al. 2021) and sample sizes were small; it is also important to note expressive language function was not examined. In contrast, another study in Cameroon found children aged 4 to 9 years who are HEU had lower cognitive scores on KABC, Second Edition, than HUU children, although differences were no longer significant after adjusting for confounding factors, suggesting the importance of contextual factors (Debeaudrap et al. 2018). One earlier study in Zambia showed a possible impact on educational achievement at school age, as determined by lower mathematic abilities (Nicholson et al. 2015). Finally the PREDICT study from Cambodia and Thailand found children who are HEU aged 2 through to 12 years of age had lower IQs and delays in language and fine motor development compared to HUU children, even after adjusting for confounding factors (Kerr et al. 2014). More research is needed from the current ART era.

The heterogeneity between studies, populations, and changing PMTCT guidelines may explain the differences in reported neurodevelopmental outcomes. Studies differ in terms of design; varying ages of the children included; neurodevelopmental tools used; population demographics in LMICs compared to high-income countries; associated coinfections and substance use; feeding practices; and ART usage. The quality of the studies also varies, and common limitations across individual studies include a lack of appropriate HUU control groups and longitudinal data, an inadequate consideration of relevant confounding factors, and small samples sizes. Differences in design and outcome measures have resulted in scarce data on ART (Sherr et al. 2014), and small sample sizes mean that studies may not be powered sufficiently to reveal subtle differences. While meta-analyses provide evidence for modest differences in neurodevelopment between HEU and HUU children early in life, particularly in language and motor domains, more work is needed to understand later outcomes. A recent systematic review highlighted methodological considerations for future research to better understand the long-term trajectories of children who are HEU (Wedderburn et al. 2022b).

FACTORS POTENTIALLY INFLUENCING THE NEURODEVELOPMENT OF CHILDREN WHO ARE HIV-EXPOSED AND UNINFECTED

Gestation and the first few years of life represent a time of substantial brain growth, where critical neural pathway development and network maturation occur (Hermoye et al. 2006). Exposures during these first 1000 days may have a lifelong impact on health outcomes. The complex processes of brain development are vulnerable to external exposures, and evidence suggests that HIV and ART exposure without infection can impact neurodevelopment during this time. Both direct effects of HIV and ART exposure on the developing nervous system, and indirect effects, including maternal physical and psychological health, maternal–child interaction, parenting decisions, feeding choices, and wider socioenvironmental factors associated with being born into a family affected by HIV, are hypothesised to impact the neurodevelopment of HEU children (le Roux et al. 2016; Wedderburn et al. 2019a). Other factors such as genetic vulnerabilities, difficulties with hearing and vision, and neurological disabilities related to birth can also play a role. In summary, the neurodevelopmental trajectory is likely to be influenced by a complex, multifactorial causal pathway. The potential roles of different exposures that may contribute to the neurodevelopment of HEU children are addressed below. A detailed conceptual framework and discussion of mechanisms can be found in Wedderburn et al. 2019a.

HIV Exposure and the Immune System

HIV infection is known to have significant effects on the neurodevelopment of children who are living with HIV. The virus has a particular affinity for the anatomy of the central nervous system (CNS). Both direct infection of the CNS by the virus and secondary effects of immunodeficiency, including coinfections, as well as complications of metabolic and endocrine systems, contribute to poor cognitive, psychological and behavioural outcomes of children living with HIV (see Chapters 11, 12, and 13 for more information).

From a biological perspective, it can be hypothesised that immune activation and chronic systemic inflammation in women living with HIV may impact foetal neurodevelopment, even without foetal HIV infection. Furthermore, HIV exposure can cause immune activation and inflammation in children who are HEU (Mofenson 2015), and the resulting effects on the foetal immune system may lead to the release of neurotoxins that cause neuronal adaptation and impaired network function (Krogh, Green, and Thayer 2015). The interactions between the nervous and immune systems are complex, and it is thought that the immune system plays a substantial role in brain development. Various immune molecules and microglial receptors have been associated with aspects of early neural development, including cell differentiation and migration (Bilbo and Schwarz 2012). Studies have described up-regulated and down-regulated pro-inflammatory cytokines in children who are HEU compared to HUU (Abu-Raya et al. 2016; Dirajlal-Fargo et al. 2019; Sevenoaks et al. 2021); and certain CNS maturation processes, such as cell migration and axonal growth, may be vulnerable to these changes at different stages of development (Bilbo and Schwarz 2012; Tran et al. 2016).

A number of studies have shown immune abnormalities among children who are HEU, including a cell profile that appears different to both HUU children and children living with HIV for T-cell activation and altered lymphocyte subsets (Abu-Raya et al. 2016). The causes of these differences are unclear and many of these immunological changes may result from exposure to HIV virions and proteins. Thus, specific responses to HIV are seen even when HIV-exposed infants remain uninfected. HEU children have also been shown to have reduced placental antibody transfer to vaccine-preventable diseases, leaving them at higher risk of other infections (Jones et al. 2011). These immunological differences put children at risk of adverse clinical outcomes, particularly in the first year of life. Literature shows that adverse birth outcomes are associated with HIV and ART exposure (Wedi et al. 2016; Uthman et al. 2017); and one South African study found HEU children born preterm are subsequently at greater risk for neurodevelopmental delays compared to those born at term (le Roux et al. 2018). A report from the same study found cumulative maternal HIV viraemia was associated with higher odds of motor and expressive language delay (le Roux et al. 2019). Separately, another South African study found an association between lower maternal CD4 counts and poorer language outcomes (Wedderburn et al. 2019b), supporting a potential relationship between maternal immune function and child neurodevelopment.

ART Exposure

Antiretroviral drugs are able to cross the placenta with varying degrees of penetration and may cause a range of side effects. Exposure to antiretrovirals may also occur through breast milk or directly as prophylaxis to the infant. Over the past decade, international policy regarding ART has changed considerably. The scale-up of ART has led to improved maternal health; however, more infants are being exposed to ART and more women are conceiving while on ART. Within the current ART era, there has been an increased focus on the potential toxic impact of exposure to antiretrovirals in utero on neonatal outcomes (Desmonde et al. 2016), including preterm delivery, low birthweight, being small-for-gestational age, and metabolic abnormalities (Jao and Abrams 2014).

It remains difficult to separate the effects of HIV and ART. Data from an early trial of zidovudine did not find any long-term consequences (PACTG 076 trial) (Connor et al. 1994). Conversely, studies in France raised concerns about mitochondrial abnormalities with exposure to nucleoside reverse transcriptase inhibitors (NRTIs) (Blanche et al. 1999; Barret et al. 2003). More recently, the US Pediatric HIV/AIDS Cohort Study (PHACS) established the SMARTT study in HEU children (Sirois et al. 2016; Williams et al. 2016). They found that children who are HEU have increased late language development at 12 months (Rice et al. 2013) and that, specifically, antenatal exposure to atazanavir was associated with delayed language development (Sirois et al. 2013). However, other papers from the same cohort did not replicate the impact of atazanavir on language outcomes at 24 months, suggesting that the effects may be transient (Rice et al. 2013; Himes et al. 2015). In addition, didanosine and stavudine appeared to impact development (Williams et al. 2016), although other antiretrovirals were not found to have any major impact on neurodevelopment at age 9 to 15 months (Sirois et al. 2013). In Botswana, efavirenz was also associated with poor language outcomes at age 24 months (Cassidy et al. 2019). However, studies comparing different regimens including zidovudine monotherapy versus triple ART (Chaudhury et al. 2018) found no differences after adjusting for potential confounders, as did a randomised controlled trial of triple NRTIs versus dual NRTIs and protease inhibitor ART (Kacanek et al. 2018). Overall, a recent systematic review found little or no effect of specific maternal ART regimens examined (Wedderburn et al. 2022b); however, the few studies and lack of consistency in treatment regimens make it difficult to draw confident conclusions. Data on the long-term safety of antiretrovirals and treatment combinations are still suboptimal (Mofenson 2015), and this is an area of research that requires further investigation. A review by Toledo and colleagues covers ART and child neurological development in more detail (Toledo et al. 2021).

Family and Caregiving Environment

There are many other factors that play a role in the early development of children who are HEU. There is extensive literature on the effect of family dynamics on childhood development. The ecological concept that child development is an ongoing biological and psychological process, influenced by the wider environment including family, school, and society, has gained particular recognition (Bronfenbrenner 1979). This supports the idea that family and social context play a critical role in long-term neurodevelopmental outcomes. These outcomes are influenced by the interaction between risk and resilience, and the accumulation of multiple risk factors puts children at higher risk for neurodevelopmental problems. Children born into families affected by HIV may face multiple adversities that differ from those of children unaffected by HIV.

Critical to neurodevelopment is the parent–child relationship, which may be impacted by HIV/AIDS through physical illness, parental death, parental separation or divorce, parental mental illness, and parental strain from emotional, financial, and social pressures (Stein et al. 2014). More than 17 million children are estimated to have lost one or both parents as a result of the HIV/AIDS epidemic (Leyenaar 2005). Parental death or illness can profoundly affect children emotionally, as well as the relationships they develop – the consequences of which can remain in adulthood. Institutionalisation of orphans and the resulting dearth of healthy primary relationships impairs neurodevelopment, and these negative consequences are widely documented (Leyenaar 2005).

Parental health and caregiving ability are known to affect children's health outcomes in both HIV-infected and uninfected populations. Additionally, in mothers living with HIV, disease severity shows distinct links to infant health outcomes (le Roux, Abrams, and Meyer 2016). A study in Uganda found that poorer caregiving environments were associated with lower language scores, indicating a key role for the home environment in determining child HEU outcomes (Familiar et al. 2018). Parental psychological health directly affects child neurodevelopment, and the stigma associated with HIV, along with financial and social pressures, can lead to both relationship and mental health problems. Depression is well documented in women with HIV and it may affect maternal–child interaction, parenting, adherence to medication, and maternal physical health (Mebrahtu et al. 2018). Exposure to gender-based violence, intimate partner violence, and abuse, have also been shown to impact child neurodevelopment (Barnett et al. 2021).

Exposure to Other Infections and Toxins

Children who are HEU are at risk of exposure to other infections early in life through living with family members with HIV. Mothers with HIV are at greater risk of contracting infectious diseases, which also increases their risks of becoming ill. Cytomegalovirus infection is found more frequently in HEU children than in HUU children, and has been separately linked to developmental delays (Gompels et al. 2012; Filteau and Rowland-Jones 2016). Cytomegalovirus is also associated with adverse birth outcomes, which are risk factors for developmental delay (Wedderburn et al. 2019a). Children who are HEU are additionally at risk of more severe infections in early life due to differences in their immune function compared to HUU children (Abu-Raya et al. 2016). Spending prolonged periods of time ill and/or hospitalised can further impair neurodevelopment (Slogrove, Reikie, and Cotton 2012).

Finally, there is an extensive literature demonstrating that maternal alcohol and illicit substance use, particularly during pregnancy, have an impact on child neurodevelopment (Donald et al. 2017; Donald et al. 2019). Increased maternal alcohol exposure has been reported in some settings (le Roux et al. 2018), and one study reported that higher maternal substance use in pregnancy had a greater (negative) effect on neurodevelopmental trajectories than infant HIV/ART exposure (Alimenti et al. 2006).

Socioeconomic Circumstances

The social and economic determinants of health have been widely documented and they include housing, nutrition, security, sanitation, and access to health care (Grantham-McGregor et al. 2007; Evans, Jones, and Prendergast 2016; Black et al. 2017). Poverty and stunting are known to impact neurodevelopment through a myriad of factors, with far-reaching effects (Filteau 2009). Living in poverty has also been negatively associated with brain volume and academic performance (Hair et al. 2015). Therefore, studies comparing HEU and HUU child outcomes from the same socioeconomic settings are necessary to fully understand this impact.

Feeding Modality and Nutrition

Breastfeeding plays a critical role in child health outcomes, providing both protection against infectious diseases and long-term health benefits (Victora et al. 2016). Breastfeeding also positively impacts cognitive outcomes and benefits child brain development (McCrory and Murray 2013; Victora et al. 2016). Feeding advice to mothers with HIV has changed over time, as our understanding of the vertical transmission risks and the benefits of breastfeeding has evolved. The current WHO guidelines for mothers with HIV advise exclusive breastfeeding for the first 6 months of life and then ongoing breastfeeding for at least 12 months, and may continue for up to 24 months or longer (WHO 2021). This advice was only introduced in 2013, and there are large numbers of children whose mothers did not breastfeed due to previous guidance. This complicates analysis of the impact of HIV exposure on neurodevelopmental outcomes (le Roux, Abrams, and Meyer 2016). Differences in neurodevelopmental outcomes between children who are HEU and HUU seen in pre-ART era studies may have been influenced by feeding modality, and further work is needed to understand the impact of feeding choice on the neurodevelopment of children who are HEU. However, more recent studies of breastfeeding populations continue to show deficits in the neurodevelopment of children who are HEU compared to HUU (le Roux et al. 2018), as do other studies controlling for breastfeeding (Wedderburn et al. 2019b).

Genetic Vulnerabilities and Epigenetic Programming

Early life programming is influenced by the uterine environment, resulting in epigenetic changes with far-reaching outcomes (Williams and Drake 2015). Epigenetic modifications in DNA methylation and gene expression are influenced by environmental events, with the potential for long-term impact on

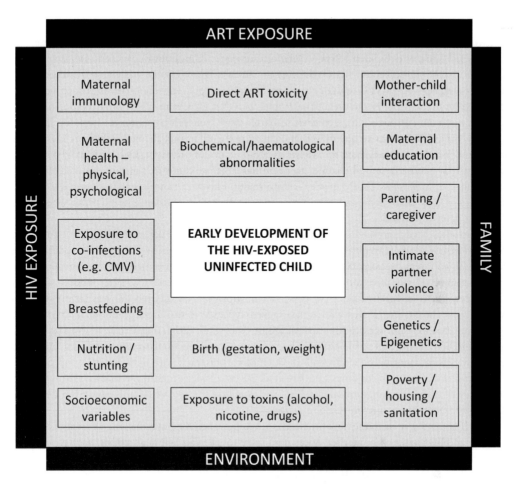

Figure 15.2 Variables potentially influencing the early development of HIV-exposed and uninfected children.
Abbreviations: ART, antiretroviral therapy; CMV, cytomegalovirus.

health outcomes. Future research will determine the role of HIV and ART exposure in epigenetic mechanisms that dictate later neurodevelopment.

Overall, further work is needed to understand the effects of HIV and ART exposure on child neurodevelopment in the context of other risk and protective factors (Figure 15.2).

THE ROLE OF NEUROIMAGING IN UNDERSTANDING THE MECHANISMS BEHIND NEURODEVELOPMENT

Advances in neuroimaging technology provide new approaches to investigating the neuronal pathways that underlie neurodevelopment, which may help explain the neurobiological mechanisms behind developmental delays. A small number of research studies have investigated the brain structure of children who are HEU, as documented in a recent review (McHenry et al. 2019a). The Drakenstein Child Health

Study (DCHS) in South Africa has used magnetic resonance imaging (MRI) to examine grey and white matter in infants at 2 to 6 weeks of age. Smaller basal ganglia nuclei and total grey matter volumes were found in HEU infants compared to HUU infants, and maternal immunosuppression in pregnancy was associated with lower volumes (Wedderburn et al. 2022a). White matter was assessed using diffusion tensor imaging, a powerful MRI tool for visualising microstructure. The results demonstrated a difference in brain white matter microstructure and neurology between HEU and HUU infants, and correlations between abnormal neurology and specific white matter tracts were evident (Tran et al. 2016). These findings suggest that HIV-associated neurological changes occur early and, therefore, that any management strategies need to be initiated early to have the greatest chance of preserving developmental potential. It also means that neuroanatomical changes are identifiable before exposure to other postnatal contextual factors, suggesting a key role for the in utero environment. However, more research is needed to ascertain whether these early changes are transient, reflecting the altered in utero environment, or whether they persist into later childhood.

Other studies have examined older children. Reports from the CHER cohort in South Africa have shown differences in white matter microstructure and neurometabolites by HIV exposure status in children aged 7 and 9 years respectively (Jankiewicz et al. 2017; Robertson et al. 2018). Another study from Thailand examined brain microstructure in 10-year-old children who are HEU and found no differences compared to HUU children (Jahanshad et al. 2015). However, the sample size was small, and subtle neurocognitive deficits in children who are HEU were reported in the larger group of children from the same cohort that were not seen in the smaller sample (Kerr et al. 2014). Separately, a study from France examined structural scans of HEU children aged 10 to 44 months for qualitative changes: 50% of the scans showed scan abnormalities, although most children presented with neurological symptoms limiting the generalisability of the findings (Tardieu et al. 2005). Critical questions remain regarding both the significance of early neuroanatomical changes over time and the role of neuroimaging in investigating neurodevelopmental outcomes in this population.

Finally, innovative tools to measure functional outcomes, including eye-tracking (Boivin et al. 2017b; Chhaya et al. 2018) and computerised assessment techniques (Van Pelt et al. 2022), have recently been pioneered with children who are HEU in SSA. These show potential for future work.

SCREENING: THE ASSESSMENT OF NEURODEVELOPMENT IN CHILDREN WHO ARE HIV-EXPOSED AND UNINFECTED

There is a considerable body of evidence to suggest that neurodevelopment should be carefully assessed in children who are HEU. In many contexts, the growth and development of all children is monitored at various intervals over the first 5 years of life. Given current concerns, any screening systems (general or specific) should consider HIV exposure as a risk factor for poor developmental outcomes, and health care professionals conducting these assessments should pay particular attention to children who are HEU.

Screening tools to effectively detect developmental problems in at-risk children need to be identified and ideally incorporated into routine childcare. Recently, there has been a request that researchers standardise tools in studies of children who are HEU to allow comparisons across regions and to monitor outcomes across populations (Slogrove, Archary, and Cotton 2016). The Bayley Infant Neurodevelopmental Screener (Aylward 1995; Bayley 2006) is one example of a screening tool. Developmental screening tools that can identify at-risk children in the community, rather than within health facility settings, are needed, as children who are HEU may not be in the medical system and screening assessments may be inconsistently performed. Assessments should be culturally and geographically appropriate for the child concerned and should be translated into the home language of the family. This improves communication and understanding while also allowing for comparison between groups and across contexts. Additionally, these tools should be sensitive enough to identify problems in domains where these children are most at risk.

INVESTIGATIONS: THE FORMAL ASSESSMENT OF THE INDIVIDUAL CHILD

Any child suspected of having developmental delay should be formally assessed to ascertain the degree and profile of developmental impairment using a tool that is feasible and culturally appropriate to the setting. Given the evidence for increased morbidity in the HEU population and the potential impacts on neurodevelopment, a thorough history and examination for infectious diseases should also be performed. Other causes of neurodevelopmental delay (see Table 5.2 in Chapter 5) should be ruled out. It is important to consider the possibility of postnatal HIV transmission, which would warrant repeat HIV testing.

Investigations should be tailored to both presentation and context, and the role of different factors that can influence the neurodevelopment of a child who is HEU should be considered. A detailed list of investigations for neurodevelopmental delay is available in Chapter 5. Initially, in a primary care consultation, the following may be conducted:

1. Routine history:
   - Complete history including developmental milestones, antenatal details (such as birth history, alcohol use, substance use, medications, maternal infections), and immunisations.
2. Clinical examination:
   - Full examination including neurological assessment.
   - Height and weight measured and plotted on a growth chart to look for stunting and wasting. Nutritional status assessed.
   - Head circumference measured and plotted on a growth chart to assess the trajectory.
   - Ear, nose, and throat examination for problems that could impact language and attention.
   - Hearing and vision assessment.
3. Home environment and family assessment.
4. Blood tests (including full blood count) to rule out treatable conditions, such as iron deficiency anaemia.
5. School reports assessed as needed and depending on the child's age.

Further assessment, referral to secondary level specialists, and decisions surrounding tertiary care, may be appropriate depending on the child. For example:

6. If there is evidence of significant developmental delay or deterioration, or problems at school, without obvious cause, then the child may be referred to a specialist paediatrician where available.
7. Further investigations, including neuroimaging and EEG, may be appropriate if abnormalities are found on neurological examination or if seizures are suspected.
8. Referral to speech and language therapy or audiology may be appropriate if there are concerns regarding language.
9. Referral to a psychologist for neuropsychological and cognitive testing may be appropriate if there are concerns regarding psychosocial and educational factors.

MANAGEMENT STRATEGIES

Programmes for optimal child development across populations where HIV is prevalent should consider the wide spectrum of risk factors in this population, including HIV and ART exposure, and should prioritise the early detection of developmental delays. A general holistic approach following the Nurturing Care Framework (https://nurturing-care.org/) should be taken, with assessments to detect problems early, and implementation of interventions to ensure all children are able to reach their full potential. Care for those children found to have developmental delay and for their families should involve a multidisciplinary team consisting of both health care professionals and educational providers. Any factors that are identified as having adverse effects should be addressed and treated where possible. If comorbidities are identified, these need to be treated as well. Advice should be offered to parents and caregivers in order to provide the best possible environment to stimulate neurodevelopment. Research suggests that children with developmental delays can benefit from early childhood education and care. Measures such as early home visits (Gardner et al. 2003), stimulation programmes (Walker et al. 2005), and interventions to optimise the home environment (Daelmans et al. 2015), should be considered.

Targeted interventions for at-risk children and their families that integrate health, nutrition, education, water, sanitation, and hygiene (WASH) initiatives are also needed to ensure optimal development. A randomised trial in rural Zimbabwe found infant and young child feeding in combination with WASH interventions improved motor, language, and behavioural scores in children who are HEU (Chandna et al. 2020). A review of interventions found massage therapy in small samples showed improvements in developmental domains measured, whereas mixed outcomes were reported for caregiver training and cognitive therapy interventions (McHenry et al. 2019b). Randomised controlled trials of early child development interventions involving training caregivers in impoverished areas of Uganda, focusing on HIV and HEU cohorts, have been conducted (Boivin et al. 2020a). While an intervention for caregivers was found to improve child language (Boivin et al. 2013), a cluster-randomised trial found caregiver training improved caregiving quality but did not significantly impact the neurodevelopment of children who are HEU compared to a health and nutrition training intervention (Boivin et al. 2017a); further research is needed.

THE PUBLIC HEALTH PERSPECTIVE

The Sustainable Development Goals have made early child development a priority on the global agenda (www.sdgs.un.org/goals). There has been a call to action to improve conditions for all children and to optimise early child development, with an emphasis on vulnerable and at-risk children. The neurodevelopment of children who are HEU has substantial public health relevance, particularly in countries where HEU children represent a significant portion of annual births. Early cognitive and behavioural skills have an impact on schooling, health, and social potential (Grantham-McGregor et al. 2007; Black et al. 2017), and therefore even minor neurodevelopmental impairment can have important long-term implications, both at the individual and societal level.

From a public health perspective, it is important to promote primary prevention of maternal HIV. Alongside, it is critical to promote ART use, optimal PMTCT care, and to maintain the health of mothers living with HIV in order to prevent HIV transmission and to ensure the best possible outcomes for children who are HEU. The neurodevelopment of children who are HEU should be monitored and any delays should be referred for management early to ensure that these vulnerable children have the greatest chance of meeting their neurocognitive potential.

FUTURE RESEARCH

Large high-quality studies are needed to follow up children who are HEU from birth to adulthood to determine the long-term outcomes and to investigate mechanisms. Surveillance of new ART regimens is also needed as many infants have been exposed to ART in utero, as prophylaxis after birth, and for up to 2+ years during breastfeeding, and the impact of this exposure remains relatively unexplored.

CONCLUSIONS

Most children born to mothers living with HIV will remain uninfected. The neurodevelopment of children who are HEU is of substantial public health importance given the growing paediatric population (Slogrove 2021). Evidence suggests that children who are HEU may be at increased risk of neurodevelopmental and neurocognitive deficits. Recent reviews have found that specific domains at risk include early language development and motor skills, although research in older children remains limited. This warrants careful monitoring of children who are HEU to ensure early detection, investigation, and management of any developmental delays. Maternal, familial, environmental, socioeconomic, nutritional, and infectious factors also play critical roles in neurodevelopmental functioning. Management strategies need to take these into account. Recent developments have been made in domain assessments, interventions, and scale-up; however, children who are HEU continue to face a multiplicity of risk factors. Future research is required to determine how exposure to HIV and/or ART without subsequent HIV infection affects long-term neurodevelopmental trajectories.

Acknowledgements

We would like to thank Professor Andrew J. Prendergast and Professor Suzanne Filteau for their valuable advice and input into this chapter. We would like to thank Ella Weldon for her help with the literature review.

REFERENCES

Abu-Raya B, KollmannTR, Marchmant A, MacGillivray DM (2016) The immune system of HIV-exposed uninfected infants. *Front Immunol*, 7: 383.

Alimenti A, Forbes JC, Oberlander TF et al. (2006) A prospective controlled study of neurodevelopment in HIV-uninfected children exposed to combination antiretroviral drugs in pregnancy. *Pediatrics*, 118: e1139–e1145.

Arikawa S, Rollins N, Newell ML, Becquet R (2016) Mortality risk and associated factors in HIV-exposed, uninfected children. *Trop Med Int Health*, 21: 720–734.

Aylward GP (1995) *Bayley Infant Neurodevelopmental Screener*. San Antonio, TX: The Psychological Corporation.

Barnett W, Halligan SL, Wedderburn C et al. (2021) Maternal emotional and physical intimate partner violence and early child development: Investigating mediators in a cross-sectional study in a South African birth cohort. *BMJ Open*, 11: e046829.

Barrett B, Tardieu M, Rustin P et al. (2003) Persistent mitochondrial dysfunction in HIV-1-exposed but uninfected infants: Clinical screening in a large prospective cohort. *AIDS*, 17: 1769–1785.

Bayley N (2006) *Bayley Scales of Infant and Toddler Development: Technical Manual*. Bloomington, IN: NCS Pearson Inc.

Bilbo SD, Schwarz JM (2012) The immune system and developmental programming of brain and behavior. *Front Neuroendocrinol*, 33: 267–286.

Black MM, Walker SP, Fernald LCH et al. (2017) Early childhood development coming of age: Science through the life course. *Lancet*, 389: 77–90.

Blanche S, Tardieu M, Rustin P et al. (1999) Persistent mitochondrial dysfunction and perinatal exposure to anti-retroviral nucleoside analogues. *Lancet*, 354: 1084–1089.

Boivin MJ, Green SD, Davies AG, Giordani B, Mokili JK, Cutting WA (1995) A preliminary evaluation of the cognitive and motor effects of pediatric HIV infection in Zairian children. *Health Psychol*, 14: 13–21.

Boivin MJ, Bangirana P, Nakasujja N et al. (2013) A year-long caregiver training program to improve neurocognition in preschool Ugandan HIV-exposed children. *J Dev Behav Pediatr*, 34: 269–278.

Boivin MJ, Nakasujja N, Familiar-Lopez I et al. (2017a) Effect of caregiver training on the neurodevelopment of HIV-exposed uninfected children and caregiver mental health: A Ugandan cluster-randomized controlled trial. *J Dev Behav Pediatr*, 38: 753–764.

Boivin MJ, Weiss J, Chhaya R et al. (2017b) The feasibility of automated eye tracking with the Early Childhood Vigilance Test of attention in younger HIV-exposed Ugandan children. *Neuropsychology*, 31: 525–534.

Boivin MJ, Barlow-Mosha L, Chernoff MC et al. (2018) Neuropsychological performance in African children with HIV enrolled in a multisite antiretroviral clinical trial. *AIDS*, 32: 189–204.

Boivin MJ, Maliwichi-Senganimalunje L, Ogwang LW et al. (2019) Neurodevelopmental effects of ante-partum and post-partum antiretroviral exposure in HIV-exposed and uninfected children versus HIV-unexposed and uninfected children in Uganda and Malawi: A prospective cohort study. *Lancet HIV*, 6: e518–e530.

Boivin MJ, Augustinavicius JL, Familiar-Lopez I et al. (2020a) Early childhood development caregiver training and neurocognition of HIV-exposed Ugandan siblings. *J Dev Behav Pediatr*, 41: 221–229.

Boivin MJ, Chernoff M, Fairlie L et al. (2020b) African multi-site 2-year neuropsychological study of school-age children perinatally infected, exposed, and unexposed to human immunodeficiency virus. *Clin Infect Dis*, 71: e105–e114.

Brennan AT, Bonawitz R, Gill CJ et al. (2016) A meta-analysis assessing all-cause mortality in HIV-exposed uninfected compared with HIV-unexposed uninfected infants and children. *AIDS*, 30: 2351–2360.

Bronfenbrenner U (1979) *The Ecology of Human Development: Experiments by Nature and Design.* Cambridge, MA: Harvard University Press.

Caniglia EC, Patel K, Huo Y et al. (2016) Atazanavir exposure in utero and neurodevelopment in infants: A comparative safety study. *AIDS*, 30: 1267–1278.

Cassidy AR, Williams PL, Leidner J et al. (2019) In utero efavirenz exposure and neurodevelopmental outcomes in HIV-exposed uninfected children in Botswana. *Pediatr Infect Dis J*, 38: 828–834.

Chandna J, Ntozini R, Evans C et al. (2020) Effects of improved complementary feeding and improved water, sanitation and hygiene on early child development among HIV-exposed children: Substudy of a cluster randomised trial in rural Zimbabwe. *BMJ Glob Health*, 5: e001718.

Chaudhury S, Williams PL, Mayondi GK et al. (2017) Neurodevelopment of HIV-exposed and HIV-unexposed uninfected children at 24 months. *Pediatrics*, 140: e20170988.

Chaudhury S, Mayondi GK, Williams PL et al. (2018) In-utero exposure to antiretrovirals and neurodevelopment among HIV-exposed-uninfected children in Botswana. *AIDS*, 32: 1173–1183.

Cheong JL, Hunt RW, Anderson PJ et al. (2008) Head growth in preterm infants: Correlation with magnetic resonance imaging and neurodevelopmental outcome. *Pediatrics*, 121: e1534–e1540.

Chhaya R, Weiss J, Seffren V et al. (2018) The feasibility of an automated eye-tracking-modified Fagan test of memory for human faces in younger Ugandan HIV-exposed children. *Child Neuropsychol*, 24: 686–701.

Connor EM, Sperling RS, Gelber R et al. (1994) Reduction of maternal–infant transmission of human immunodeficiency virus type 1 with zidovudine treatment. Pediatric AIDS Clinical Trials Group Protocol 076 Study Group. *N Engl J Med*, 331: 1173–1180.

Daelmans B, Black MM, Lombardi J et al. (2015) Effective interventions and strategies for improving early child development. *BMJ*, 351: h4029.

Debeaudrap P, Bodeau-Livinec F, Pasquier E et al. (2018) Neurodevelopmental outcomes in HIV-infected and uninfected African children. *AIDS*, 32: 2749–2757.

Desmonde S, Goetghebuer T, Thorne C, Leroy V (2016) Health and survival of HIV perinatally exposed but uninfected children born to HIV-infected mothers. *Curr Opin HIV AIDS*, 11: 465–476.

Dirajlal-Fargo S, Mussi-Pinhata MM, Weinberg A et al. (2019) HIV-exposed-uninfected infants have increased inflammation and monocyte activation. *AIDS*, 33: 845–853.

Donald KAM, Fernandez A, Claborn K et al. (2017) The developmental effects of HIV and alcohol: A comparison of gestational outcomes among babies from South African communities with high prevalence of HIV and alcohol use. *AIDS Res Ther*, 14: 28.

Donald KA, Weddrrburn CJ, Barnett W et al. (2019) Risk and protective factors for child development: An observational South African birth cohort. *PLoS Med*, 16: e1002920.

Evans C, Jones CE, Prendergast AJ (2016) HIV-exposed, uninfected infants: New global challenges in the era of paediatric HIV elimination. *Lancet Infect Dis*, 16: e92–e107.

Evans C, Chasekwa B, Ntozini R, Humphrey JH, Prendergast AJ (2016) Head circumferences of children born to HIV-infected and HIV-uninfected mothers in Zimbabwe during the preantiretroviral therapy era. *AIDS*, 30: 2323–2328.

Familiar I, Collins SM, Sikorskii A et al. (2018) Quality of caregiving is positively associated with neurodevelopment during the first year of life among HIV-exposed uninfected children in Uganda. *J Acquir Immune Defic Syndr*, 77: 235–242.

Filteau S (2009) The HIV-exposed, uninfected African child. *Trop Med Int Health*, 14: 276–287.

Filteau S, Rowland-Jones S (2016) Cytomegalovirus infection may contribute to the reduced immune function, growth, development, and health of HIV-exposed, uninfected African children. *Front Immunol*, 7: 257.

Gardner JM, Walker SP, Powell CA, Grantham-McGregor S (2003) A randomized controlled trial of a home-visiting intervention on cognition and behavior in term low birth weight infants. *J Pediatr*, 143: 634–639.

Gompels UA, Larke N, Sanz-Ramos M et al. (2012) Human cytomegalovirus infant infection adversely affects growth and development in maternally HIV-exposed and unexposed infants in Zambia. *Clin Infect Dis*, 54: 434–442.

Gonzalez R, Ruperez M, Sevene E et al. (2017) Effects of HIV infection on maternal and neonatal health in southern Mozambique: A prospective cohort study after a decade of antiretroviral drugs roll out. *PLoS One*, 12: e0178134.

Grantham-McGregor S, Cheung YB, Cueto S et al. (2007) Developmental potential in the first 5 years for children in developing countries. *Lancet*, 369: 60–70.

Hair NL, Hanson JL, Wolfe BL, Pollak SD (2015) Association of child poverty, brain development, and academic achievement. *JAMA Pediatr*, 169: 822–829.

Hermoye L, Saint-Martin C, Cosnard G et al. (2006) Pediatric diffusion tensor imaging: Normal database and observation of the white matter maturation in early childhood. *Neuroimage*, 29: 493–504.

Himes SK, Huo Y, Siberry GK et al. (2015) Meconium atazanavir concentrations and early language outcomes in HIV-exposed uninfected infants with prenatal atazanavir exposure. *J Acquir Immune Defic Syndr*, 69: 178–186.

Jahanshad N, Couture MC, Prasitsuebsai W et al. (2015) Brain imaging and neurodevelopment in HIV-uninfected Thai children born to HIV-infected mothers. *Pediatr Infect Dis J*, 34: e211–e216.

Jankiewicz M, Holmes MJ, Taylor PA et al. (2017) White matter abnormalities in children with HIV infection and exposure. *Front Neuroanat*, 11: 88.

Jao J, Abrams EJ (2014) Metabolic complications of in utero maternal HIV and antiretroviral exposure in HIV-exposed infants. *Pediatr Infect Dis J*, 33: 734–740.

Jones CE, Naidoo S, De Beer C, Esser M, Kampmann B, Hesseling AC (2011) Maternal HIV infection and antibody responses against vaccine-preventable diseases in uninfected infants. *JAMA*, 305: 576–584.

Kacanek D, Williams PL, Mayondi G et al. (2018) Pediatric neurodevelopmental functioning ater in utero exposure to triple-NRTI vs. dual-NRTI + PI ART in a randomized trial, Botswana. *J Acquir Immune Defic Syndr*, 79: e93–e100.

Kerr SJ, Puthanakit T, Vibol U et al. (2014) Neurodevelopmental outcomes in HIV-exposed-uninfected children versus those not exposed to HIV. *AIDS Care*, 26: 1327–1335.

Krogh K, Green M, Thayer S (2015) HIV-1 tat-induced changes in synaptically-driven network activity adapt during prolonged exposure. *Current HIV Research*, 12: 406.

Laughton B, Cornell M, Kidd M et al. (2018) Five-year neurodevelopment outcomes of perinatally HIV-infected children on early limited or deferred continuous antiretroviral therapy. *J Int AIDS Soc*, 21: e25106.

Le Doare K, Bland R, Newell ML (2012) Neurodevelopment in children born to HIV-infected mothers by infection and treatment status. *Pediatrics*, 130: e1326–e1344.

Le Roux SM, Abrams EJ, Myer L (2016) Rethinking the HIV-exposed, uninfected child: Epidemiologic perspectives. *Future Microbiol*, 11: 717–720.

Le Roux SM, Abrams EJ, Nguyen K, Myer L (2016) Clinical outcomes of HIV-exposed, HIV-uninfected children in sub-Saharan Africa. *Trop Med Int Health*, 21: 829–845.

Le Roux SM, Donald KA, Brittain K et al. (2018) Neurodevelopment of breastfed HIV-exposed uninfected and HIV-unexposed children in South Africa. *AIDS*, 32: 1781–1791.

Le Roux SM, Donald KA, Kroon M. et al. (2019) HIV viremia during pregnancy and neurodevelopment of HIV-exposed uninfected children in the context of universal antiretroviral therapy and breastfeeding: A prospective study. *Pediatr Infect Dis J*, 38: 70–75.

Leyenaar JK (2005) HIV/AIDS and Africa's orphan crisis. *Paediatr Child Health*, 10: 259–260.

McCrory C, Murray A (2013) The effect of breastfeeding on neuro-development in infancy. *Matern Child Health J*, 17: 1680–1688.

McHenry MS, McAteer CI, Oyungu E et al. (2018) Neurodevelopment in young children born to HIV-infected mothers: A meta-analysis. *Pediatrics*, 141: e20172888.

McHenry MS, Balogun KA, McDonald BC, Vreeman RC, Whipple EC, Serghides L (2019a) In utero exposure to HIV and/or antiretroviral therapy: A systematic review of preclinical and clinical evidence of cognitive outcomes. *J Int AIDS Soc*, 22: e25275.

McHenry MS, McAteer CI, Oyungu E, Deathe AR, Vreeman RC (2019b) Interventions for developmental delays in children born to HIV-infected mothers: A systematic review. *AIDS Care*, 31: 275–282.

Mebrahtu H, Simms V, Chingono R et al. (2018) Postpartum maternal mental health is associated with cognitive development of HIV-exposed infants in Zimbabwe: A cross-sectional study. *AIDS Care*, 30: 74–82.

Mofenson LM (2015) Editorial commentary: New challenges in the elimination of pediatric HIV infection: The expanding population of HIV-exposed but uninfected children. *Clin Infect Dis*, 60: 1357–1360.

Newell ML, Coovadia H, Cortina-Borja M et al. (2004) Mortality of infected and uninfected infants born to HIV-infected mothers in Africa: A pooled analysis. *Lancet*, 364: 1236–1243.

Nicholson L, Chisenga M, Siame J, Kasonka L, Filteau S (2015) Growth and health outcomes at school age in HIV-exposed, uninfected Zambian children: Follow-up of two cohorts studied in infancy. *BMC Pediatr*, 15: 66.

Nozyce ML, Huo Y, Williams PL et al. (2014) Safety of in utero and neonatal antiretroviral exposure: Cognitive and academic outcomes in HIV-exposed, uninfected children 5-13 years of age. *Pediatr Infect Dis J*, 33: 1128–1133.

Ntozini R, Chandna J, Evans C et al. (2020) Early child development in children who are HIV-exposed uninfected compared to children who are HIV-unexposed: Observational sub-study of a cluster-randomized trial in rural Zimbabwe. *J Int AIDS Soc*, 23: e25456.

Redmond SM, Yao TJ, Russell JS et al. (2016) Longitudinal evaluation of language impairment in youth with perinatally acquired human immunodeficiency virus (HIV) and youth with perinatal HIV exposure. *J Pediatric Infect Dis Soc*, 5: S33–S40.

Rice ML, Zeldow B, Siberrty GK et al. (2013). Evaluation of risk for late language emergence after in utero antiretroviral drug exposure in HIV-exposed uninfected infants. *Pediatr Infect Dis J*, 32: e406–e413.

Robertson FC, Holmes MJ, Cotton MF et al. (2018) Perinatal HIV infection or exposure is associated with low N-acetylaspartate and glutamate in basal ganglia at age 9 but not 7 years. *Front Hum Neurosci*, 12: 145.

Ruperez M, Gonzalez R, Maculuve S et al. (2017) Maternal HIV infection is an important health determinant in non-HIV-infected infants. *AIDS*, 31: 1545–1553.

Sevenoaks T, Wedderrburn CJ, Donald KA et al. (2021) Association of maternal and infant inflammation with neurodevelopment in HIV-exposed uninfected children in a South African birth cohort. *Brain Behav Immun*, 91: 65–73.

Sherr L, Croome N, Parra Castaneda K, Bradshaw K (2014) A systematic review of psychological functioning of children exposed to HIV: Using evidence to plan for tomorrow's HIV needs. *AIDS Behav*, 18: 2059–2074.

Sirois PA, Huo Y, Williams PL et al. (2013) Safety of perinatal exposure to antiretroviral medications: Developmental outcomes in infants. *Pediatr Infect Dis J*, 32: 648–655.

Sirois PA, Chernoff MC, Malee KM et al. (2016) Associations of memory and executive functioning with academic and adaptive functioning among youth with perinatal HIV exposure and/or infection. *J Pediatric Infect Dis Soc*, 5: S24–S32.

Slogrove A, Reikie B, Naidoo S et al. (2012) HIV-exposed uninfected infants are at increased risk for severe infections in the first year of life. *J Trop Pediatr*, 58: 505–508.

Slogrove AL, Archary M, Cotton MF (2016) Optimizing research methods to understand HIV-exposed uninfected infant and child morbidity: Report of the second HEU infant and child workshop. *Front Immunol*, 7: 576.

Slogrove AL, Powis KM, Johnson LF, Stover J, Mahy M (2020) Estimates of the global population of children who are HIV-exposed and uninfected, 2000-18: a modelling study. *Lancet Glob Health*, 8: e67–e75.

Slogrove AL (2021) It is a question of equity: Time to talk about children who are HIV-exposed and 'HIV-free'. *J Int AIDS Soc*, 24: e25850.

Stein A, Desmond C, Garbarino J et al. (2014) Predicting long-term outcomes for children affected by HIV and AIDS: Pperspectives from the scientific study of children's development. *AIDS*, 28(Suppl 3): S261–S268.

Tardieu M, Brunelle F, Raybaud C et al. (2005) Cerebral MR imaging in uninfected children born to HIV-seropositive mothers and perinatally exposed to zidovudine. *AJNR Am J Neuroradiol*, 26: 695–701.

Taron-Brocard C, Le Chenadec J, Faye A et al. (2014) Increased risk of serious bacterial infections due to maternal immunosuppression in HIV-exposed uninfected infants in a European country. *Clin Infect Dis*, 59: 1332–1345.

Toledo G, Côté HCF, Adler C, Thorne C, Goetghebuer T (2021) Neurological development of children who are HIV-exposed and uninfected. *Developmental Medicine & Child Neurology*, 63, 1161–1170.

Tran LT, Roos A, Fouche JP et al. (2016) White matter microstructural integrity and neurobehavioral outcome of HIV-exposed uninfected neonates. *Medicine (Baltimore)*, 95: e2577.

UNAIDS (2021) *AIDSinfo* [Online]. Available: http://aidsinfo.unaids.org [Accessed 12 February 2022].

UNICEF (2016) *Children and AIDS Seventh Stocktaking Report.*

Uthman OA, Nachega JB, Anderson J et al. (2017) Timing of initiation of antiretroviral therapy and adverse pregnancy outcomes: A systematic review and meta-analysis. *Lancet HIV*, 4: e21–e30.

Van Pelt AE, Scott JC, Morales KH et al. (2022) Structural validity of a computerized neurocognitive battery for youth affected by human immunodeficiency virus in Botswana. *Psychol Assess*, 34: 139–146.

Van Rie A, Mupuala A, Dow A (2008) Impact of the HIV/AIDS epidemic on the neurodevelopment of preschool-aged children in Kinshasa, Democratic Republic of the Congo. *Pediatrics*, 122: e123–e128.

van Wyhe KS, Van de Water T, Boivin MJ, Cotton MF, Thomas KG (2017) Cross-cultural assessment of HIV-associated cognitive impairment using the Kaufman assessment battery for children: A systematic review. *J Int AIDS Soc*, 20: 21412.

van Wyhe KS, Laughton B, Cotton MF et al. (2021) Cognitive outcomes at ages seven and nine years in South African children from the children with HIV early antiretroviral (CHER) trial: A longitudinal investigation. *J Int AIDS Soc*, 24: e25734.

Victora CG, Bahl R, Barros AJ et al. (2016) Breastfeeding in the 21st century: Epidemiology, mechanisms, and lifelong effect. *Lancet*, 387: 475–490.

von Mollendorf C, Von Gottberg A, Tempia S et al. (2015) Increased risk for and mortality from invasive pneumococcal disease in HIV-exposed but uninfected infants aged <1 year in South Africa, 2009–2013. *Clin Infect Dis*, 60: 1346–1356.

Walker SP, Chang SM, Powell CA, Grantham-McGregor SM (2005) Effects of early childhood psychosocial stimulation and nutritional supplementation on cognition and education in growth-stunted Jamaican children: Prospective cohort study. *Lancet*, 366: 1804–1807.

Wedderburn CJ, Evans C, Yeung S, Gibb DM, Donald KA, Prendergast AJ (2019a) Growth and neurodevelopment of HIV-exposed uninfected children: A conceptual framework. *Curr HIV/AIDS Rep*, 16: 501–513.

Wedderburn CJ, Yeung S, Rehman AM et al. (2019b) Neurodevelopment of HIV-exposed uninfected children in South Africa: Outcomes from an observational birth cohort study. *Lancet Child Adolesc Health*, 3: 803–813.

Wedderburn CJ, Groenewold NA, Roos A et al. (2022a) Early structural brain development in infants exposed to HIV and antiretroviral therapy in utero in a South African birth cohort. *J Int AIDS Soc*, 25: e25863.

Wedderburn CJ, Weldon E, Bertran-Cobo C et al. (2022b) Early neurodevelopment of HIV-exposed uninfected children in the era of antiretroviral therapy: A systematic review and meta-analysis. *Lancet Child Adolesc Health*, 6: 393–408.

Wedi CO, Kirtley S, Hopewell S, Corrigan R, Kennedy SH, Hedmelaar J (2016) Perinatal outcomes associated with maternal HIV infection: A systematic review and meta-analysis. *Lancet HIV*, 3: e33–e48.

White M, Connor KL (2020) In utero HIV exposure and the early nutritional environment influence infant neuro-development: Findings from an evidenced review and meta-analysis. *Nutrients*, 12: 3375.

WHO (2015) *Guideline on When to Start Antiretroviral Therapy and on Pre-exposure Prophylaxis for HIV.* Geneva: World Health Organization.

WHO (2016) *What's New in HIV Infant Diagnosis.* Fact sheet: HIV treatment and care. Geneva: World Health Organization.

WHO (2017) Mother-to-child transmission of HIV [Online]. Available: https://www.who.int/teams/global-hiv-hepatitis-and-stis-programmes/hiv/prevention/mother-to-child-transmission-of-hiv [Accessed 24 July 2023].

WHO (2021) *Consolidated Guidelines on HIV Prevention, Testing, Treatment, Service Delivery and Monitoring: Recommendations for a Public Health Approach.* Geneva: World Health Organization.

Williams PL, Hazra R, Van Dyke RB et al. (2016) Antiretroviral exposure during pregnancy and adverse outcomes in HIV-exposed uninfected infants and children using a trigger-based design. *AIDS*, 30: 133–144.

Williams TC, Drake AJ (2015) What a general paediatrician needs to know about early life programming. *Arch Dis Child*, 100: 1058–1063.

CHAPTER 16

Antiretroviral Therapy and the Nervous System in Perinatally Infected Children

Eric Decloedt and Karen Cohen

INTRODUCTION

Untreated human immunodeficiency virus (HIV) infection has a significant impact on early neurocognitive development. In the pre-antiretroviral therapy (ART) era, up to a third of children infected with HIV-1 developed progressive HIV encephalopathy (Chiriboga et al. 2005). Untreated HIV infection is associated with cognitive deficits and developmental delay.

For more than a decade, treatment guidelines have recommended that all children under 12 months of age commence ART immediately at the time of diagnosis (WHO 2008). From 2015, the World Health Organization (WHO) guidelines moved to recommend ART for all children irrespective of age or disease stage (WHO 2016a). The incidence of HIV encephalopathy has decreased dramatically with introduction of combination antiretroviral therapy (cART) (Vreeman et al. 2015).

However, despite guidelines recommending universal access to ART, coverage is not always optimal. Coverage is lower among children than among adults. In 2021, global ART coverage was 75% but only 52% of children living with HIV infection and requiring ART globally were receiving ART (WHO 2022).

ART reduces, but does not remove, the risk of neurocognitive sequelae of HIV infection. Many children perinatally infected with HIV and treated with ART will have neurocognitive complications with developmental delay, motor deficits, and cognitive impairment (Crowell et al. 2014; Vreeman et al. 2015). There is evidence that early initiation of ART is protective of neurocognitive development (Laughton et al. 2012). However, a study in Thai children who were at an older age at ART initiation (median age 6 years 4 months) found no neurodevelopmental or cognitive difference between the immediate and the deferred ART groups (Puthanakit et al. 2013). This suggests that very early initiation of ART – ideally in infancy – is necessary for the optimal neuroprotective effects of ART to be realised (Vreeman et al. 2015).

There have been a few reports of suspected 'cures' of HIV in children started on ART very early in life: for example, the 'Mississippi baby', who was perinatally infected and started on ART 30 hours after birth. ART was interrupted at 18 months, after which viral load was undetectable for 2 years before relapse. Relapse is likely due to persistence of HIV in reservoir sites. The central nervous system (CNS) is a potential reservoir for HIV. Before the ART era, HIV was shown to infect cells in the brain, including microglial cells, astrocytes, macrophages, and neurons (Cantó-Nogués et al. 2005). Studies generally look at autopsy specimens as it is difficult to study the presence and replication of HIV in brain tissue in living people. It remains unknown whether an HIV reservoir persists in brain tissue during ART (Luzuriaga et al. 2015; Henderson et al. 2020). Extrapolation is made from findings in the cerebrospinal fluid (CSF), which suggest that there is a separate population of infected cells in the CNS, established early on in HIV-infection (Dahl et al. 2014). Eradicating such a reservoir will be important in achieving a cure for HIV, which is the subject of ongoing research (Deeks et al. 2021).

Several reasons have been suggested as to why children perinatally infected with HIV may still develop neurocognitive impairment. Neuronal injury may predate initiation of ART or may result from inflammatory responses post-ART initiation (Vreeman et al. 2015). The introduction of ART, however, does not reverse pre-existing neurological manifestations of HIV infection (Puthanakit et al. 2013). It has also been postulated that antiretrovirals with poor CNS penetration results in poorer neurocognitive outcomes because replication of the HIV virus in the CNS is not suppressed (Letendre et al. 2008; Vreeman et al. 2015). In addition, concerns have been raised about both short- and long-term neurological toxicities of antiretroviral medicines, particularly with exposure at times of intense neurocognitive development.

NEUROLOGICAL AND NEUROPSYCHIATRIC ADVERSE EFFECTS OF ANTIRETROVIRAL MEDICINES

A range of both short- and long-term neuropsychiatric adverse effects has been attributed to antiretroviral medication. The bulk of the data on adverse drug reactions comes from studies in adults, with fewer data on children. Studying neuropsychiatric effects in infants and young children is particularly challenging.

Nucleoside and Nucleotide Reverse Transcriptase Inhibitors

The nucleoside and nucleotide reverse transcriptase inhibitors (NRTIs) as a class inhibit the mitochondrial enzyme DNA polymerase gamma. This causes mitochondrial toxicity (Birkus, Hitchcock, and Cihlar 2002). Mitochondrial toxicity results in several clinical manifestations, including lactic acidaemia and acidosis, lipoatrophy, and peripheral neuropathy. The extent of mitochondrial toxicity varies between NRTIs. The most mitochondrially toxic NRTIs are zalcitabine, stavudine, and didanosine. Lamivudine, abacavir, and the nucleotide analogue reverse transcriptase inhibitor tenofovir have the least mitochondrial toxicity. Zalcitabine, stavudine, and didanosine are no longer recommended and, because of their toxicity, very rarely used. In a prospective Paediatric AIDS Clinical Trial Group cohort study of children in the USA, peripheral neuropathy developed in 13 out of 1154 (1.1%) children treated with stavudine in combination with lamivudine and in 8 out of 1336 (0.6%) children treated with zidovudine in combination with lamivudine (Van Dyke et al. 2008). In a cross-sectional study of 182 South African children who were systematically assessed for neuropathy, 24% were found to have a peripheral neuropathy (95% confidence interval 18–30%) (Peters et al. 2014). The majority (86%) of these children were taking stavudine and lamivudine, with 6.6% taking abacavir and lamivudine, and 2.7% taking zidovudine and didanosine (Peters et al. 2014). Cotrimoxazole prophylaxis and didanosine exposure were independent risk factors for neuropathy in this study (Peters et al. 2014).

Stavudine was previously recommended by the WHO as a component of standard first-line ART for children (WHO 2006). In a South African observational cohort study including 3579 children, followed up for a median of 41 months, the incidence of treatment-limiting toxicity due to stavudine was 50.6 (95% confidence interval 46.2–55.4) per 1000 patient years (Fortuin-de Smidt et al. 2017). Abacavir, which replaced stavudine in South African treatment guidelines, is much better tolerated, with an incidence of treatment-limiting toxicity of 1.6 (95% confidence interval 0.5–4.8) per 1000 patient years (Fortuin-de Smidt et al. 2017). The vast majority of stavudine substitutions in this cohort were due to lipodystrophy (Fortuin-de Smidt et al. 2017). Peripheral neuropathy is a rare cause of stavudine substitution in children; only 2 out of 96 NRTI substitutions (2%) in an earlier South African paediatric observational cohort analysis were for neuropathy (Palmer et al. 2013).

Increasing concerns regarding stavudine toxicity resulted in it being removed from first-line ART recommendations (WHO 2016b). The current WHO guidelines stipulate that stavudine should no longer be prescribed or procured (WHO 2021).

Non-nucleoside Reverse Transcriptase Inhibitors: Efavirenz

The non-nucleoside reverse transcriptase inhibitor (NNRTI) efavirenz was widely used in first-line ART, particularly in resource-limited settings. The 2016 WHO consolidated antiretroviral guidelines recommended efavirenz-containing ART for first-line treatment of HIV in both adults and children from 3 years of age (WHO 2016b). However, because of growing NNRTI resistance, the WHO now recommends that the integrase strand transfer inhibitor (INSTI) dolutegravir be used in first-line therapy regimens in place of efavirenz (WHO 2021). However, there are still many patients – both children and adults – taking efavirenz, particularly in resource-limited settings.

Efavirenz is known to cause several neuropsychiatric side effects, including sleep disturbance, vivid nightmares, insomnia, headache, and dizziness (Kenny et al. 2012). Efavirenz can also occasionally precipitate severe psychiatric symptoms, including depression, suicidal ideation, and psychosis (Kenny et al. 2012) and should be avoided in patients with a history of severe psychiatric illness with psychotic features. There are case reports of children with cerebellar dysfunction, generalised seizures, and absence seizures caused by efavirenz (Strehlau et al. 2011; Pinillos et al. 2016).

CNS side effects are commonly found in adult patients. A systematic review found that a third of adults who commence efavirenz-containing ART report CNS side effects, which are severe in 6.1% of cases (Ford et al. 2015). It is very challenging to assess for presence of CNS side effects in young children and infants (Tukei et al. 2012). In a Ugandan prospective observational cohort of children and adolescents receiving ART, 25 out of 177 (14.1%) of those receiving efavirenz experienced CNS adverse effects; this may underestimate prevalence as children under age 5 years could not report CNS side effects (Tukei et al. 2012). The most commonly reported side effects in this cohort were dizziness, anxiety, and nightmares (Tukei et al. 2012).

Neuropsychiatric side effects are frequently reported immediately after efavirenz initiation and tend to wane as time passes (Apostolova et al. 2015). However, there is an increasing appreciation that some patients experience ongoing and persistent CNS side effects while taking efavirenz.

Neuropsychiatric adverse effects experienced by patients taking efavirenz are frequently associated with high plasma efavirenz concentrations (Marzolini et al. 2001; Gallego et al. 2004). A 12-year-old child developed psychotic symptoms on efavirenz and was found to have markedly elevated efavirenz concentrations (Lowenhaupt et al. 2007). Her symptoms resolved with withdrawal of efavirenz. Four children with severe neurotoxicity on efavirenz (cerebellar dysfunction, generalised seizures, and absence seizures) were found to have a markedly elevated efavirenz concentration, ranging from 20mg/L to 60mg/L, which is up to 15 times higher than the upper limit of the suggested target therapeutic range

(1–4mg/L) (Pinillos et al. 2016). In all four children the symptoms resolved after efavirenz was discontinued (Pinillos et al. 2016).

Efavirenz is hepatically metabolised. The primary cytochrome enzyme responsible for efavirenz metabolism is cytochrome P450 isoenzyme 2B6 (CYP2B6). The primary metabolite is 8-hydroxy efavirenz. Polymorphisms of CYP2B6 may result in a loss of isoenzyme function, which slows down the metabolism of efavirenz. Single nucleotide polymorphisms CYP2B6 516G→T, 983T→C, and 15582C→T are frequent in sub-Saharan African patients (Sinxadi et al. 2015). In South Africa, 20% of African patients treated with efavirenz were found to be slow metabolisers because of these single nucleotide polymorphisms (Sinxadi et al. 2015). Slow metabolisers have markedly higher plasma concentrations of efavirenz than extensive metabolisers with standard dosing. In a cohort study, all adult patients presenting with late-onset efavirenz neurotoxicity syndrome were genotyped as slow CYP2B6 metabolisers (van Rensburg et al. 2022). Slow metabolisers may, therefore, require lower doses of efavirenz than are standard. The slow metabolising phenotype is common in Africa. In a systematic review of randomised controlled trials of standard dose efavirenz, reduced dose efavirenz was found to have improved tolerability with less CNS adverse effects and to be non-inferior to standard dose (Amin et al. 2014, 2015; Ford et al. 2015; Chen et al. 2020). The WHO currently recommends efavirenz at low dose (400mg) as the alternative first-line regimen for adults and adolescents initiating ART, in settings where pre-treatment HIV drug resistance to NNRTs is <10% (WHO 2021).

The risk of active tuberculosis is increased in HIV-infected patients, frequently requiring concomitant treatment for both tuberculosis and HIV infection. Drug interactions between antiretrovirals and antituberculosis treatment need to be taken into account when prescribing for HIV and tuberculosis coinfected patients. Rifampicin is known to induce the metabolism of many drugs, including protease inhibitors, NNRTIs, and dolutegravir. There were concerns that efavirenz concentrations would be decreased with tuberculosis treatment, but this was not confirmed in South African patients, where efavirenz concentrations were similar with and without tuberculosis treatment (Cohen et al. 2009). A study conducted in South African coinfected children found that first-line antituberculosis treatment has little effect on efavirenz concentrations in children who were extensive or intermediate efavirenz metabolisers (McIlleron et al. 2013). However, in slow metabolisers efavirenz concentrations were increased in the presence of first-line antituberculosis treatment (McIlleron et al. 2013). The mechanism for this differential effect is thought to be due to inhibition of the CYP2A6 accessory metabolic pathways by isoniazid, which generates the 7-hydroxyefavirenz metabolite (di Iulio et al. 2009). The CYP2A6 accessory metabolic pathway is important for efavirenz metabolism in slow metabolisers who have impaired CYP2B6 function (McIlleron et al. 2013). Slow metabolisers already have higher concentrations of efavirenz than intermediate and extensive metabolisers. Slow metabolisers may be at increased risk of developing CNS side effects during tuberculosis treatment due to efavirenz concentrations being further increased by isoniazid inhibition (McIlleron et al. 2013). In fact, isoniazid coadministration is an associated risk factor for the development of late-onset efavirenz neurotoxicity syndrome in a cohort of genotypically confirmed efavirenz slow metabolisers (van Rensburg et al. 2022).

A systematic review of four AIDS Clinical Trial group studies, including data on more than 5000 adult patients, compared rates of suicidality between patients initiated on efavirenz and those initiated on non-efavirenz-containing ART regimens (Mollan et al. 2014). Worryingly, this study found a two-fold increase in suicidality in patients initiated on efavirenz (Mollan et al. 2014). The investigators explored association between efavirenz-metaboliser status and suicidality and found that slow metabolisers were at increased risk (Mollan et al. 2017). This association was seen amongst white participants but not black participants – reasons for this are unclear. In adult patients there is some evidence from cross-sectional studies that prolonged exposure to efavirenz is associated with poorer cognitive outcomes than with alternative ART options. It is postulated that efavirenz may exacerbate HIV-associated neurocognitive disorder due to neuronal toxicity of both the parent drug and the 8-hydroxy metabolite. The long-term effects of efavirenz on cognition in children require further study (Underwood, Robertson, and Winston 2015).

Integrase Strand Transfer Inhibitors: Dolutegravir

Dolutegravir potently and rapidly suppresses HIV-1 viral replication and has a high barrier to the development of resistance. Dolutegravir was found to have superior tolerability to efavirenz in a systematic review and network meta-analysis of randomised controlled trials (Kanters et al. 2016). Dolutegravir is an attractive option for first-line ART because of its potency and tolerability. The WHO now recommends dolutegravir-containing first-line ART regimens for adults and adolescents, as well as for infants and children for whom dolutegravir dosing has been approved. There are ongoing studies of the use of dolutegravir in children. As of July 2021 dolutegravir is approved by the European Medicines Agency and the United States Food and Drug Administration for infants and children older than 4 weeks and weighing at least 3kg. The pharmacokinetics of dolutegravir are being evaluated in neonates (NCT05590325).

There were concerns regarding teratogenicity in patients taking dolutegravir at the time of conception and in very early pregnancy due to a signal from a pregnancy cohort study in Botswana where early surveillance results suggested an increase in the risk of neural tube defects associated with dolutegravir exposure (Mosime and Abrams 2018; Zash, Makhema, and Shapiro 2018). However, as more data from that cohort have accrued, the difference observed in the rate of neural tube defects between females taking dolutegravir-based regimens at the time of conception compared to other antiretroviral drugs has shrunk (Zash et al. 2019, 2021). In the most recent analysis, the prevalence estimate for neural tube defects in infants born to mothers taking dolutegravir in very early pregnancy had stabilised at approximately 2 per 1000, and does not differ significantly from the rate in infants born to mothers taking non-dolutegravir-based ART regimens at conception. Dolutegravir-containing ART is now the preferred first-line regimen for all patients initiating ART, including females of childbearing potential (WHO 2021). Dolutegravir in combination with an optimised NRTI backbone is also recommended for second-line therapy in adults, adolescents, and children failing non-dolutegravir-based regimens.

In patients taking dolutegravir, neuropsychiatric adverse events were reported in the phase 3 randomised clinical trials, as well as in post-marketing observational cohorts (Cailhol et al. 2017; Fettiplace et al. 2017; Kheloufi et al. 2017; Menard et al. 2017; Scheper et al. 2017). Insomnia (including grade 3 and 4 severity), headache, and irritability are the most frequently reported neuropsychiatric adverse events (Walmsley et al. 2013; Fettiplace et al. 2017; Menard et al. 2017). There are reports of dolutegravir treatment discontinuations due to significant neuropsychiatric adverse effects in patients with no previous psychiatric history (Kheloufi et al. 2015; Scheper et al. 2017). Serious neuropsychiatric symptoms described in patients taking dolutegravir include severe depression, suicidal ideation, feelings of being 'high', and feeling 'dissociated' from the world. Dolutegravir discontinuation rates due to neuropsychiatric adverse events range from 3.5% to 8% (Scheper et al. 2017). Symptoms tend to appear early, typically within 4 weeks of initiating dolutegravir. Adverse effects may be concentration related since dolutegravir trough concentrations were significantly higher in adult patients with neuropsychiatric adverse events than in those without (1.31µg/mL vs 1.01µg/mL, $p = 0.0013$) (Yagura et al. 2017).

PENETRATION OF ANTIRETROVIRALS INTO THE CENTRAL NERVOUS SYSTEM

The concentration of HIV within the CSF correlates with the degree of cognitive impairment (Brew et al. 1997). Early ART has been associated with improved neurodevelopmental outcomes in children (Laughton et al. 2012). However, HIV-1 RNA+ cell frequency is increased in the brain tissue of simian immunodeficiency virus-infected rhesus macaques receiving ART compared to untreated rhesus macaques (0.04% vs 0.38%). This presumably reflects poor penetration of antiretrovirals, resulting in persistent HIV-1 viral replication (Estes et al. 2017). Suboptimal penetration of antiretrovirals into the CNS with ongoing viral replication is considered to be a risk factor for ongoing neuronal damage and cognitive impairment (Nightingale et al. 2014). CSF discordance or compartmentalisation with ongoing viral replication despite suppressed plasma viraemia has been described in 10% of adult patients (Edén et al. 2010). Data on children are limited but compartmentalised CSF virus was detected in up to 50% of treatment-naïve children (Sturdevant et al. 2012).

CSF antiretroviral concentration measurements are frequently used as a proxy for CNS antiretroviral exposure. However, the CSF may be a poor predictor of brain concentrations and may under-estimate exposure (Curley et al. 2017). In addition, distribution of ART is not homogenous in the brain: for example, efavirenz concentrations were up to threefold higher in the white matter versus the grey matter of rhesus macaques (Srinivas, Rosen, and Gilliland 2019). In vitro 50% inhibitory concentration (IC_{50}) is used to estimate the CNS efficacy of antiretroviral drugs. The IC_{50} is the concentration that yields 50% of maximal inhibition of viral replication when the antiretroviral is used as a monotherapy. One should be aware of the limitations of the IC_{50} when drawing conclusions (Yilmaz, Price, and Gisslén 2012; Decloedt et al. 2015). The primary target for HIV in the brain is the macrophages and microglia, which may not be the cell type in which the particular IC_{50} has been established, and the IC_{50} in HIV-infected microglia is higher compared to bone marrow-derived macrophages and peripheral blood mononuclear cells (Asahchop et al. 2017). In addition, the IC_{50} does not take into account synergistic effects of combination ART. Furthermore, it is unclear by how much an antiretroviral should exceed the IC_{50} to achieve 100% viral replication inhibition, since IC_{100} is not usually determined. Finally, the CSF and extracellular concentrations may not necessarily correlate with brain parenchyma viral suppression, which may in part explain the lack of correlation between CSF antiretroviral concentrations and neurocognitive outcomes in clinical trials (Letendre et al. 2008; Ellis et al. 2014; Asahchop et al. 2017).

Nucleoside and Nucleotide Reverse Transcriptase Inhibitors

Most NRTIs penetrate the CNS well, with low protein binding that allows for easy diffusion across the blood–brain barrier (Table 16.1) (Yilmaz, Price, and Gisslén 2012b). At standard doses, CSF NRTI concentrations will generally exceed the in vitro IC_{50}. Zidovudine is considered to achieve the best CNS exposure in the NRTI class, with 75% of plasma exposure (Fischl et al. 1987; Rolinski et al. 1997). Zidovudine improved neurocognitive performance in patients with complex HIV-associated dementia when it was used as monotherapy during the early treatment years of HIV (Sidtis et al. 1993). Abacavir concentrations in the CSF are approximately 35% of total abacavir plasma concentration (McDowell et al. 1999, 2000). Lamivudine CSF concentrations are 12% of total plasma concentrations in children (Mueller et al. 1998). Tenofovir penetrates the CNS very poorly, requiring active transport, with concentrations well below the in vitro IC_{50} to suppress viral replication at standard therapeutic doses (Best et al. 2012). NRTIs are prodrugs that require intracellular phosphorylation into active metabolites which have longer half-lives than the parent compound (Bazzoli et al. 2010). Tenofovir, the parent drug, may

Table 16.1 Summary of antiretroviral cerebrospinal fluid exposure data.

Antiretroviral	Estimated CSF exposure compared to plasma	Target concentration	CSF viral suppression data	Reference
Nucleoside reverse transcriptase inhibitors				
Abacavir	*Ratio of* AUC_{CSF}/AUC_{plasma} 36±5%[a] ,95% CI 28–46)	IC_{50} 17 ng/ml	Abacavir (300 mg 12 hourly) CSF concentrations exceed IC_{50} for 85% of the dosing interval in adult patients. Once daily administered abacavir provides similar CSF concentrations and CSF to plasma ratio.	Capparelli et al. (2005b); Calcagno et al. (2018)
Emtricitabine	*Ratio of pharmacokinetic time points* 26%[b] (range 5–41%)	IC_{50} 70 ng/ml		Calcagno et al. (2011)
Lamivudine	*Ratio of* AUC_{CSF}/AUC_{plasma} 15.1±1.3%[a] (range 12.4–17.5%)	IC_{50} 549.6 ng/ml	Lamivudine (150 mg 12 hourly) CSF concentrations exceed the IC_{50} in adult patients.	Foudraine et al. (1998); Haas et al. (2000); Yilmaz, Price, and Gisslén (2012)
Zidovudine	*Ratio of* AUC_{CSF}/AUC_{plasma} 75±26%[a]	IC_{50} 0.002–2.400 μmol/l	Zidovudine CSF concentrations exceed the IC_{50} in adult patients.	Rolinski et al. (1997); Foudraine et al. (1998)
Nucleotide reverse transcriptase inhibitor				
Tenofovir disoproxil fumerate	*Ratio of pharmacokinetic time points* 5.7%[b] (range 0.12–0.66%)	IC_{50} 11.5 ng/ml	Tenofovir disoproxil fumerate (300 mg daily) CSF concentrations exceed the IC_{50} in 23% of adult patients, suggesting limited CSF transfer.	Best et al. (2012)
Integrase inhibitor				
Dolutegravir	*Ratio of pharmacokinetic time points* 0.52%[b] IQR (3.0–10.0%) (range 0.4–84%)	IC_{50} 0.2 ng/ml	Dolutegravir (50 mg 12 hourly) CSF concentrations exceed IC_{50} by 90-fold in adult patients with rapid reduction of CSF HIV-1.	Letendre et al. (2014)

(Continued)

Table 16.1 Continued

Antiretroviral	Estimated CSF exposure compared to plasma	Target concentration	CSF viral suppression data	Reference
Protease inhibitors				
Atazanavir	*Ratio of AUC$_{CSF}$/AUC$_{plasma}$* 0.74%	IC$_{50}$ 1ng/ml	Atazanavir (with or without ritonavir) CSF concentrations do not exceed IC$_{50}$ in more than 80% of adult patients.	Best et al. (2009); Cusini et al. (2013)
Lopinavir/ ritonavir	*Ratio of pharmacokinetic time points* 0.23%[b] IQR (0.12–0.75%)	IC$_{50}$ 1.9ng/ml	Lopinavir/ritonavir CSF concentrations exceed the IC$_{50}$ in adult patients 5-fold.	Capparelli et al. (2005a); DiCenzo et al. (2009)
Darunavir/ ritonavir	*Ratio of pharmacokinetic time points* 1.4%[b] IQR (0.9–1.8%)	IC$_{50}$ 1.78ng/ml	Darunavir CSF concentrations exceed the IC$_{50}$ and IC$_{90}$ by >20-fold respectively.	Croteau et al. (2013)
Non-nucleoside reverse transcriptase inhibitors				
Efavirenz	*Ratio of pharmacokinetic time points* Unbound 120%[b] IQR (97–212%)	IC$_{50}$ 0.36–1.3ng/ml	Efavirenz unbound concentrations exceed the IC$_{50}$ in adult patients.	Avery et al. (2013a, 2013b); Yilmaz et al. (2012)
Nevirapine	*Ratio of pharmacokinetic time points* 62.6%[b] (range 41–77%)	IC$_{50}$ 32.0ng/ml	Data on CSF viral suppression limited.	Antinori et al. (2005); Yilmaz, Price, and Gisslén (2012)

Concentrations are total concentrations unless otherwise specified.

[a] Mean ± standard deviation

[b] Median

Abbreviations: AUC, area under the concentration time curve; IC$_{50}$, in vitro 50% inhibitory concentration; IQR, interquartile range.

predict pharmacological activity poorly as it is phosphorylated intracellularly to the active metabolite tenofovir diphosphate and the intracellular concentrations of tenofovir diphosphate are non-linear to tenofovir (Duwal, Schütte, and von Kleist 2012). There are fewer data on intracellular concentrations of phosphorylated pharmacologically active NRTI metabolites in macrophages (Bazzoli et al. 2010). Paired plasma-CSF concentrations of various antiretrovirals were evaluated in 20 HIV-infected children (aged 8–18 years on treatment), with a high degree of pharmacokinetic variability and low CSF NRTI concentrations that were below the IC_{50} (Van den Hof et al. 2018). Despite pharmacokinetic variability and low CSF NRTI concentrations, all patients had CSF viral suppression. This suggests that NRTI concentrations in the CSF do not reflect active phosphorylated intracellular concentrations.

Non-nucleoside Reverse Transcriptase Inhibitors

Efavirenz is highly protein bound (>99.5%) and efavirenz CSF exposure is less than 1% of plasma exposure. However, the protein-free efavirenz fraction penetrates easily into the CSF and, thus, the protein-free concentrations in the CSF and plasma are similar (Yilmaz et al. 2012; Avery et al. 2013b). The protein-free concentration is pharmacologically active. Both total and protein-free efavirenz concentrations in the CSF exceed the IC_{50} in the majority of patients studied (Best et al. 2011; Yilmaz et al. 2012; Avery et al. 2013a, 2013b; Cusini, Vernazza, and Yerly 2013). Efavirenz is predominantly metabolised by CYP2B6 into several metabolites, of which 8-hydroxy-efavirenz is the main metabolite (di Iulio et al. 2009; Avery et al. 2013a). Efavirenz metabolites do not seem to inhibit viral replication but may play a role in the agent's CNS adverse event profile (Kenedi and Goforth 2011; Tovar-y-Romo et al. 2012; Avery et al. 2013a, 2013b). Eight-hydroxy efavirenz has been hypothesised to play a role in neurotoxicity and CSF 8-hydroxy efavirenz has been associated with an increase in patient neurocognitive symptoms (Tovar-y-Romo et al. 2012; Winston et al. 2015). Extensive metabolisers may generate more 8-hydroxy-efavirenz and be predisposed to develop more neurotoxicity (Vujkovic et al. 2018). However, the association between extensive metabolisers and high 8-OH-efavirenz has not been found by others (Winston et al. 2015). Nevirapine has limited CSF penetration data, although it is considered to have the best characteristics for blood–brain barrier passage among the NNRTIs (van Praag et al. 2002; Antinori et al. 2005; Saitoh et al. 2007). Nevirapine is the least protein-bound NNRTI (60% protein binding) and has a low molecular weight of 266.6g/mol. The effect of nevirapine on CSF viral suppression has not been studied.

Protease Inhibitors

The CNS penetration of the protease inhibitors is limited by their large molecular size (molecular weight above 500Da) and their affinity to bind to plasma proteins (Yilmaz, Price, and Gisslén 2012). The protease inhibitor ritonavir is added to other protease inhibitors to inhibit the P-glycoprotein efflux pump and cytochrome P450 enzyme. Both the P-glycoprotein efflux pump and the cytochrome P450 enzyme reduce protease inhibitor concentrations significantly if not inhibited. When boosted with ritonavir, lopinavir reaches therapeutic concentrations in plasma. Lopinavir is 97% to 99% protein bound, with less than 0.5% of total lopinavir concentrations reaching the CSF (Lafeuillade et al. 2002; Solas et al. 2003; Capparelli et al. 2005a; DiCenzo et al. 2009; Cusini, Vernazza, and Yerly 2013). However, the total lopinavir CSF concentrations exceed in vitro IC_{50} (Capparelli et al. 2005a; DiCenzo et al. 2009; Cusini et al. 2013). Ritonavir added to atazanavir increases plasma total atazanavir concentrations by more than double, while CSF concentrations only increase slightly (Best et al. 2009). The estimate of total atazanavir penetration when boosted with ritonavir in the CSF is 0.74% of plasma concentrations

(Best et al. 2009). CSF atazanavir concentrations are not above the in vitro IC_{50} in many patients and may not inhibit CNS viral replication. Darunavir is considered to have adequate CSF exposure at the dose of darunavir/ritonavir 600/100mg (Calcagno et al. 2014).

Integrase Strand Transfer Inhibitors

The integrase strand transfer inhibitors are considered to penetrate the CSF well. CSF dolutegravir concentrations exceed the IC_{50} by 66 to 90 times (Letendre et al. 2014). Raltegravir total CSF concentrations are approximately 6.0% that of plasma and exceed the IC_{50} in all patients (Yilmaz et al. 2009; Johnson et al. 2013).

Clinical Data Evaluating High Central Nervous System Penetrating Antiretroviral Therapy

Clinical neurocognitive endpoints and the relationship with antiretroviral pharmacokinetics has been best described by the CNS penetration-effectiveness (CPE) score hypothesis studies. Antiretroviral CPE ranking has been proposed based on the chemical properties, CSF pharmacology, and effectiveness in the CNS (Letendre et al. 2008). Antiretrovirals with a high CPE rank have been proposed to penetrate the CNS better and to treat ongoing residual CNS viral replication; however, it has not been conclusively shown that ART regimens with high CPE result in improved cognitive function in adult patients with HIV-associated neurocognitive disorder (Letendre et al. 2008; Ellis et al. 2014). Inversely, high CPE antiretroviral regimens have been associated with an increased risk of dementia with a hazard ratio of 1.74 (confidence interval 1.15–2.65), perhaps indicating a threshold at which CNS ART concentrations contribute to neurotoxicity (Caniglia et al. 2014). Additionally, various confounders should be controlled for, including patient demographics, comorbidities, antiretroviral experience, and standardisation of neuropsychological assessments and normative data (Arentoft et al. 2022). Neuroimaging, specifically blood oxygenation level dependent (BOLD) functional magnetic resonance imaging (fMRI), may be more sensitive in detecting abnormal brain function compared to neuropsychological assessment. The amplitude of the BOLD fMRI response to a task is associated with regional changes in cerebral blood flow and metabolism. In adult patients the amplitude of the BOLD fMRI response was significantly greater in participants treated with low CPE ART (Ances et al. 2008). The investigators hypothesised that high CPE ART reduces the metabolic demand in brain microenvironments with a more normalised BOLD fMRI response.

There have been limited and also conflicting studies evaluating high CNS penetrating antiretroviral regimens in HIV-infected children. Patel et al. found that CNS-penetrating regimens in perinatally HIV-infected children did not result in a statistically significant reduction in the incidence of HIV encephalopathy but were associated with a survival benefit (74% reduction in the risk of death, 95% confidence interval 39–89%) after HIV encephalopathy diagnosis compared with low CNS-penetrating regimens (Patel et al. 2009). Crowell et al. found that, rather than CPE scores, virological suppression during infancy is associated with improved neurocognitive outcomes in children (Crowell et al. 2015). Of note, blood–brain barrier permeability is different in children compared to adults and the CPE score has been developed and evaluated in adults. The efflux transporter, P-glycoprotein, which is also expressed at the blood–brain barrier, has limited expression at birth, and adult levels of expression of P-glycoprotein were only reached at 6 months (Lam et al. 2015). While the CPE studies are interesting, randomised controlled trials comparing high CPE to low CPE antiretrovirals are needed to determine whether CPE has a real role in routine paediatric practice.

REFERENCES

Amin J, Becker S, Beloso W et al. (2014) Efficacy of 400 mg efavirenz versus standard 600 mg dose in HIV-infected, antiretroviral-naive adults (ENCORE1): A randomised, double-blind, placebo-controlled, non-inferiority trial. *Lancet* (London, England) [online], 383(9927): 1474–1482. Available from: https://pubmed.ncbi.nlm.nih.gov/24522178/ [accessed 29 November 2022].

Amin J, Becker S, Beloso W et al. (2015) Efficacy and safety of efavirenz 400 mg daily versus 600 mg daily: 96-week data from the randomised, double-blind, placebo-controlled, non-inferiority ENCORE1 study. *The Lancet Infectious Diseases* [online], 15(7): 793–802.

Ances BM, Roc AC, Korczykowski M, Wolf RL, Kolson DL (2008) Combination antiretroviral therapy modulates the blood oxygen level-dependent amplitude in human immunodeficiency virus-seropositive patients. *Journal of Neurovirology,* 14(8): 418–424.

Antinori A, Perno CF, Giancola ML et al. (2005) Efficacy of cerebrospinal fluid (CSF)-penetrating antiretroviral drugs against HIV in the neurological compartment: Different patterns of phenotypic resistance in CSF and plasma. *Clinical Infectious Diseases: An Official Publication of the Infectious Diseases Society of America*, 41(12): 1787–1793.

Apostolova N, Funes HA, Blas-Garcia A, Galindo MJ, Alvarez A and Esplugues JV (2015) Efavirenz and the CNS: What we already know and questions that need to be answered. *The Journal of Antimicrobial Chemotherapy*, 70(10): 2693–2708.

Arentoft A, Troxell K, Alvarez K et al. (2022) HIV antiretroviral medication neuropenetrance and neurocognitive outcomes in HIV+ adults: A review of the literature examining the central nervous system penetration effectiveness score. *Viruses* [online], 14(6). Available from: https://www.ncbi.nlm.nih.gov/pmc/articles/PMC9227894/ [accessed 29 November 2022].

Asahchop EL, Meziane O, Mamik MK et al. (2017) Reduced antiretroviral drug efficacy and concentration in HIV-infected microglia contributes to viral persistence in brain. *Retrovirology*, 14(1): 47.

Avery LB, VanAusdall JL, Hendrix CW, Bumpus NN (2013a) Compartmentalization and antiviral effect of efavirenz metabolites in blood plasma, seminal plasma, and cerebrospinal fluid. *Drug Metabolism and Disposition: The Biological Fate of Chemicals*, 41(2): 422–429.

Avery LB, Sacktor N, McArthur JC, Hendrix CW (2013b) Protein-free efavirenz concentrations in cerebrospinal fluid and blood plasma are equivalent: Applying the law of mass action to predict protein-free drug concentration. *Antimicrobial Agents and Chemotherapy*, 57(3): 1409–1414.

Bazzoli C, Jullien V, Le Tiec C, Rey E, Mentré F, Taburet A-M (2010) Intracellular pharmacokinetics of antiretroviral drugs in HIV-infected patients, and their correlation with drug action. *Clinical Pharmacokinetics*, 49(1): 17–45.

Best BM, Letendre SL, Brigid E et al. (2009) Low atazanavir concentrations in cerebrospinal fluid. *AIDS* (London, England), 23(1): 83–87.

Best BM, Koopmans PP, Letendre SL et al. (2011) Efavirenz concentrations in CSF exceed IC50 for wild-type HIV. *The Journal of Antimicrobial Chemotherapy*, 66(2): 354–357.

Best BM, Letendre SL, Koopmans P et al. (2012) Low cerebrospinal fluid concentrations of the nucleotide HIV reverse transcriptase inhibitor, tenofovir. *Journal of Acquired Immune Deficiency Syndromes (1999)*, 59(4): 376–381.

Birkus G, Hitchcock MJM, Cihlar T (2002) Assessment of mitochondrial toxicity in human cells treated with tenofovir: Comparison with other nucleoside reverse transcriptase inhibitors. *Antimicrobial Agents and Chemotherapy*, 46(3): 716–723.

Brew BJ, Pemberton L, Cunningham P, Law MG (1997) Levels of human immunodeficiency virus type 1 RNA in cerebrospinal fluid correlate with AIDS dementia stage. *The Journal of Infectious Diseases*, 175(4): 963–966.

Cailhol J, Rouyer C, Alloui C, Jeantils V (2017) Dolutegravir and neuropsychiatric adverse events. *Aids*, 31(14): 2023–2024.

Calcagno A, Bonora S, Simiele M et al. (2011) Tenofovir and emtricitabine cerebrospinal fluid-to-plasma ratios correlate to the extent of blood-brain barrier damage. *AIDS* (London, England), 25(11): 1437–1439.

Calcagno A, Simiele M, Alberione MC et al. (2014) Cerebrospinal fluid inhibitory quotients of antiretroviral drugs in HIV-infected patients are associated with compartmental viral control. *Clinical Infectious Diseases*, 60: 311–317.

Calcagno A, Pinnetti C, De Nicolò A et al. (2018) Cerebrospinal fluid abacavir concentrations in HIV-positive patients following once-daily administration. *British Journal of Clinical Pharmacology*, 84(6): 1380–1383.

Caniglia EC, Cain LE, Justice A et al. (2014) Antiretroviral penetration into the CNS and incidence of AIDS-defining neurologic conditions. *Neurology* [online], 83(2): 134. Available from: https://www.ncbi.nlm.nih.gov/pmc/articles/PMC4117168/ [accessed 29 November 2022].

Cantó-Nogués C, Sánchez-Ramón S, Álvarez S, Lacruz C, Muñóz-Fernández MÁ (2005) HIV-1 infection of neurons might account for progressive HIV-1-associated encephalopathy in children. *Journal of Molecular Neuroscience* [online], 27(1): 79–89. Available from: https://link.springer.com/article/10.1385/JMN:27:1:079 [accessed 29 November 2022].

Capparelli EV, Holland D, Okamoto C et al. (2005a) Lopinavir concentrations in cerebrospinal fluid exceed the 50% inhibitory concentration for HIV. *AIDS (London, England)*, 19(9): 949–952.

Capparelli EV, Letendre SL, Ellis RJ, Patel P, Holland D, Mccutchan JA (2005b) Population pharmacokinetics of abacavir in plasma and cerebrospinal fluid. *Antimicrobial Agents and Chemotherapy*, 49(6): 2504–2506.

Chen J, Chen R, Shen Y et al. (2020) Efficacy and safety of lower dose tenofovir disoproxil fumarate and efavirenz versus standard dose in HIV-infected, antiretroviral-naive adults: A multicentre, randomized, noninferiority trial. *Emerging Microbes & Infections* [online], 9(1): 843. Available from: https://www.ncbi.nlm.nih.gov/pmc/articles/PMC7241516/ [accessed 29 November 2022].

Chiriboga CA, Fleishman S, Champion S, Gaye-Robinson L, Abrams EJ (2005) Incidence and prevalence of HIV encephalopathy in children with HIV infection receiving highly active anti-retroviral therapy (HAART). *The Journal of Pediatrics*, 146(3): 402–407.

Cohen K, Grant A, Dandara C et al. (2009) Effect of rifampicin-based antitubercular therapy and the cytochrome P450 2B6 516G>T polymorphism on efavirenz concentrations in adults in South Africa. *Antiviral Therapy*, 14(5): 687–695.

Croteau D, Rossi SS, Best BM et al. (2013) Darunavir is predominantly unbound to protein in cerebrospinal fluid and concentrations exceed the wild-type HIV-1 median 90% inhibitory concentration. *The Journal of Antimicrobial Chemotherapy*, 68(3): 684–689.

Crowell CS, Malee KM, Yogev R, Muller WJ (2014) Neurologic disease in HIV-infected children and the impact of combination antiretroviral therapy. *Reviews in Medical Virology*, 24(5): 316–331.

Crowell CS, Huo Y, Tassiopoulos K et al. (2015) Early viral suppression improves neurocognitive outcomes in HIV-infected children. *AIDS (London, England)*, 29(3): 295–304.

Curley P, Rajoli RKR, Moss DM et al. (2017) Efavirenz is predicted to accumulate in brain tissue: An *in silico, in vitro*, and *in vivo* investigation. *Antimicrobial Agents and Chemotherapy*, 61(1): e01841–16.

Cusini A, Vernazza PL, Yerly S (2013) Higher CNS penetration-effectiveness of long-term combination antiretroviral therapy is associated with better HIV-1 viral suppression in cerebrospinal fluid. *Journal of Acquired Immune Deficiency Syndromes (1999)*, 62(1): 28–35.

Dahl V, Gisslen M, Hagberg L et al. (2014) An example of genetically distinct HIV type 1 variants in cerebrospinal fluid and plasma during suppressive therapy. *The Journal of Infectious Diseases* [online], 209(10): 1618. Available from: https://www.ncbi.nlm.nih.gov/pmc/articles/PMC3997583/ [accessed 29 November 2022].

Decloedt EHEH, Rosenkranz B, Maartens G, Joska J (2015) Central nervous system penetration of antiretroviral drugs: Pharmacokinetic, pharmacodynamic and pharmacogenomic considerations. *Clinical Pharmacokinetics*, 54(6): 581–598.

Deeks SG, Archin N, Cannon P et al. (2021) Research priorities for an HIV cure: International AIDS Society Global Scientific Strategy 2021. *Nature Medicine* [online], 27(12): 2085–2098. Available from: https://www.nature.com/articles/s41591-021-01590-5 [accessed 6 December 2022].

DiCenzo R, DiFrancesco R, Cruttenden K, Donnelly J, Schifitto G (2009) Lopinavir cerebrospinal fluid steady-state trough concentrations in HIV-infected adults. *The Annals of Pharmacotherapy*, 43(12): 1972–1977.

di Iulio J, Fayet A, Arab-Alameddine M et al (2009) In vivo analysis of efavirenz metabolism in individuals with impaired CYP2A6 function. *Pharmacogenetics and Genomics* [online], 19(4): 300–309. Available from: http://www.ncbi.nlm.nih.gov/pubmed/19238117 [accessed 9 June 2014].

Duwal S, Schütte C, von Kleist M (2012) Pharmacokinetics and pharmacodynamics of the reverse transcriptase inhibitor tenofovir and prophylactic efficacy against HIV-1 infection. *PloS One*, 7(7): e40382.

Edén A, Fuchs D, Hagberg L et al. (2010) HIV-1 viral escape in cerebrospinal fluid of subjects on suppressive antiretroviral treatment. *The Journal of Infectious Diseases*, 202(12): 1819–1825.

Ellis RJ, Letendre S, Vaida F et al. (2014) Randomized trial of central nervous system-targeted antiretrovirals for HIV-associated neurocognitive disorder. *Clinical Infectious Diseases: An Official Publication of the Infectious Diseases Society of America*, 58(7): 1015–1022.

Estes JD, Kityo C, Ssali F et al. (2017) Defining total-body AIDS-virus burden with implications for curative strategies. *Nature Medicine*, 23(11): 1271–1276.

Fettiplace A, Stainsby C, Winston A et al. (2017) Psychiatric symptoms in patients receiving dolutegravir. *Journal of Acquired Immune Deficiency Syndromes (1999)*, 74(4): 423–431.

Fischl MA, Richman DD, Grieco MH et al. (1987) The efficacy of azidothymidine (AZT) in the treatment of patients with AIDS and AIDS-related complex. A double-blind, placebo-controlled trial. *The New England Journal of Medicine*, 317(4): 185–191.

Ford N, Shubber Z, Pozniak A et al. (2015) Comparative safety and neuropsychiatric adverse events associated with efavirenz use in first-line antiretroviral therapy: A systematic review and meta-analysis of randomized trials. *Journal of Acquired Immune Deficiency Syndromes (1999)*, 69(4): 422–429.

Fortuin-de Smidt M, de Waal R, Cohen K et al. (2017) First-line antiretroviral drug discontinuations in children. *PloS One*, 12(2): e0169762.

Foudraine NA, Hoetelmans RM, Lange JM et al. (1998) Cerebrospinal-fluid HIV-1 RNA and drug concentrations after treatment with lamivudine plus zidovudine or stavudine. *Lancet*, 351(9115): 1547–1551.

Gallego L, Barreiro P, del Río R et al. (2004) Analyzing sleep abnormalities in HIV-infected patients treated with Efavirenz. *Clinical Infectious Diseases: An Official Publication of the Infectious Diseases Society of America*, 38(3): 430–432.

Haas DW, Clough LA, Johnson BW et al. (2000) Evidence of a source of HIV type 1 within the central nervous system by ultraintensive sampling of cerebrospinal fluid and plasma. *AIDS Research and Human Retroviruses*, 16(15): 1491–1502.

Henderson LJ, Reoma LB, Kovacs JA, Nath A (2020) Advances toward curing HIV-1 infection in tissue reservoirs. *Journal of Virology* [online], 94(3). Available from: https://pubmed.ncbi.nlm.nih.gov/31694954/ [accessed 29 November 2022].

Johnson DH, Sutherland D, Acosta EP, Erdem H, Richardson D, Haas DW (2013) Genetic and non-genetic determinants of raltegravir penetration into cerebrospinal fluid: A single-arm pharmacokinetic study. *PloS One*, 8(12): e82672.

Kanters S, Vitoria M, Doherty M et al. (2016) Comparative efficacy and safety of first-line antiretroviral therapy for the treatment of HIV infection: A systematic review and network meta-analysis. *The Lancet. HIV*, 3(11): e510–e520.

Kenedi CA, Goforth HW (2011) A systematic review of the psychiatric side-effects of efavirenz. *AIDS and Behavior*, 15(8): 1803–1818.

Kenny J, Musiime V, Judd A, Gibb D (2012) Recent advances in pharmacovigilance of antiretroviral therapy in HIV-infected and exposed children. *Current Opinion in HIV and AIDS*, 7(4): 305–316.

Kheloufi F, Allemand J, Mokhtari S, Default A (2015) Psychiatric disorders after starting dolutegravir: Report of four cases. *AIDS (London, England)*, 29(13): 1723–1725.

Kheloufi F, Boucherie Q, Blin O, Micallef J (2017) Neuropsychiatric events and dolutegravir in HIV patients: A worldwide issue involving a class effect. *AIDS (London, England)*, 31: 1775–1777.

Lafeuillade A, Solas C, Halfon P, Chadapaud S, Hittinger G, Lacarelle B (2002) Differences in the detection of three HIV-1 protease inhibitors in non-blood compartments: Clinical correlations. *HIV Clinical Trials*, 3(1): 27–35.

Lam J, Baello S, Iqbal M et al. (2015) The ontogeny of P-glycoprotein in the developing human blood–brain barrier: Implication for opioid toxicity in neonates. *Pediatric Research*, 78(4): 417–421.

Laughton B, Cornell M, Grove D et al. (2012) Early antiretroviral therapy improves neurodevelopmental outcomes in infants. *AIDS (London, England)*, 26(13): 1685–1690.

Letendre S, Marquie-Beck J, Capparelli E et al. (2008) Validation of the CNS penetration-effectiveness rank for quantifying antiretroviral penetration into the central nervous system. *Archives of Neurology*, 65(1): 65–70.

Letendre SL, Mills AM, Tashima KT et al. (2014) ING116070: A study of the pharmacokinetics and antiviral activity of dolutegravir in cerebrospinal fluid in HIV-1-infected, antiretroviral therapy-naive subjects. *Clinical Infectious Diseases: An Official Publication of the Infectious Diseases Society of America*, 59(7): 1032–1037.

Lowenhaupt EA, Matson K, Qureishi B, Saitoh A, Pugatch D (2007) Psychosis in a 12-year-old HIV-positive girl with an increased serum concentration of efavirenz. *Clinical Infectious Diseases: An Official Publication of the Infectious Diseases Society of America*, 45(10): e128-30.

Luzuriaga K, Gay H, Ziemniak C et al. (2015) Viremic relapse after HIV-1 remission in a perinatally infected child. *New England Journal of Medicine* [online], 372(8): 786–788. Available from: https://www.nejm.org/doi/10.1056/NEJMc1413931 [accessed 29 November 2022].

Marzolini C, Telenti A, Decosterd LA, Greub G, Biollaz J, Buclin T (2001) Efavirenz plasma levels can predict treatment failure and central nervous system side effects in HIV-1-infected patients. *AIDS (London, England)*, 15(1): 71–75.

McDowell JA, Chittick GE, Ravitch JR, Polk RE, Kerkering TM, Stein DS (1999) Pharmacokinetics of [14C] abacavir, a human immunodeficiency virus type 1 (HIV-1) reverse transcriptase inhibitor, administered in a single oral dose to HIV-1-infected adults: A mass balance study. *Antimicrobial Agents and Chemotherapy*, 43: 2855–2861.

McDowell JA, Lou Y, Symonds WS, Stein DS (2000) Multiple-dose pharmacokinetics and pharmacodynamics of abacavir alone and in combination with zidovudine in human immunodeficiency virus-infected adults. *Antimicrobial Agents and Chemotherapy*, 44(8): 2061–2067.

McIlleron HM, Schomaker M, Ren Y et al. (2013) Effects of rifampin-based antituberculosis therapy on plasma efavirenz concentrations in children vary by *CYP2B6* genotype. *AIDS (London, England)*, 27(12): 1933–1940.

Menard A, Montagnac C, Solas C et al. (2017) Neuropsychiatric adverse effects on dolutegravir: An emerging concern in Europe. *AIDS (London, England)*, 31(8): 1201–1203.

Mollan KR, Smurzynski M, Eron JJ et al. (2014) Association between efavirenz as initial therapy for HIV-1 infection and increased risk for suicidal ideation or attempted or completed suicide: An analysis of trial data. *Annals of Internal Medicine*, 161(1): 1–10.

Mollan KR, Tierney C, Hellwege JN et al. (2017) Race/ethnicity and the pharmacogenetics of reported suicidality with efavirenz among clinical trials participants. *The Journal of Infectious Diseases*, 216(5): 554–564.

Mosime W, Abrams EJ (2018) Safety of dolutegravir in pregnancy: Late breaking findings, interpretations, and implications. In: *AIDS*. Amsterdam. 23–27 July. Available from: https://programme.aids2018.org/Programme/Session/1589 [accessed 18 August 2023].

Mueller BU, Lewis LL, Yuen GJ et al. (1998) Serum and cerebrospinal fluid pharmacokinetics of intravenous and oral lamivudine in human immunodeficiency virus-infected children. *Antimicrobial Agents and Chemotherapy*, 42(12): 3187–3192.

Nightingale S, Winston A, Letendre S et al. (2014) Controversies in HIV-associated neurocognitive disorders. *The Lancet. Neurology*, 13(11): 1139–1151.

Palmer M, Chersich M, Moultrie H, Kuhn L, Fairlie L, Meyers T (2013) Frequency of stavudine substitution due to toxicity in children receiving antiretroviral treatment in sub-Saharan Africa. *AIDS (London, England)*, 27(5): 781–785.

Patel K, Ming X, Williams PL et al. (2009) Impact of HAART and CNS-penetrating antiretroviral regimens on HIV encephalopathy among perinatally infected children and adolescents. *AIDS (London, England)*, 23(14): 1893–1901.

Peters RPH, Van Ramshorst MS, Struthers HE, McIntyre JA (2014) Clinical assessment of peripheral neuropathy in HIV-infected children on antiretroviral therapy in rural South Africa. *European Journal of Pediatrics*, 173(9): 1245–1248.

Pinillos F, Dandara C, Swart M et al. (2016) Case report: Severe central nervous system manifestations associated with aberrant efavirenz metabolism in children: The role of *CYP2B6* genetic variation. *BMC Iinfectious Diseases*, 16: 56.

Puthanakit T, Ananworanich J, Vonthanak S et al. (2013) Cognitive function and neurodevelopmental outcomes in HIV-infected children older than 1 year of age randomized to early versus deferred antiretroviral therapy: The PREDICT neurodevelopmental study. *The Pediatric Infectious Disease Journal*, 32(5): 501–508.

Rolinski B, Bogner JR, Sadri I, Wintergerst U, Goebel FD (1997) Absorption and elimination kinetics of zidovudine in the cerebrospinal fluid in HIV-1-infected patients. *Journal of Acquired Immune Deficiency Syndromes and Human Retrovirology: Official Publication of the International Retrovirology Association*, 15(3): 192–197.

Saitoh A, Sarles E, Capparelli E et al. (2007) *CYP2B6* genetic variants are associated with nevirapine pharmacokinetics and clinical response in HIV-1-infected children. *AIDS* (London, England), 21(16): 2191–2199.

Scheper H, van Holten N, Hovens J, de Boer M (2017) Severe depression as a neuropsychiatric side effect induced by dolutegravir. Published online 2017; *HIV Medicine*, April 2018, 19(4): e58–e59.

Sidtis JJ, Gatsonis C, Price RW et al. (1993) Zidovudine treatment of the AIDS dementia complex: Results of a placebo-controlled trial. AIDS Clinical Trials Group. *Annals of Neurology*, 33(4): 343–349.

Sinxadi PZ, Leger PD, McIlleron HM et al. (2015) Pharmacogenetics of plasma efavirenz exposure in HIV-infected adults and children in South Africa. *British Journal of Clinical Pharmacology*, 80(1): 146–156.

Solas C, Lafeuillade A, Halfon P, Chadapaud S, Hittinger G, Lacarelle B (2003) Discrepancies between protease inhibitor concentrations and viral load in reservoirs and sanctuary sites in human immunodeficiency virus-infected patients. *Antimicrobial Agents and Chemotherapy*, 47(1): 238–243.

Srinivas N, Rosen EP, Gilliland WM (2019) Antiretroviral concentrations and surrogate measures of efficacy in the brain tissue and CSF of preclinical species. *Xenobiotica: The Fate of Foreign Compounds in Biological Systems*, 49(10): 1192–1201.

Strehlau R, Martens L, Coovadia A et al. (2011) Absence seizures associated with efavirenz initiation. *The Pediatric Infectious Disease Journal*, 30(11): 1001–1003.

Sturdevant CB, Dow A, Jabara CB et al. (2012) Central nervous system compartmentalization of HIV-1 subtype C variants early and late in infection in young children. *PLoS Pathogens*, 8(12): e1003094.

Tovar-y-Romo LB, Bumpus NN, Pomerantz D et al. (2012) Dendritic spine injury induced by the 8-hydroxy metabolite of efavirenz. *The Journal of Pharmacology and Experimental Therapeutics*, 343(3): 696–703.

Tukei VJ, Asiimwe A, Maganda A et al. (2012) Safety and tolerability of antiretroviral therapy among HIV-infected children and adolescents in Uganda. *Journal of Acquired Immune Deficiency Syndromes (1999)*, 59(3): 274–280.

Underwood J, Robertson KR, Winston A (2015) Could antiretroviral neurotoxicity play a role in the pathogenesis of cognitive impairment in treated HIV disease? *AIDS* (London, England), 29(3): 253–261.

Van den Hof M, Blokhuis C, Cohen S et al. (2018) CNS penetration of ART in HIV-infected children. *The Journal of Antimicrobial Chemotherapy*, 73(2): 484–489.

Van Dyke RB, Wang L, Williams PL et al. (2008) Toxicities associated with dual nucleoside reverse-transcriptase inhibitor regimens in HIV-infected children. *The Journal of Infectious Diseases*, 198(11): 1599–1608.

van Praag RME, van Weert ECM, van Heeswijk RPG et al. (2002) Stable concentrations of zidovudine, stavudine, lamivudine, abacavir, and nevirapine in serum and cerebrospinal fluid during 2 years of therapy. *Antimicrobial Agents and Chemotherapy*, 46(3): 896–899.

van Rensburg R, Nightingale S, Brey N et al. (2022) Pharmacogenetics of the late-onset efavirenz neurotoxicity syndrome (LENS). *Clinical Infectious Diseases*, 75(3): 399–405. Available from: https://doi.org/10.1093/cid/ciab961 [accessed 29 November 2022].

Vreeman RC, Scanlon ML, McHenry MS, Nyandiko WM (2015) The physical and psychological effects of HIV infection and its treatment on perinatally HIV-infected children. *Journal of the International AIDS Society*, 18(Suppl 6): 20258.

Vujkovic M, Bellamy SL, Zuppa AF et al. (2018) Polymorphisms in cytochrome P450 are associated with extensive efavirenz pharmacokinetics and CNS toxicities in an HIV cohort in Botswana. *The Pharmacogenomics Journal*, 1 June 2018.

Walmsley SL, Antela A, Clumeck N et al. (2013) Dolutegravir plus abacavir-lamivudine for the treatment of HIV-1 infection. *The New England Journal of Medicine*, 369(19): 1807–1818.

WHO (2006) *Antiretroviral Therapy for HIV Infection in Adults and Adolescents* [online]. Available from: http://www.who.int/hiv/pub/arv/adult/en/ [accessed 18 September 2018].

WHO (2008) *Report of the WHO Technical Reference Group, Paediatric HIV/ART Care Guideline Group Meeting* [online]. Available from: http://www.who.int/hiv/pub/paediatric/WHO_Paediatric_ART_guideline_rev_mreport_2008.pdf [accessed 18 September 2018].

WHO (2016a) *Consolidated Guidelines on the Use of Antiretroviral Drugs for Treating and Preventing HIV Infection. Recommendations for a Public Health Approach.* [online]. *Second Edition* [online]: 480. Available from: http://www.who.int/hiv/pub/arv/arv-2016/en/ [accessed 22 October 2017].

WHO (2016b) *Consolidated Guidelines on the Use of Antiretroviral Drugs for Treating and Preventing HIV Infection. Recommendations for a Public Health Approach. Second Edition.* Geneva: WHO Press.

WHO (2021) *Consolidated Guidelines on HIV Prevention, Testing, Treatment, Service Delivery and Monitoring: Recommendations for a Public Health Approach.* 16 July 2021: 548.

WHO (2022) *HIV* [online]. Available from: https://www.who.int/news-room/fact-sheets/detail/hiv-aids [accessed 29 November 2022].

Winston A, Amin J, Clarke A et al. (2015) Cerebrospinal fluid exposure of efavirenz and its major metabolites when dosed at 400 mg and 600 mg once daily: A randomized controlled trial. *Clinical Infectious Diseases: An Official Publication of the Infectious Diseases Society of America*, 60(7): 1026–1032.

Yagura H, Watanabe D, Kushida H et al. (2017) Impact of UGT1A1 gene polymorphisms on plasma dolutegravir trough concentrations and neuropsychiatric adverse events in Japanese individuals infected with HIV-1. *BMC Infectious Diseases*, 17(1): 622.

Yilmaz A, Gisslén M, Spudich S et al. (2009) Raltegravir cerebrospinal fluid concentrations in HIV-1 infection. *PLoS One*, 4(9): 1–5.

Yilmaz A, Watson V, Dickinson L, Back D (2012) Efavirenz pharmacokinetics in cerebrospinal fluid and plasma over a 24-hour dosing interval. *Antimicrobial Agents and Chemotherapy*, 56(9): 4583–4585.

Yilmaz A, Price RW, Gisslén M (2012) Antiretroviral drug treatment of CNS HIV-1 infection. *The Journal of Antimicrobial Chemotherapy*, 67(2): 299–311.

Zash R, Makhema J, Shapiro RL (2018) Neural-tube defects with dolutegravir treatment from the time of conception. *The New England Journal of Medicine* [online], 379(10): 979–981. Available from: https://pubmed.ncbi.nlm.nih.gov/30037297/ [accessed 29 November 2022].

Zash R, Holmes L, Diseko M et al. (2019) Neural-tube defects and antiretroviral treatment regimens in Botswana. *The New England Journal of Medicine* [online], 381(9): 827–840. Available from: https://pubmed.ncbi.nlm.nih.gov/31329379/ [accessed 29 November 2022].

Zash R, Holmes LB, Diseko M et al. (2021) 23rd International AIDS Conference. Update on neural tube defects with antiretroviral exposure in the Tsepamo study, Botswana. Available from: https://theprogramme.ias2021.org/PAGMaterial/PPT/3301_4869/IAS2021_TsepamoUpdate_final.pdf [accessed 24 August 2023].

Interventions to Enhance Developmental Outcomes of HIV-affected Children and Adolescents

Amina Abubakar, Moses K Nyongesa, Stanley W Wanjala, Micaela Rice, Sevil Ozdemir, Patrick N Mwangala, Judith K Bass, and Michael J Boivin

INTRODUCTION

Millions of children and adolescents globally are directly affected by the human immunodeficiency virus (HIV) pandemic. These children present with multiple developmental delays and impairments as well as difficulties in psychological adjustment. The pathways to poor outcomes are both biomedical (e.g. disease progression and nutrition) and psychosocial (parental physical and mental health, stigma and poverty). This chapter highlights some of the interventions that have been observed to ameliorate the adverse effects of HIV infection in the affected paediatric population. Research gaps, such as the potential benefits of combined interventions, the need for pragmatic evaluation of long-term benefits of these interventions, and their scalability and sustainability, are discussed.

INTERVENTIONS TO ENHANCE THE DEVELOPMENTAL OUTCOMES OF HIV-AFFECTED CHILDREN AND ADOLESCENTS

Millions of children globally are adversely affected by the HIV pandemic (UNAIDS 2012). In this chapter, the term HIV-affected children refers to children directly infected by the virus, children who have been orphaned by HIV infection, and children living with an HIV-infected parent or caregiver (UNAIDS 2012). HIV-affected children are potentially at risk of suboptimal psychological functioning (Abubakar et al. 2008; Sherr, Mueller, and Varrall 2009; Le Doaré, Bland, and Newell 2012). This chapter summarises evidence on the impact of the HIV pandemic on children's psychological functioning; explores pathways through which HIV impacts psychological functioning; and presents evidence on ways to support psychological functioning in this population. Understanding how best to stimulate development among HIV-affected children is crucial, since it can facilitate the planning and scale-up of targeted intervention programmes.

WHAT IS THE IMPACT OF HIV ON PAEDIATRIC PSYCHOLOGICAL FUNCTIONING?

Reviews indicate that HIV-positive children suffer mild to severe impairments in motor, cognitive, and language functioning (Sherr, Mueller, and Varrall 2009). Additionally, mental health problems such as depression, anxiety, and suicidal ideation have also been reported among this population (Musisi and Kinyanda 2009; Kamau et al. 2012). The adverse effects of HIV infection begin early in life and may persist into early and middle childhood. In a systematic review of the literature, Le Doaré, Bland, and Newell (2012) noted that the mean motor and cognitive scores of infants who acquired HIV infection early in life were between 1 and 2 standard deviations below that of the general population, although this changed when they were started on antiretroviral therapy (ART).

Evidence indicates that HIV-affected adolescents also suffer developmental problems such as cognitive delays and mental health problems (Abubakar 2012). In their review, Le Doaré and colleagues noted that the delays among older HIV-infected children are much subtler and differentiated, with some developmental domains more severely affected than others. Noteworthy is that during adolescence, apart from a continuation of challenges that HIV-infected children experience from early childhood, new challenges related to growing up emerge. Among the most salient of these challenges is the handling of disclosure (Vaz et al. 2010; Brown et al. 2011). Some of the critical questions when handling disclosure include when and whom to disclose the HIV status to. During adolescence, HIV-infected children are also expected to become more autonomous and to ensure they adhere to the prescribed treatment; at this point, suboptimal adherence to therapy could pose a big problem. Both caregivers and health care providers face challenges in enforcing adherence among HIV-infected adolescents. Because of poor adherence, higher rates of treatment failure and acquisition of resistance mutations conferring reduced susceptibility to antiretrovirals (ARVs) have been reported among HIV-infected adolescents compared to adults. Lastly, HIV-infected adolescents have to deal with issues around their sexuality and reproductive health. These additional worries and challenges can adversely affect their quality of life.

Children who are perinatally or postnatally exposed to parental HIV illness have also been observed to present with poor developmental and mental health outcomes, although the evidence is less consistent. In a systematic review of the literature on the psychological functioning of HIV-exposed uninfected children, Sherr et al. (2014) identified 11 studies of which six reported data from sub-Saharan Africa (SSA). The review reported that seven studies observed delays in at least one psychological functioning domain among HIV-exposed but uninfected children. Affected domains included language, mental and motor development, processing speed and general IQ. As access to prevention of mother-to-child transmission interventions becomes more widespread, understanding the developmental needs of HIV-exposed uninfected children will become increasingly important.

WHICH FACTORS HAVE BEEN ASSOCIATED WITH AN INCREASED RISK OF POOR OUTCOMES AMONG HIV-AFFECTED CHILDREN?

The association between HIV exposure and poor neurobehavioural outcomes has been consistently demonstrated; however, there is significant variability in the developmental outcomes of HIV-affected children. This brings into focus one crucial question: What factors exacerbate the level of risk among HIV-affected children? Research indicates that both biomedical and psychosocial factors contribute to poor outcomes in HIV-affected children. Moreover, these risk factors tend to cluster within the same children, i.e. many children affected by HIV also experience a host of other risk factors.

HIV has neurotropic features; consequently, it directly impacts the central nervous system (CNS). Earlier studies have isolated HIV from CNS components such as cerebrospinal fluid, brain tissues, and the spinal cord. HIV damages the CNS, causing inflammation which partially contributes to the neuro-behavioural impairments observed among infected children and adolescents (Smith and Wilkins 2014). Before the introduction of ARVs, HIV was associated with progressive encephalopathy in up to 50% of infected children and static encephalopathy in up to 90% of infected children. With the scale-up of ARVs, severe encephalopathies are less frequent; nevertheless, neurobehavioural impairments persist and become more pronounced with disease progression. It therefore follows that children and adolescents presenting with advanced HIV/AIDS are also likely to present with more severe developmental delays and impairments (Abubakar et al. 2009).

Additionally, HIV-infected children are likely to experience nutritional compromise (Kuona et al. 2014). In general, nutritional deficiencies have been associated with compromised neurobehavioural outcomes in various contexts (Abubakar and van de Vijver 2012) and seem to exacerbate the adverse effects of HIV infection on neurodevelopmental outcomes, since earlier studies indicate that children who are infected and malnourished experience a higher degree of neurodevelopmental impairments compared to their peers who are only HIV positive or only malnourished (Abubakar et al. 2009; Ruel et al. 2012). HIV-infected females are also at increased risk of adverse perinatal outcomes such as low birth weight, and low gestational age; in turn, these factors have independently been observed to lead to poor neurodevelopmental outcomes (Brocklehurst and French 1998; Dos Reis et al. 2015).

HIV infection also compromises the caregiving context (see Figure 17.1 for a summary of these). HIV-infected parents are likely to have more medical bills than families that do not have a person with a chronic illness, a situation that severely depletes income and contributes to familial poverty; and children growing up in families experiencing socioeconomic strain are more likely to experience poor neurodevelopmental outcomes compared to their peers. Moreover, HIV-infected adults may experience significantly more mental health problems such as depression, and anxiety (Marwick and Kaaya 2010; Andersen et al. 2015), which have been associated with compromised parenting behaviour thus lowering psychosocial stimulation in their children. Compromised parenting behaviour and suboptimal psycho-social stimulation have been associated with poor neurobehavioural outcomes both in HIV-infected and HIV-affected children (Allen et al. 2014). Other psychosocial factors that may compromise child development in the context of HIV include stigma, low social support, and orphanhood, among others (Cluver et al. 2012; Nachega et al. 2012; Boyes and Cluver 2013).

Longitudinal studies in low- and middle-income countries demonstrate that children born into poverty are more likely to experience impairments in cognitive development (Grantham-McGregor 2007; Walker et al. 2011), particularly in SSA (Sigman et al. 1989; Escueta et al. 2014). Exposure to poverty-related cumulative risk in early childhood appears to affect brain development, with detrimental impact on cognitive and emotional developmental trajectory (Walker et al. 2011). An impoverished context limits opportunities for cognitive stimulation and can lead to inadequate nutrition that can impair development (Walker et al. 2011; Britto et al. 2013). It follows that, in a review of risk for adverse child development outcomes in low- and middle-income countries, Walker et al. (2011) identified inadequate cognitive stim-ulation as one of four key risk factors in need of urgent intervention with children up to 5 years of age. In particular, children from low socioeconomic backgrounds can experience diminished language inputs and enter school at a disadvantage, with disparities persisting throughout their education, leading to reduced future earnings and adult poverty (Grantham-McGregor et al. 2007; Leffel and Suskind 2013).

As conceived by Goffman (2009), stigma arises when negative meanings attached to a discrediting trait, such as HIV/AIDS, result in avoidance, less than full acceptance, and discrimination of people with that trait. Stigma has been shown to have a raft of disadvantages, especially on children and adolescents

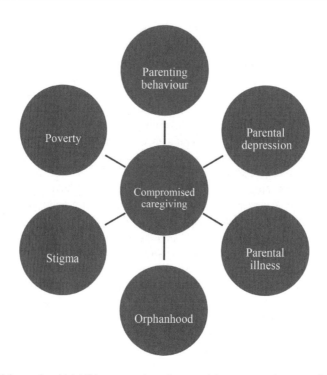

Figure 17.1 Potential ways in which HIV compromises the caregiving context, thus contributing to compromised psychological functioning.

as this is a period of physical, pubertal, and cognitive maturation in addition to psychosocial changes, including identity formation and the development of independent social relationships (Taddeo, Egedy, and Frappier 2008). Stigma compromises child development, as it has been shown to have negative impacts on prevention, diagnosis, and treatment of HIV/AIDS, leading to self-stigmatisation (Simbayi et al. 2007) exacerbating the impacts of the AIDS pandemic.

From the evidence base, children affected by HIV/AIDS are more likely than their unaffected peers to encounter stigma, including overt discriminatory behaviours, as well as stereotyped attitudes (Wei et al. 2016) and they face more significant challenges to their psychosocial well-being compared to their peers, thereby affecting their growth and development (Forsyth et al. 1996; Makame, Ani, and Grantham-McGregor 2002; Andrews, Skinner, amd Zuma 2006; Thurman et al. 2015). Studies in China report that children's school adjustment (peer relationships, school interest, anxiety, rule compliance), social adjustment (hopefulness and sense of control over future, future expectations, self-esteem), and internalising problems (loneliness, depressive symptoms) have been associated with stigma among HIV/AIDS-affected children (Lin et al. 2010; Zhao et al. 2010, 2012). Forehand and colleagues in the USA (Forehand et al. 1998) report that HIV-affected children exhibit poor psychosocial adjustment and greater delinquent behaviour. In light of this, child-friendly interventions need to be developed to address the psychosocial needs of HIV-affected children.

HIV-affected children experience a range of negative effects associated with AIDS among family members, including having to care for ill and dying caregivers (Nyambedha, Wandibba, and Aagaard-Hansen 2003), reduced access to health care and other services (Andrews, Skinner, and Zuma 2006; Miller et al. 2006), reduced access to school (Kamali et al. 1996; Nyambedha, Wandibba, Aagaard-Hansen

2003), lack of adult care (Heymann et al. 2007), unstable living situations (Ntozi 1997), loss of social support (Cluver and Orkin 2009), and stigma (Cluver, Gardner, and Operario 2008; Nyamukapa et al. 2010). This type of contextual adversity, and for HIV-infected children the virus itself, places HIV-affected children at risk of multiple poor developmental outcomes (Engle et al. 2007; Fernald et al. 2011; Walker et al. 2011; Wachs and Rahman 2013).

WHAT CAN WE DO TO ENHANCE THE PSYCHOLOGICAL OUTCOMES OF HIV-AFFECTED CHILDREN?

The evidence base shows that HIV-affected children experience poor psychological outcomes due to both direct and indirect effects of the virus. These risk factors usually co-occur, and their cumulative effects have the greatest neurocognitive and psychological impact. Consequently, addressing the psychological needs of these children will require a multifaceted, and multisectoral, approach. Figure 17.2 summarises a set of interventions that seem to be important in addressing the psychological needs of HIV-affected children.

Biomedical Interventions

When HIV-infected mothers receive adequate medical care that improves their physical health, the positive effects seem to translate into better psychological functioning for their children. Two areas have received specific attention: nutritional supplementation and treatment with ARVs.

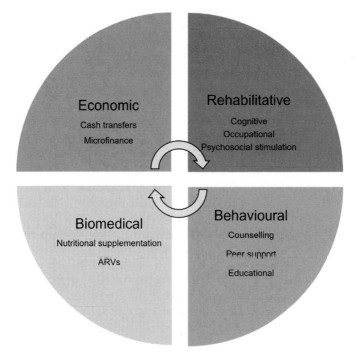

Figure 17.2   Potential interventions for HIV-affected children.
Abbreviation: ARV, antiretrovirals.

When investigating the impact of ARVs, one of the critical questions has been to what extent the use of ARVs has contributed to better neurodevelopmental and psychosocial functioning in the paediatric population. For instance, Brahmbhatt and colleagues investigated the potential benefits of ARV use on children's functioning in various neurodevelopmental domains, including motor, language, cognitive, and social–emotional development (Brahmbhatt et al. 2014). Their study was conducted in Uganda among 329 children aged between 0 and 6 years. They observed that, among HIV-infected children (n = 116), long-term use of ARVs was associated with decreased impairments in fine motor function, receptive language, and expressive language among others. However, the positive effects of ARV use have not always been consistent, as reported by another study (Smith and Wilkins 2014).

Maternal nutritional supplementation also enhances neurodevelopmental outcomes of both HIV-infected and HIV-exposed but uninfected children, although these effects have not been consistently reported (Duggan et al. 2012). Methodological shortfalls associated with several of the current studies, for example, small sample sizes, short-term follow-up, and the lack of consideration of the potentially powerful moderating influence of psychosocial factors, may contribute to the reported inconsistencies.

Interventions to Enhance Motor Development

Potterson and colleagues reported the effectiveness of a basic psychosocial stimulation approach in enhancing cognitive and motor development among South African HIV-infected infants who were assessed at 6, 12, and 18 months of age (Potterton et al. 2010). Another study by Perez and colleagues looked at the potential benefits of massage therapy on growth and development of neonates born to HIV-infected mothers in South Africa (Perez et al. 2015). In this study, mothers in the intervention group were trained to massage their infants daily for 15 minutes. The study reported that massage therapy contributed to the overall improvement in the developmental outcomes of HIV-exposed infants

Behavioural Interventions

These interventions aim at identifying strategies that can be implemented to encourage HIV-affected children to embrace adaptive coping strategies while avoiding maladaptive coping strategies. Behavioural interventions cover a wide range of issues, including handling disclosure, coping with loss, making life choices such as proper sexual behaviour, and enhancing mental health outcomes.

In South Africa, several family-based programmes have been implemented to mitigate the effects of HIV exposure on behavioural and mental health outcomes. One such programme is the VUKA family programme, which uses a community-based approach to address the psychological and medical needs of HIV-infected adolescents and their caregivers (Bhana et al. 2014). In this programme, a 10-session intervention of approximately 3 months duration is delivered. In a pilot study evaluating its efficacy, it was reported that VUKA contributed to enhanced adherence to ART and to enhanced communication between adolescents and caregivers. However, the intervention did not seem to improve mental health and behavioural outcomes as measured by Child Depression Inventory (Kovacs 1978) and the Strengths and Difficulties Questionnaire (Goodman 2001). The Collaborative HIV Prevention and Adolescent Mental Health Project-South Africa (CHAMP+ SA) is another example of a family-based intervention programme (Small et al. 2014). The intervention attempts to strengthen familial relationships as a mechanism for addressing risk-taking behaviours of young people. CHAMP+ multi-family meetings act as forums for safe communication about sensitive topics found hard to discuss (e.g. related to puberty, sexuality, sexual and drug risk-taking), within and across families. Family decision-making and parental monitoring skills are also emphasised to create a strong adult protective shield for young people living in HIV-endemic neighbourhoods.

Other family-based interventions have been reported elsewhere in SSA. In Rwanda, Betancourt and others have provided a preliminary evaluation of the short-term impact of the Family Strengthening Intervention (FSI-HIV) (Betancourt et al. 2014, 2017), a family home-visiting intervention aimed at promoting mental health and improving parent–child relationships in families with caregivers living with HIV. The FSI-HIV is structured consisting of four core components: building parenting skills and improving family communication; enhancing family connectedness and hope; providing psychoeducation on HIV; and strengthening problem-solving skills. The authors' study evaluating the acceptability and feasibility of the FSI-HIV reported that it enhanced family connectedness and improved parenting behaviour (Betancourt et al. 2014). Their pilot trial results (Cavazos-Rehg et al. 2021) showed that children in the FSI-HIV intervention had fewer depressive symptoms compared to those receiving usual care from social work services, at 3-month follow-up. In Uganda, Cavazos-Rehg and colleagues conducted a randomised controlled trial to evaluate the impact of a family-based economic strengthening intervention on the mental health of adolescents living with HIV (Cavazos-Rehg et al. 2021). The intervention comprised of four family financial management sessions (delivered by a finance mentor), support for ART, micro-enterprises for family income (over 24 months), plus 12 educational sessions and adherence counselling (delivered by lay counsellors). The intervention group reported lower hopelessness scores (at 24 weeks) and lower depression scores (at 36 months). Other research groups have evaluated the potential role of using peer groups as a vehicle for implementing interventions aimed at enhancing psychological outcomes. In South Africa, Snyder and colleagues developed and piloted a programme known as Hlanganani (coming together) (Snyder et al. 2014). This programme involves laypersons who facilitate a brief cognitive behavioural support group targeting recently diagnosed (within the past 12 months) HIV-infected young people. Based on data from 109 participants, the programme was associated with an increase in safe sex practices and higher adherence to ARV treatment regimen. In Zimbabwe, Willis and colleagues evaluated the effectiveness of using community adolescent treatment supporters to improve linkage and retention in care, adherence to ART, and the psychosocial well-being of adolescents living with HIV (Willis et al. 2019). Community adolescent treatment supporters were young people, aged 18 to 24 years, trained and mentored to offer ART adherence and psychosocial support counselling. Trial results (at 12 months) showed significant improvements in the psychosocial well-being of these adolescents, i.e. confidence, self-esteem, and self-worth, but also in their quality of life.

Interventions primarily addressing mental health issues such as psychological distress, depression, and anxiety in children and adolescents (collectively referred to as young people) living with HIV are limited (Bhana et al. 2021). In part, this is because of the limited epidemiological data to inform such interventions (Mellins and Malee 2013; Vreeman, McCoy, and Lee 2017). Incorporation of mental health components (but not as a primary focus) into family-based programmes such as the VUKA and CHAMPS+, described above, may also explain the dearth of mental health-specific interventions for young people living with HIV. Nevertheless, the few mental health-specific trials that have been conducted on young people living with HIV report promising findings (Bhana et al. 2021). Brown and colleagues in the USA, tested the preliminary effect of a combination of cognitive behavioural therapy and medication management algorithm against treatment as usual among 44 young people living with HIV (Brown et al. 2016). The authors report that those on a combination of cognitive behavioural therapy and medication management algorithm, compared to those on treatment as usual, reported significantly fewer depressive symptoms (as measured by the Quick Inventory for Depression Symptomatology) and were more likely to be in remission at the end of treatment (week 24; 65% vs 10%) and at the final follow-up (week 48; 71% vs 7%).

Informed by primary mental health needs and worries expressed by Tanzanian young people living with HIV, Dow and colleagues investigated the feasibility and acceptability of Sauti ya Vijana (The Voice of Youth) intervention (Dow et al. 2018). This intervention, consisting of 10 group sessions and

2 individual sessions, each lasting approximately 90 minutes, targets to reduce mental health symptoms and increase resilience among young people 12 to 24 years old living with HIV. The authors found the intervention highly feasible and acceptable among these Tanzanian youths. In Uganda, Senyonyi and colleagues conducted a cognitive behavioural therapy group intervention trial aiming to reduce HIV transmission risk behaviour, depression, anxiety, and alcohol use in perinatally HIV-infected adolescents, age 12 to 18 years (Senyonyi et al. 2012). Even though there were no significant between-group differences in the outcomes of interest, the authors report a general reduction in levels of HIV sexual transmission risk behaviour, depression, and alcohol use levels among study participants.

To build the evidence base, there is a need for more, perhaps transdiagnostic, interventional research involving children and adolescents living with HIV and mental comorbidities. Innovative treatment alternatives to the regular face-to-face psychological treatment are more attractive to young people in general. This includes internet- and computer-based cognitive behavioural therapy. Ebert and colleagues, in a meta-analysis of these technology-based approaches to intervention delivery, report that they are efficacious in the treatment of anxiety and depressive symptoms in young people (Ebert et al. 2015). Given the increased internet coverage and mobile use in Africa (GSMA 2016; Akamai 2017) and the general internet savviness of the younger generations (Ebert et al. 2015), it is time to explore computer-based cognitive behavioural therapy as a platform of intervention delivery for young people living with HIV, the majority of whom live in SSA (UNAIDS 2018).

Cognitive Interventions

These interventions usually include programmes that specifically train neurocognition through teaching skills and through strategies for improving functioning in one or several cognitive domains, such as executive function, in addition to other essential well-being outcomes (Martin et al. 2011). To date, few studies have explored the application and benefits of such interventions among children and adolescents affected by HIV, especially in the context of SSA. One such intervention is the application of cognitive supports through the visualisation of future task performance to improve naturalistic prospective memory in HIV-infected young people (Faytell et al. 2017, 2018; Pennar et al. 2018). Findings on this intervention suggest that it could benefit HIV-infected young people specifically on their treatment outcomes such as viral load reduction (Pennar et al. 2018). However, more trials are needed to further evaluate its efficacy and effectiveness. Another intervention is the Mindfulness instruction for HIV-infected young people, which was evaluated in the USA (Kerrigan et al. 2018; Webb et al. 2018). In one of these studies, the programme was associated with increased mindfulness, problem-solving coping styles, and increased regulation of negative emotional stimuli, hence suggesting that the programme has potential benefits on various cognitive and emotional outcomes (Webb et al. 2018). Elsewhere, in India Sinha and Kumar evaluated mindfulness-based cognitive behaviour therapy with emotionally disturbed adolescents affected by HIV/AIDS (Sinha and Kumar 2010). Though the results were promising, more research was recommended to test further the efficacy of the intervention with larger samples of adolescents.

In Uganda, a computerised cognitive rehabilitation training (CCRT) intervention was found to be potentially useful in improving neurocognition, especially on clinically stable children living with HIV (Boivin et al. 2016). In field tests with HIV-positive rural Ugandan children, Boivin and colleagues have used CCRT programmes to evaluate the neurocognitive benefits of weekly training sessions over the course of several months (Boivin et al. 2010, 2016; Boivin, Ruisenor-Escudero, and Familiar-Lopez 2016). These were proprietary commercially available programmes used for helping school-age children with idiopathic or acquired (e.g. traumatic brain injury) neurocognitive disabilities. When selected so as to be adaptable to the cultural context for Ugandan children, CCRT intervention could be of neuro-psychological benefit for children living with HIV (Boivin and Giordani 2009; Bangirana, Boivin, and Giordani 2013; Boivin and Giordani 2013; Boivin et al. 2006).

The Games for Entertainment and Learning laboratory at Michigan State University developed a cog-nitive games package designed to be available for scale-up on tablets maintained on a mobile network in the SSA context. This game package is called African Brain Powered Games and was designed as a CCRT intervention available as an app for tablets or smart phones. In pilot testing and preliminary clinical trials evaluation in Uganda (Giordani et al. 2015; Novak et al. 2017), Giordani et al. demonstrated that Brain Powered Games achieves significant neuropsychological change in computerised attention and cognitive performance outcomes (Giordani et al. 2015).

Economic Interventions

Children living in poverty are at a high risk of experiencing poor psychological outcomes. In various African countries, conditional and unconditional cash transfers are being implemented to provide a buffer against the harsh economic circumstances that are likely to exacerbate the negative impact of HIV in children's lives (Schubert et al. 2007; Crea et al. 2015). Few of these cash-transfer studies have reported the impact of these interventions on developmental outcomes; however, for the studies that have reported an impact, cash transfers have been associated with reduction in risky sexual behaviour, enhanced school attendance, and better psychosocial adjustment (Baird et al. 2012; Cluver et al. 2013).

Cash transfers are not the only form of economic intervention to have been evaluated. Other research-ers have looked at family economic empowerment intervention to address mental health functioning of HIV-affected children (Han, Ssewamala, and Wang 2013). The intervention comprised matched chil-dren's savings accounts, financial management workshops, and mentorship. Using a cluster randomised controlled trial, it was reported that children in the intervention clusters reported a reduction in hope-lessness and depression levels, leading to significant improvement in their mental health functioning (Han, Ssewamala, and Wang 2013).

FUTURE DIRECTIONS

This chapter shows the multiple impacts of HIV infection resulting from multiple influences. Interventions that have been implemented so far indicate that there is need to develop programmes that target nutrition, ensure early and adequate medical care, and provide social protection measures, in order to enhance psychological functioning of HIV-affected children. Data indicate that inter-ventions targeting each of these areas are likely to contribute to positive neurodevelopmental and psychosocial outcomes. What largely remains unknown is the potential impact of carefully combined intervention programmes.

A study in South Africa evaluated what was referred to as Cash Plus – a combination of cash trans-fers with enhanced caregiving practices (Cluver et al. 2012). The authors reported that Cash Plus had higher returns in terms of improved psychosocial outcomes compared to cash transfers alone. In Uganda, Ssewamala and colleagues examined whether a comprehensive microfinance intervention could help reduce the rates of depression among AIDS-orphaned young people (Ssewamala et al. 2012). The authors noted that a comprehensive microfinance intervention (involving savings accounts, financial management workshops, and mentorship) in addition to the traditional services for AIDS orphans (these services included counselling and the provision of school supplies) would contribute to better mental health outcomes. These pioneering multifaceted intervention programmes provide initial data on the value of combined interventions for enhancing neurological and psychosocial outcomes among HIV-affected children and adolescents.

Most of the studies included in the current review were small-scale randomised controlled studies with short follow-up periods. The long-term impact of the interventions highlighted in this chapter has yet to be evaluated. For these interventions to be considered worthwhile by policymakers there is a need to evaluate the extent to which the positive impact is sustained in the long term.

Given the magnitude of the HIV pandemic and the sheer numbers of HIV-affected children and adolescents, there is a need for scaling up intervention programmes that show the most benefit. Moreover, evaluating the pragmatic conditions under which these benefits could be sustained needs to be prioritised. The scalability of most of the studies is also yet to be evaluated. However, it is only when there is sufficient evidence of the long-term impact, sustainability, and fidelity of the interventions that scaling up is most likely to happen. Studies that investigate the scalability of the most promising interventions are recommended.

CONCLUSIONS

The existing evidence base clearly illustrates that HIV infection impairs neurodevelopment and psychosocial functioning of both infected and affected children and adolescents. Given the complex causal pathways between HIV infection and poor psychosocial outcomes, there is a need to implement multifaceted evidence-based interventions. Further, evaluations of pragmatic, useful, scalable, and sustainable multifaceted programmes are urgently required.

REFERENCES

Abubakar A, Van Baar A, Van de Vijver FJ, Holding P, Newton CR (2008) Paediatric HIV and neurodevelopment in sub-Saharan Africa: A systematic review. *Tropical Medicine International Health* 13(7): 880–887.

Abubakar A, Holding P, Newton CR, van Baar A, van de Vijver FJ (2009) The role of weight for age and disease stage in poor psychomotor outcome of HIV-infected children in Kilifi, Kenya. *Developmental Medicine & Child Neurology,* 51(12): 968–973.

Abubakar A (2012) Growing up positive: Opportunities and challenges faced by Kenyan adolescents living with HIV. *International Journal of Psychology* 47(Suppl): 476.

Abubakar A, van de Vijver F (2012) Socioeconomic status, anthropometric status and developmental outcomes of East African children. In: Preedy VR, editor, *Handbook of Anthropometry: Physical Measures of Human Form in Health and Disease.* New York: Springer, 2012, pp. 2679–2693.

Akamai (2017) *State of the Internet Connectivity: Q1 2017 Report.* Available at https://www.akamai.com/fr/fr/multimedia/documents/state-of-the-internet/q1-2017-state-of-the-internet-connectivity-report.pdf.

Allen A, Finestone M, Eloff I et al. (2014) The role of parenting in affecting the behavior and adaptive functioning of young children of HIV-infected mothers in South Africa. *AIDS and Behavior,* 2014; 18(3): 605–616.

Andersen L, Kagee A, O'Cleirigh C, Safren S, Joska J (2015) Understanding the experience and manifestation of depression in people living with HIV/AIDS in South Africa. *AIDS Care,* 27(1): 59–62.

Andrews G, Skinner D, Zuma K (2006) Epidemiology of health and vulnerability among children orphaned and made vulnerable by HIV/AIDS in sub-Saharan Africa. *AIDS Care,* 8(3): 269–276.

Baird SJ, Garfein RS, McIntosh CT, Özler B (2012) Effect of a cash transfer programme for schooling on prevalence of HIV and herpes simplex type 2 in Malawi: A cluster randomised trial. *Lancet,* 379(9823): 1320–1329.

Bangirana P, Boivin MJ, Giordani B (2013) Computerized cognitive rehabilitation therapy (CCRT) for African children: Evidence for neuropsychological benefit and future directions. In: Boivin MJ, Giordani B, editors, *Neuropsychology of Children in Africa: Perspectives on Risk and Resilience. Volume 1.* New York: Springer, pp. 277–298.

Betancourt TS, Ng LC, Kirk CM et al. (2014) Family-based prevention of mental health problems in children affected by HIV and AIDS: An open trial. *AIDS*, 28: S359–S368.

Betancourt TS, Ng LC, Kirk CM et al. (2017) Family-based promotion of mental health in children affected by HIV: A pilot randomized controlled trial. *Journal of Child Psychology and Psychiatry*, 58(8): 922–930.

Bhana A, Mellins CA, Petersen I et al. (2014) The VUKA family program: Piloting a family-based psychosocial intervention to promote health and mental health among HIV infected early adolescents in South Africa. *AIDS Care*, 2014; 26(1): 1–11.

Bhana A, Kreniske P, Pather A, Abas MA, Mellins CA (2021) Interventions to address the mental health of adolescents and young adults living with or affected by HIV: State of the evidence. *Journal of the International AIDS Society*, 24: e25713.

Boivin MJ, Giordani B (2009) Neuropsychological assessment of African children: Evidence for a universal basis to cognitive ability. In: Chiao JY, editor, *Cultural Neuroscience: Cultural Influences on Brain Function. Volume 178.* New York: Elsevier, pp. 113–135.

Boivin MJ, Busman RA, Parikh SM et al. (2010) A pilot study of the neuropsychological benefits of computerized cognitive rehabilitation in Ugandan children with HIV. *Neuropsychology*, 24(5): 667–673.

Boivin MJ, Giordani B (eds) (2013) *Neuropsychology of Children in Africa: Perspectives on Risk and Resilience.* New York: Springer.

Boivin MJ, Nakasujja N, Sikorskii A, Opoka RO, Giordani B (2016) A randomized controlled trial to evaluate if computerized cognitive rehabilitation improves neurocognition in Ugandan children with HIV. *AIDS Research & Human Retroviruses*, 32(8): 743–755.

Boivin MJ, Ruisenor-Escudero H, Familiar-Lopez I (2016) CNS impact of perinatal HIV infection and early treatment: The need for behavioral rehabilitative interventions along with medical treatment and care. *Curr HIV/AIDS Rep*, 13(6): 318–327.

Boyes ME, Cluver LD (2013) Relationships among HIV/AIDS orphanhood, stigma, and symptoms of anxiety and depression in South African youth: A longitudinal investigation using a path analysis framework. *Clinical Psychological Science*, 1(3): 323–330.

Brahmbhatt H, Boivin M, Ssempijja V et al. (2014) Neurodevelopmental benefits of anti-retroviral therapy in Ugandan children 0–6 Years of age with HIV. *Journal of Acquired Immune Deficiency Syndromes (1999)*, 67(3): 316.

Britto RPdA, Florêncio TMT, Benedito Silva AA, Sesso R, Cavalcante JC, Sawaya AL (2013) Influence of maternal height and weight on low birth weight: A cross-sectional study in poor communities of northeastern Brazil. *PLoS One*, 8(11): e80159.

Brocklehurst P, French R (1998) The association between maternal HIV infection and perinatal outcome: A systematic review of the literature and meta-analysis. *BJOG: An International Journal of Obstetrics & Gynaecology*, 105(8): 836–848.

Brown BJ, Oladokun RE, Osinusi K, Ochigbo S, Adewole IF, Kanki P (2011) Disclosure of HIV status to infected children in a Nigerian HIV Care Programme. *AIDS Care*, 23(9): 1053–1058.

Brown LK, Kennard BD, Emslie GJ et al. (2016) Effective treatment of depressive disorders in medical clinics for adolescents and young adults living with HIV: A controlled trial. *Journal of Acquired Immune Deficiency Syndromes (1999)*, 71(1): 38–46.

Cavazos-Rehg P, Byansi W, Xu C et al. (2021) The impact of a family-based economic intervention on the mental health of HIV-infected adolescents in Uganda: Results from Suubi + Adherence. *Journal of Adolescent Health*, 68(4): 742–749.

Cluver LD, Gardner F, Operario D (2008) Effects of stigma on the mental health of adolescents orphaned by AIDS. *Journal of Adolescent Health*, 42(4): 410–417.

Cluver L, Orkin M (2009) Cumulative risk and AIDS-orphanhood: Interactions of stigma, bullying and poverty on child mental health in South Africa. *Social Science & Medicine*, 69(8): 1186–1193.

Cluver LD, Orkin M, Gardner F, Boyes ME (2012) Persisting mental health problems among AIDS-orphaned children in South Africa. *Journal of Child Psychology and Psychiatry, and Allied Disciplines*, 53(4): 363–370.

Cluver L, Boyes M, Orkin M, Pantelic M, Molwena T, Sherr L (2013) Child-focused state cash transfers and adolescent risk of HIV infection in South Africa: A propensity-score-matched case-control study. *The Lancet Global Health*, 1(6): e362–e370.

Crea TM, Reynolds AD, Sinha A et al. (2015) Effects of cash transfers on children's health and social protection in Sub-Saharan Africa: Differences in outcomes based on orphan status and household assets. *BMC Public Health*, 15(1): 511.

Dos Reis HLB, Araujo KDS, Ribeiro LP et al. (2015) Preterm birth and fetal growth restriction in HIV-infected Brazilian pregnant women. *Revista do Instituto de Medicina Tropical de São Paulo*, 57(2): 111–120.

Dow DE, Mmbaga BT, Turner EL et al. (2018) Building resilience: A mental health intervention for Tanzanian youth living with HIV. *AIDS Care*, 30(Suppl 4): 12–20.

Duggan C, Manji KP, Kupka R et al. (2012) Multiple micronutrient supplementation in Tanzanian infants born to HIV-infected mothers: A randomized, double-blind, placebo-controlled clinical trial. *The American Journal of Clinical Nutrition*, 96(6): 1437–1446.

Ebert DD, Zarski AC, Christensen H et al. (2015) Internet and computer-based cognitive behavioral therapy for anxiety and depression in youth: A meta-analysis of randomized controlled outcome trials. *PLoS One*, 10(3): e0119895.

Engle PL, Black MM, Behrman JR et al. (2007) Strategies to avoid the loss of developmental potential in more than 200 million children in the developing world. *Lancet*, 369(9557): 229–242.

Escueta M, Whetten K, Ostermann J, O'Donnell K (2014) Adverse childhood experiences, psychosocial well-being and cognitive development among orphans and abandoned children in five low income countries. *BMC International Health and Human Rights*, 14(1): 6.

Faytell MP, Doyle KL, Naar-King S et al. (2017) Visualisation of future task performance improves naturalistic prospective memory for some younger adults living with HIV disease. *Neuropsychological Rehabilitation*, 27(8): 1142–1155.

Faytell MP, Doyle K, Naar-King S et al. (2018) Calendaring and alarms can improve naturalistic time-based prospective memory for youth infected with HIV. *Neuropsychological Rehabilitation*, 28(6): 1038–1051.

Fernald LC, Weber A, Galasso E, Ratsifandrihamanana L (2011) Socioeconomic gradients and child development in a very low income population: Evidence from Madagascar. *Developmental Science*, 14(4): 832–847.

Forehand R, Steele R, Armistead L, Morse E, Simon P, Clark L (1998) The Family Health Project: Psychosocial adjustment of children whose mothers are HIV infected. *Journal of Consulting and Clinical Psychology*, 66(3): 513.

Forsyth BW, Damour L, Nagler S, Adnopoz J (1996) The psychological effects of parental human immunodeficiency virus infection on uninfected children. *Archives of Pediatrics & Adolescent Medicine*, 150(10): 1015–1020.

Giordani B, Novak B, Sikorskii A et al. (2015) Designing and evaluating Brain Powered Games for cognitive training and rehabilitation in at-risk African children. *Global Mental Health*, 2(e6): 1–14.

Goffman E (2009) *Stigma: Notes on the Management of Spoiled Identity*. New York: Simon & Schuster.

Goodman R (2001) Psychometric properties of the Strengths and Difficulties Questionnaire. *Journal of the American Academy of Child & Adolescent Psychiatry*, 40(11): 1337–1345.

Grantham-McGregor S (2007) Early child development in developing countries. *Lancet*, 369(9564): 824.

Grantham-McGregor S, Cheung YB, Cueto S et al. (2007) Developmental potential in the first 5 years for children in developing countries. *Lancet*, 369(9555): 60–70.

GSMA (2016) *The Mobile Economy: Africa 2016*. Available at https://www.gsma.com/mobileeconomy/africa/.

Han C-K, Ssewamala FM, Wang JS-H (2013) Family economic empowerment and mental health among AIDS-affected children living in AIDS-impacted communities: Evidence from a randomised evaluation in southwestern Uganda. *Journal of Epidemiology and Community Health*, 67(3): 225–230.

Heymann J, Earle A, Rajaraman D, Miller C, Bogen K (2007) Extended family caring for children orphaned by AIDS: Balancing essential work and caregiving in a high HIV prevalence nation. *AIDS Care*, 19(3): 337–345.

Kamali A, Seeley JA, Nunn AJ, Kengeya-Kayondo JF, Ruberantwari A, Mulder DW (1996) The orphan problem: Experience of a sub-Saharan Africa rural population in the AIDS epidemic. *AIDS Care*, 8(5): 509–515.

Kamau JW, Kuria W, Mathai M, Atwoli L, Kangethe R (2012) Psychiatric morbidity among HIV-infected children and adolescents in a resource-poor Kenyan urban community. *AIDS Care*, 24(7): 836–842.

Kerrigan D, Grieb SM, Ellen J, Sibinga E (2018) Exploring the dynamics of ART adherence in the context of a mindfulness instruction intervention among youth living with HIV in Baltimore, Maryland. *AIDS Care*, 30(11): 1400–1405.

Kovacs M (1978) Children's Depression Inventory (CDI). Unpublished manuscript, University of Pittsburgh.

Kuona P, Kandawasvika G, Gumbo F, Nathoo K, Stray-Pedersen B (2014) Growth and development of the HIV exposed uninfected children below 5 years in developing countries: Focus on nutritional challenges, mortality and neurocognitive function. *Food and Nutrition Sciences*, 5(20): 2000.

Le Doaré K, Bland R, Newell M-L (2012) Neurodevelopment in children born to HIV-infected mothers by infection and treatment status. *Pediatrics*, 130(5): e1326–e1344.

Leffel KS, Suskind D (2013) Parent-directed approaches to enrich the early language environments of children living in poverty. *Seminars in Speech and Language*, 34(4): 267–278.

Lin X, Zhao G, Li X et al. (2010) Perceived HIV stigma among children in a high HIV-prevalence area in central China: Beyond the parental HIV-related illness and death. *AIDS Care*, 22(5): 545–555.

Makame V, Ani C, Grantham-McGregor S (2002) Psychological well-being of orphans in Dar El Salaam, Tanzania. *Acta Paediatrica*, 91(4): 459–465.

Martin M, Clare L, Altgassen AM, Cameron MH, Zehnder F (2011) Cognition-based interventions for healthy older people and people with mild cognitive impairment. *Cochrane Database of Systematic Reviews*, (1): CD006220.

Marwick KF, Kaaya SF (2010). Prevalence of depression and anxiety disorders in HIV-positive outpatients in rural Tanzania. *AIDS Care* 22(4): 415–419.

Mellins CA, Malee KM (2013) Understanding the mental health of youth living with perinatal HIV infection: Lessons learned and current challenges. *Journal of the International AIDS Society*, 16: 18593.

Miller CL, Spittal PM, Wood E et al. (2006) Inadequacies in antiretroviral therapy use among Aboriginal and other Canadian populations. *AIDS Care*, 18(8): 968–976.

Musisi S, Kinyanda E (2009) Emotional and behavioral disorders in HIV seropositive adolescents in urban Uganda. *East African Medical Journal*, 86: 16–24.

Nachega JB, Morroni C, Zuniga JM et al. (2012) HIV-related stigma, isolation, discrimination, and serostatus disclosure: A global survey of 2035 HIV-infected adults. *Journal of the International Association of Physicians in AIDS Care (JIAPAC)*, 11(3): 172–178.

Novak B, Giordani B, Boivin MJ, Winn B (2017) Potential uses of computer-based cognitive rehabilitation programs. In: Abubakar A, van de Vijver FJR, editors, *Handbook of Applied Developmental Science in Sub-Saharan Africa*. New York: Springer, pp. 281–290.

Ntozi J (1997) Effect of AIDS on children: The problem of orphans in Uganda. *Health Transitions Review*, 7(Suppl): 23–40.

Nyambedha EO, Wandibba S, Aagaard-Hansen J (2003) Changing patterns of orphan care due to the HIV epidemic in western Kenya. *Social Science & Medicine*, 57(2): 301–311.

Nyamukapa CA, Gregson S, Wambe M et al. (2010) Causes and consequences of psychological distress among orphans in eastern Zimbabwe. *AIDS Care*, 22(8): 988–996.

Pennar A, Naar S, Woods S, Nichols S, Outlaw A, Ellis D (2018) Promoting resilience through neurocognitive functioning in youth living with HIV. *AIDS Care*, 30(Suppl 4): 59–64.

Perez E, Carrara H, Bourne L, Berg A, Swanevelder S, Hendricks M (2015) Massage therapy improves the development of HIV-exposed infants living in a low socio-economic, peri-urban community of South Africa. *Infant Behavior and Development*, 38: 135–146.

Potterton J, Stewart A, Cooper P, Becker P (2010) The effect of a basic home stimulation programme on the development of young children infected with HIV. *Developmental Medicine & Child Neurology*, 52(6): 547–551.

Ruel TD, Boivin MJ, Boal HE et al. (2012) Neurocognitive and motor deficits in HIV-infected Ugandan children with high CD4 cell counts. *Clinical Infectious Diseases*, 54(7): 1001–1009.

Schubert B, Webb D, Temin M, Masabane P (2007) *The Impact of Social Cash Transfers on Children Affected by HIV and AIDS: Evidence from Zambia Malawi and South Africa*. Lilongwe, Malawi: UNICEF ESARO.

Senyonyi RM, Underwood LA, Suarez E, Musisi S, Grande TL (2012) Cognitive behavioral therapy group intervention for HIV transmission risk behavior in perinatally infected adolescents. *Health*, 4(12): 12.

Sherr L, Mueller J, Varrall R (2009) A systematic review of cognitive development and child human immunodeficiency virus infection. *Psychology, Health & Medicine*, 14(4): 387–404.

Sherr L, Croome N, Castaneda KP, Bradshaw K (2014) A systematic review of psychological functioning of children exposed to HIV: Using evidence to plan for tomorrow's HIV needs. *AIDS and Behavior*, 18: 2059–2074.

Sigman M, Neumann C, Jansen AA, Bwibo N (1989) Cognitive abilities of Kenyan children in relation to nutrition, family characteristics, and education. *Child Development*, 60(6): 1463–1474.

Simbayi LC, Kalichman S, Strebel A, Cloete A, Henda N, Mqeketo A (2007) Internalized stigma, discrimination, and depression among men and women living with HIV/AIDS in Cape Town, South Africa. *Social Science & Medicine*, 64(9): 1823–1831.

Sinha UK, Kumar D (2010) Mindfulness-based cognitive behaviour therapy with emotionally disturbed adolescents affected by HIV/AIDS. *Journal of Indian Association for Child and Adolescent Mental Health*, 6(1): 19–30.

Small L, Mercado M, Gopalan P, Pardo G, Mellins C, McKay MM (2014) Enhancing the emotional wellbeing of peri-natally HIV infected youth across global contexts. *Global Social Welfare: Research, Policy & Practice*, 1(1): 25–35.

Smith R, Wilkins M (2014) Perinatally acquired HIV infection: Long-term neuropsychological consequences and challenges ahead. *Child Neuropsychology*, (ahead-of-print): 1–35.

Snyder K, Wallace M, Duby Z et al. (2014) Preliminary results from Hlanganani (Coming Together): A structured support group for HIV-infected adolescents piloted in Cape Town, South Africa. *Children and Youth Services Review*, 45: 114–121.

Ssewamala FM, Neilands TB, Waldfogel J, Ismayilova L (2012) The impact of a comprehensive microfinance intervention on depression levels of AIDS-orphaned children in Uganda. *Journal of Adolescent Health*, 50(4): 346–352.

Taddeo D, Egedy M, Frappier J (2008) Adherence to treatment in adolescents. *Paediatrics & Child Health*, 13(1): 19–24.

Thurman TR, Kidman R, Nice J, Ikamari L (2015) Family functioning and child behavioral problems in households affected by HIV and AIDS in Kenya. *AIDS and Behavior*, 19(8): 1408–1414.

UNAIDS (2012) Core Slides: Global Summary of the AIDS Epidemic.

UNAIDS (2018) *Youth and HIV: Mainstreaming a Three-lens Approach to Youth Participation*. Geneva: UNAIDS Joint United Nations Programme on HIV/AIDS. Available at https://www.unaids.org/sites/default/files/media_asset/youth-and-hiv_en.pdf

Vaz LM, Eng E, Maman S, Tshikandu T, Behets F (2010) Telling children they have HIV: Lessons learned from findings of a qualitative study in sub-Saharan Africa. *AIDS Patient Care and STDs*, 24(4): 247–256.

Vreeman RC, McCoy BM, Lee S (2017) Mental health challenges among adolescents living with HIV. *Journal of the International AIDS Society*, 20(Suppl 3): 21497–21497.

Wachs TD, Rahman A (2013) The nature and impact of risk and protective influences on children's development in low-income countries. In: Britto PR, Engle PL, Super CM, editors, *Handbook of Early Childhood Development Research and its Impact on Global Policy*. New York: Oxford University Press, pp. 85–122.

Walker SP, Wachs TD, Grantham-McGregor S et al. (2011) Inequality in early childhood: Risk and protective factors for early child development. *Lancet*, 378(9799): 1325–1338.

Webb L, Perry-Parrish C, Ellen J, Sibinga E (2018) Mindfulness instruction for HIV-infected youth: A randomized controlled trial. *AIDS Care*, 30(6): 688–695.

Wei W, Li X, Harrison S, Zhao J, Zhao G (2016) The relationships between HIV stigma, emotional status, and emotional regulation among HIV-affected children in rural China. *AIDS Care*, 28(Suppl 2): 161–167.

Willis N, Milanzi A, Mawodzeke M et al. (2019) Effectiveness of community adolescent treatment supporters (CATS) interventions in improving linkage and retention in care, adherence to ART and psychosocial well-being: A randomised trial among adolescents living with HIV in rural Zimbabwe. *BMC Public Health*, 19(1): 1–9.

Zhao J, Li X, Fang X et al. (2010) Stigma against children affected by AIDS (SACAA): Psychometric evaluation of a brief measurement scale. *AIDS and Behavior*, 14(6): 1302–1312.

Zhao G, Li X, Zhao J, Zhang L, Stanton B (2012) Relative importance of various measures of HIV-related stigma in predicting psychological outcomes among children affected by HIV. *Community Mental Health Journal*, 48(3): 275–283.

CHAPTER 18

Conclusions and Future Directions

Jo M Wilmshurst and Amina Abubakar

This book has illustrated the diversity and extent of neurological and neurodevelopmental complications that children infected with human immunodeficiency virus (HIV) are at risk of. The landscape of neuroHIV is changing rapidly as interventions are commenced earlier and more aggressively, and the care is more comprehensive and targeted. As these children survive longer – often into adolescence and adulthood – the sequelae are far different from 20 years ago, when many children died from progressive encephalopathy and linked systemic complications (Thakur et al. 2019). HIV-infected children now face complications well recognised in adults but with expression that is altered by the influence of the HIV infection on the maturing brain. Nuances of care for these children are additionally complicated both by the challenges of drug-to-drug interactions but also the implications of the often unknown impact of antiretroviral therapy (ART) on the maturing brain.

Although guidelines support universal access to ART, this is far from the case and coverage is lower among children than among adults. In 2017, just over half the 1.8 million HIV-infected children who required ART globally were receiving this therapy. Marked improvement or remission of progressive and non-progressive encephalopathy is evident following the roll-out of combination antiretroviral therapy (cART) treatment (Czornyj 2006). However, the decline in the incidence of HIV encephalopathy since the introduction of cART surpasses access to cART. Other influences such as improved global health care are suggested but not fully delineated (Donald et al. 2015). A greater understanding of these processes would be an important contribution to developing improved approaches to care.

Guidelines are needed to clarify the preferred antiseizure medications in the care of HIV-infected children with seizures and epilepsy. Some drugs, such as carbamazepine, are recommended to be contraindicated due to drug-to-drug interactions. However, there are situations where this needs to be balanced against an optimal outcome for seizure control and quality of life, such as for children with subacute sclerosing panencephalitis where carbamazepine can be highly effective. In this setting, generally carbamazepine has been continued with ART levels carefully monitored and adjusted accordingly (Kija et al. 2015). Research in this area is very limited and this management recommendation is based on observational case studies. As newer generation ARTs roll out, these interactions are envisioned to be more manageable.

The silent progression of neuroHIV disease is compounded by lack of access to screening tools and to expertise in the settings where most children with HIV live. There is a case to advocate for serial imaging to monitor silent progression, especially of cerebrovascular disease, and there should be a low threshold to perform at least baseline neuroimaging in all HIV-infected children (Hammond et al. 2016).

Studies in children with central nervous system (CNS) immune reconstitution inflammatory syndrome are required in order to understand the incidence of, as well as to clarify, clinical case definitions. These studies need to be applicable to children in resource-constrained settings. Furthermore, what are the optimal immunomodulatory agents to use requires further research.

Whether HIV-infected children are at risk of the same chronic form of T-cell encephalitis expressed in adult patients associated with absence of CNS infections other than HIV itself, needs to be established. The role of new experimental therapeutic modalities – for example, natalizumab – that block T-cell entry into the CNS and HIV Tat protein antagonists remains an area for further research.

The World Health Organization interim guidance recommendation that the integrase inhibitor dolutegravir be used in first-line therapy regimens in place of efavirenz, has not been universally accepted (Nakkazi 2018). The risks of dolutegravir in pregnancy need to be elucidated (Rasmussen, Barfield, and Honein 2018; Zash, Makhema, and Shapiro 2018). Additionally, reported neuropsychiatric adverse events in patients taking dolutegravir need further clarification (Cuzin et al. 2018). So, whilst efavirenz is also associated with neuropsychiatric complications, replacing it with dolutegravir may not resolve this issue.

Children who are 'slow metabolisers' are at greater risk of adverse outcomes. They typically have residual viral activity in their CNS virus reservoir which persists and remains resistant to current ART. Understanding this pathogenesis and devising better targeted interventions is needed.

Antiretrovirals with a high CNS penetration effectiveness rank are proposed as resulting in more effective targeting of residual CNS viral replication. Limited and conflicting studies that evaluate high CNS penetrating antiretroviral regimens in HIV-infected children have been unable to conclude whether these agents are causal in resultant improved neurocognition (Patel et al. 2009; Crowell et al. 2015). Randomised controlled trials are needed to determine whether CNS penetration effectiveness has a role in routine paediatric practice.

HIV-infected children and adults continue to be at risk of a wide spectrum of neuroinfections. Some neuroinfections that were rare before the emergence of the HIV pandemic are now more common in HIV-infected individuals, including cryptococcal meningitis, cerebral toxoplasmosis, and progressive multifocal encephalopathy (Bowen et al. 2016). Management can be complex and ideal guidelines are still needed. Even in common conditions such as bacterial meningitis, there is insufficient evidence to direct clinical practice regarding restricted versus maintenance fluid therapy (Maconochie and Bhaumik 2016).

Future innovations that could lead to improved care for HIV-infected children include access to affordable and accurate rapid diagnostic tests as well as cost-effective neuroimaging modalities. Without inclusion of these modalities, understanding of the epidemiology and impact of neuroinfections in the setting of an HIV-infected child is limited. New classes of antimicrobial agents need to be developed. Supportive interventions such as fluid therapy, nutrition, and immunomodulatory agents, as well as the timing of cART, should be evaluated to improve the overall care and outcome of HIV-infected children with neuroinfections. Improved preventative measures, such as new vaccines and vector control programmes, are also required (John et al. 2015). Advances in knowledge will depend on collaborative, multi-centre studies in children, and improvement in care will continue to rely on adult studies (Thakur et al. 2019).

The widespread access to ARTs has improved longevity and has contributed to a reduction in the prevalence and severity of disability in HIV-infected people. However, data show that even in the presence of ARTs neurodevelopmental outcomes remain compromised (Benki-Nugent and Boivin 2019). In this book we have seen that HIV-infected people experience a host of physical, mental, cognitive, and psychosocial challenges. However, the challenges faced seem to change across the different developmental stages. For example, while children largely experience challenges around cognitive, language, and mental function, at adolescence the challenges are broader, focusing on issues such a medical adherence as they become more autonomous as well as issues on sexuality and disclosure.

As children survive through adolescence and into adulthood the complexity of their neuropsychological and neuropsychiatric states is significant (Laughton et al. 2013). Future care must focus on their psychological needs, with early detection of depression, anxiety, and executive function challenges.

Poor outcomes associated with different developmental stages result from both biomedical, for example, disease progression, drug resistance and nutritional deficiency, and psychosocial factors, such as stigma and the home environment (Abubakar 2014; Abubakar et al. 2017; Benki-Nugent and Boivin 2019). The Mediational Intervention for Sensitizing Caregivers, early childhood development and computerised cognitive rehabilitation training intervention (school age) studies highlight the need for dissemination and implementation scale-up research in HIV-affected communities (Boivin et al. 2020; Wei et al. 2022). This is especially the case for orphaned and vulnerable children (in the context of HIV) whose developmental well-being has been further compromised by the COVID pandemic, conflict and migration, and intensifying natural disasters. All these aspects have negatively affected the progress made in HIV prevention and care in the most at-risk populations globally. Bundling services in prenatal care so as to implement treatment for mothers living with HIV is recommended. The bundled services can be customised to be contextually relevant. For instance in sub-Saharan Africa some of the services that can be bundled up include quality of prenatal and postnatal care, micronutrient supplementation (e.g. vitamin D3, iron, zinc), and antimalarial prophylaxis among others. Mobile health interventions can help support these care bundles remotely.

Recent studies have tried to look at more complex biological pathways to poor outcomes such as micronutrient deficiencies, exposure to air pollution, and genetic factors (Suter et al. 2018; Yakah et al. 2019).

The advent of artificial intelligence and machine learning to digest big data sets is leading to an explosion of research on the interrelationships among complex variables. For instance, the gut, brain, and immunity axes in the context of HIV noted over past decades are currently drawing interest (Rich et al. 2020; Carrico et al. 2022). The association with mental health and cognition is becoming apparent but needs further study.

Given the complexities of the aetiology and manifestations of neurodevelopmental impairments in both children and adults, many interventions have been tested (McHenry et al. 2019). While many of these interventions seem promising, there remains a challenge since most have focussed largely on addressing a single problem. For example, there have been several interventions focusing only on the behavioural aspects. Future efforts need to focus on testing more integrated interventions that aim at addressing multiple dimensions of the challenges faced by HIV-infected people, as well as understanding multigenerational risk through epigenetic factors.

REFERENCES

Abubakar A (2014) Biomedical risk, psychosocial influences, and developmental outcomes: Lessons from the pediatric HIV population in Africa. *New Dir Child Adolesc Dev*, 146(Special Issue): 23–41. doi: 10.1002/cad.20071.

Abubakar A, Van de Vijver FJR, Hassan AS et al. (2017) Cumulative psychosocial risk is a salient predictor of depressive symptoms among vertically HIV-infected and HIV-affected adolescents at the Kenyan coast. *Ann Glob Health*, 83(5–6): 743–752. doi: 10.1016/j.aogh.2017.10.024.

Benki-Nugent S, Boivin MJ (2019) Neurocognitive complications of pediatric HIV infections. *Curr Top Behav Neurosci*, doi: 10.1007/7854_2019_102.

Boivin MJ, Augustinavicius JL, Familiar-Lopez I et al. (2020) Early childhood development caregiver training and neurocognition of HIV-exposed Ugandan siblings. *J Dev Behav Pediatr*, 41(3): 221–229. doi: 10.1097/DBP.0000000000000753.

Bowen LN, Smith B, Reich D, Quezado M, Nath A (2016) HIV-associated opportunistic CNS infections: Pathophysiology, diagnosis and treatment. *Nat Rev Neurol*, 12(11): 662–674. doi: 10.1038/nrneurol.2016.149.

Carrico AW, Cherenack EM, Rubin LH et al. (2022) Through the looking-glass: Psychoneuroimmunology and the microbiome-gut-brain axis in the modern antiretroviral therapy era. *Psychosom Med*, 84(8): 984–994. doi: 10.1097/PSY.0000000000001133.

Crowell CS, Huo Y, Tassiopoulos K et al. (2015) Early viral suppression improves neurocognitive outcomes in HIV-infected children. *AIDS*, 29(3): 295–304. doi: 10.1097/QAD.0000000000000528.

Cuzin L, Pugliese P, Katlama C et al. (2018) Integrase strand transfer inhibitors and neuropsychiatric adverse events in a large prospective cohort. *J Antimicrob Chemother*, 74(3): 754–760. doi: 10.1093/jac/dky497.

Czornyj LA (2006) Encephalopathy in children infected by vertically transmitted human immunodeficiency virus. *Revista de neurologia*, 42(12): 743–753.

Donald KA, Walker KG, Kilborn T et al. (2015) HIV Encephalopathy: Pediatric case series description and insights from the clinic coalface. *AIDS Research and Therapy*, 12(1): 2. eCollection 2015. doi: 10.1186/s12981-014-0042-7.

Hammond CK, Eley B, Wieselthaler N, Ndondo A, Wilmshurst JM (2016) Cerebrovascular disease in children with HIV-1 infection. *Dev Med Child Neurol*, 58(5): 452–460. doi: 10.1111/dmcn.13080.

John CC, Carabin H, Montano SM, Bangirana P, Zunt JR, Peterson PK (2015) Global research priorities for infections that affect the nervous system. *Nature*, 527(7578): S178–S186. doi: 10.1038/nature16033.

Kija E, Ndondo A, Spittal G, Hardie DR, Eley B, Wilmshurst JM (2015) Subacute sclerosing panencephalitis in South African children following the measles outbreak between 2009 and 2011. *S Afr Med J*, 105(9): 713–718. Retrieved from http://www.ncbi.nlm.nih.gov/pubmed/26428963.

Laughton B, Cornell M, Boivin M, Van Rie A (2013) Neurodevelopment in perinatally HIV-infected children: A concern for adolescence. *Journal of the International AIDS Society*, 16(1): 18603. doi: 10.7448/IAS.16.1.18603.

Maconochie IK, Bhaumik S (2016) Fluid therapy for acute bacterial meningitis. *Cochrane Database Syst Rev*, 11: CD004786. doi: 10.1002/14651858.CD004786.pub5.

McHenry MS, McAteer CI, Oyungu E, Deathe AR, Vreeman RC (2019) Interventions for developmental delays in children born to HIV-infected mothers: A systematic review. *AIDS Care*, 31(3): 275–282. doi: 10.1080/09540121.2018.1533629.

Nakkazi E (2018) Changes to dolutegravir policy in several African countries. *Lancet*, 392(10143): 199. doi: 10.1016/S0140-6736(18)31641-6.

Patel K, Ming X, Williams PL, Robertson K, Oleske J, Saege GR (2009) Impact of HAART and CNS-penetrating antiretroviral regimens on HIV-encephalopathy among perinatally infected children and adolescents. *AIDS*, 23(14): 1893-1901. doi: 10.1097/QAD.0b013e32832dc041.

Rasmussen SA, Barfield W, Honein MA (2018) Protecting mothers and babies – A delicate balancing act. *N Engl J Med*, 379(10): 907–909. doi: 10.1056/NEJMp1809688.

Rich S, Klann E, Bryant V et al. (2020) A review of potential microbiome-gut-brain axis mediated neurocognitive conditions in persons living with HIV. *Brain Behav Immun Health*, 9: 100168. doi: 10.1016/j.bbih.2020.100168.

Suter MK, Karr CJ, John-Stewart GC et al. (2018) Implications of combined exposure to household air pollution and HIV on neurocognition in children. *Int J Environ Res Public Health*, 15(1): 163. doi: 10.3390/ijerph15010163.

Thakur KT, Boubour A, Saylor D, Das M, Bearden DR, Birbeck GL (2019) Global HIV neurology: A comprehensive review. *AIDS*, 33(2): 163–184. doi: 10.1097/QAD.0000000000001796.

Wei J, Hou J, Mu T et al. (2022) Evaluation of computerized cognitive training and cognitive and daily function in patients living with HIV: A meta-analysis. *JAMA Netw Open*, 5(3): e220970. doi: 10.1001/jamanetworkopen.2022.0970.

Yakah W, Fenton JI, Sikorskii A et al. (2019) Serum vitamin D is differentially associated with socioemotional adjustment in early school-aged Ugandan children according to perinatal HIV status and in utero/peripartum antiretroviral exposure history. *Nutrients*, 11(7). doi: 10.3390/nu11071570.

Zash R, Makhema J, Shapiro RL (2018) Neural-tube defects with dolutegravir treatment from the time of conception. *N Engl J Med*, 379(10): 979–981. doi: 10.1056/NEJMc1807653.

Index